A Practical Approach To
The Science of Ayurveda

A Comprehensive Guide For Healthy Living

Acharya Balkrishna

LOTUS PRESS
Box 325, Twin Lakes, WI 53181 USA
email: lotuspress@lotuspress.com
website: www.LotusPress.com

ISBN: 978-0-9406-7631-2
Library of Congress Number: 2015941181

First USA edition 2015

Published by:

LOTUS PRESS

Lotus Press
P.O. Box 325
Twin Lakes, WI 53181 USA
800-824-6396 (toll free order phone)
262-889-8561 (office phone)
262-889-2461 (office fax)
www.lotuspress.com (website)
lotuspress@lotuspress.com (email)

Printed In USA

The Science of *Āyurveda*: In a Nutshell

Everybody wants to know about one's body type, the basic nature or constitution, the status of *Tridoṣa, Saptadhātu* and *Ojas* in their bodies. How to maintain *tridoṣa* in a state of equilibrium and the many ways of increasing *saptadhātu* and *ojas*? How to use rejuvenation therapy and the nature of the rejuvenator to be used in order to achieve good health and longevity and what measures should be taken for virilification to increase the body strength? There are innumerable such questions and one seeks authentic and scientific answers for them all.

Every mind is curious about the root cause of disease and the method of its eradication. It is not possible for the each person to study medical science for many years or to read *Caraka*, *Suśruta*, *Dhanvantari, Nighaṇṭus* and other *Āyurvedic* literatures and *Vedas*.

In the present era, Acharya Balkrishna is the most renowned and authentic savant who has carried out the revival and propagation of *Āyurveda*. The knowledge of *Maharṣi Caraka*, *Suśruta*, *Dhanvantari* and all other saints is completely and intimately compounded within him. As a representative of a saintly-tradition respected *Acharyashri* is sincerely working in the service of millions of people. He has efficiently compiled the essence of *Āyurveda* in the book "The Science of *Āyurveda*". It is like filling an ocean in a pot (*gāgar me sāgara*). By going through this book one can easily understand one's basic constitution, ailments in the body and effective methods of eradication. The basic principles of *Āyurveda* have been illustrated and artistically rendered in pictures in an aesthetic yet vibrant manner for the first time. I completely believe that once a person goes through this book thoroughly, she/he can certainly achieve a life-span up to a hundred years. For the basic knowledge regarding constitution, food, lifestyle and health, every person should read this book.

The aim of this book is to reach out to each and every home and family. Hence, efforts are made, so that the maximum number of people can benefit from this book. Today, millions of people are experiencing untimely death due to innumerable diseases, wherein expensive and unwanted medicines, unnecessary and costly surgeries, expensive diagnostic tests and hospitals have taken treatment away from the common man. Moreover, for the sake of treatment the patient is dragged into a vicious cycle, which ends only after death. After understanding the knowledge and information shared in this book, people will be able to save themselves from the atrocities which are being done in the name of treatment. With this, people would also be medically self-sustained. We proclaim that - "*Ārogya* (Health) is our birth right". You go through this book, and by inspiring others to do so, you must gain the blessings of good health.

"Sarve bhavantu sukhinaḥ, Sarve santu nirāmayāḥ."

Let all be healthy, let all be disease-free, with wish for happiness, health and well-being to all.

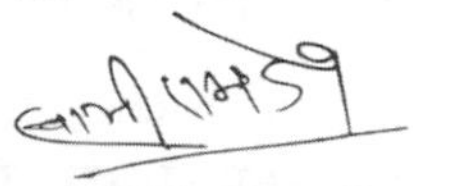

Swami Ramdev

Author's Notes

Indian civilization is not only ancient but also unique. The *Vedas* are the root and basis of our culture and civilization. They are perhaps the oldest scriptures in any heritage library. There are four *Vedas*: *Ṛgveda, Yajurveda, Sāmaveda* and *Atharvaveda*. *Āyurveda* is the oldest treatise on health and treatment; it is primarily considered be a part of *Atharvaveda*. This book provides a useful, reliable and evidence-based information about the mysteries behind the principles of an oldest and greatest treatise, *Āyurveda*. The ancient learned sages described *Āyurveda* as 'immortal.' In support of their statement they have given three reasons which cannot be ruled out, these are:

"Soya, māyurvedaḥ śāśvato nirdiśyate, anāditvāt,
Svabhāvasaṁsidhalakṣaṇatvāt, bhāvasvabhāvanityatvācca"

(*Caraka Saṁhitā*-Percept 30/26)

'That which is *Āyurveda*, in itself is complete, eternal and immortal. It regulates the behavior of the mind and emotions.' This immortal treatise *Āyurveda* was studied by *Prajāpati* through *Brahmā*, followed by *Aświni Kumars* through *Prajāpati*, from whom *Indra* learned it and from Indra sage *Bhāradwaj* studied and passed on this knowledge to *Punarvasu, Ātreya, Agniveṣa, Jatūkarṇa, Pārāśara, Hārīta, Kṣāra Pāṇi, Suśruta, Dhanvantri, Vāgbhaṭa* and many other famous sages.

In Indian culture, the four most valuable objectives of human life are *dharma, artha, kāma and mokṣa* - duty, wealth, desire and liberation, which helps to attain self-realization and gain freedom from the cycle of birth and death and getting closer to God. The actual source or base for the attainment and accomplishment of these four great objectives is a healthy body, because **"*Śarīrmādhyaṁ khalu dharma sādhanam*"**, 'the means by which one can achieve ones own duty resides only in a healthy body'. A healthy person, free from all ailments can work harder, follow the daily routine in a proper manner and perform his daily work more efficiently. He can derive pleasure and joy from any means of luxury, earn his living by any enterprise or business, and serve the family, society and the nation in a better way. In addition, one can meditate and worship The God for one's own welfare. This specifies that having a healthy body is the first among the seven pleasures that have been stated. *Āyurveda* also states the same:

"Dharmārtha kāmamokṣāṇāmārogyaṁ mūlamuttamam"

(*Caraka Saṁhitā*-Percept 1/15)

which means 'health is the base of duty, wealth, desire and liberation'.

The importance and utility of an *Āyurveda* treatise has been questioned as **"*Kimarthamāyurvedaḥ*"** which means - 'what is the objective of *Āyurveda?*' The answer is:

"Prayojanaṁ cāsya svasthasya svāsthyarakṣaṇamāturaṣya vikārapraśamanam ca"

(*Caraka Saṁhitā*-Percept 30/26)

'The objective of *Āyurveda* is to protect the health of a healthy person and cure all the ailments of a sick person'. The most important aim is that *Āyurveda* is not merely to earn profit or gain, but is meant for the benefit of humanity with a feeling of kindness and compassion, that is:

"Dharmārthaṁ nārthakāmārthamāyurvedo mahariṣibhiḥ.
prakāśito dharmaparairicchadbhiḥ sthānamakṣaram"

(*Caraka Saṁhitā Cikitsā* 1-4/57)

This states that 'the sages engaged in religious activities and who desired to attain salvation propagated the knowledge of *Āyurveda* as their duty towards the religion and not for their earnings or fulfillment of any specific personal desires.' *Āyurveda* defined the practitioner as:

"Nāthārtha nāpi kāmātharthamatha bhūta dayāṁaprati
vartate yaścikitsāyāṁ sa sarvamativartate"

(*Caraka Saṁhitā Cikitsā* 1-4/58)

'The best practitioner is that *vaidya* who performs his duty without earning money or seeking any specific reward, but only due to the compassion and sympathy for the patient'. *Āyurveda* is a practice of principles of high idealism. It is an exceptional system of medicine which lays significant emphasis on diet, what to eat and what not to eat, and explains that eradicating the cause of a disease is the first step to cure it. ***"Saṁkṣepataḥ kriyāyogo nidana parivarjanam"*** which means 'first of all eliminate the cause of the disease.' To prove its objective *Āyurveda* describes the ways and means to safeguard the health and also the reasons due to which diseases develop in the body. While explaining the modes of safeguarding health, *Āyurveda* states:

"Traya upastambhā iti - āhāraḥ svapno brahmacaryamiti"

(*Carak Saṁhitā*-Percept 11/35)

It means that 'food, sleep and celibacy (sexual restraint) are the three pillars that support stability, firmness and perfection to the body.' By utilizing these three assisting pillars in accordance with the prescribed methods, the health can be safeguarded. Along with this the cause of illness have been discussed, that is:

"Dhīdhṛtismṛtivībhraṣṭaḥ karma yat kurute, śubham.
Prajñāparādhaṁ taṁ vidyāt sarvadoṣa prakopaṇam"

(*Caraka Saṁhitā Śarīra* 1/102)

It emphasizes that 'when a person performs inauspicious activities that destroy *dhī* (intelligence), *dhṛti* (patience) and *smṛti* (memorizing power), then all the physical and mental defects provocate.' These inauspicious deeds are known as the intellectual offences. One who commits intellectual offences will suffer loss of health and his body will be disease-struck. *Āyurveda* while describing itself says:

"Tadāyurvedayatītyāyurvedaḥ"

(*Caraka Saṁhitā*-Percept 30/23)

which means that 'what imparts knowledge about the life-span is known as *Āyurveda*.' It is also said:

"Hitāhitaṁ sukhaṁ duḥkhamāyustasya hitāhitam.
mānaṁ ca tacca yatroktamāyurvedaḥ sa ucyate"

(*Caraka Saṁhitā*-Percept 1/41)

which means 'the science that describes the diet to be taken and not to be taken, as well as the good duration of life, bad duration of life, happy span of life and unhappy span of life is termed as *Āyurveda*.' Actually, *Āyurveda* is the name given to an optimal and healthy lifestyle. It is the knowledge of life and the science which makes human life healthy and happy on all levels.

We can conclude that *Āyurveda* is not merely the science that gives knowledge of treatment through herbal medicines, but it is a complete guide, an overview and a philosophy leading towards a healthy human life. *Āyurveda* not only describes the medicines for the well-being of a patient, but it also maintains and safeguards the health of a healthy person by describing daily habits in accordance with seasonal variations and providing detailed information about appropriate and beneficial food habits in different seasons as per the three body constitutions - *Vāta*, *Pitta* and *Kapha*. Descriptions have been given about foods that are mutually incompatible and unsuitable for consumption. Also mentioned are the micro-forces or subtle energies working in the body. The actual fact is that *Āyurveda* is such a vast subject that it cannot be limited within a boundary. In *Āyurveda* plants, leaves, seeds and fruits are all considered as medicines. That is:

"Anenopadeśena nānauṣadhibh ūtaṁ jagati kiñcid
dravyamupalabhyate tāṁ tāṁ yuktimarthṁ ca taṁ tamabhipretya"

(*Caraka Saṁhitā*-Percept 26/12)

It emphasizes that, 'in this universe there is no such substance which cannot act as a medicine.' According to the different uses and requirements every substance functions as a medicine. Each and every mineral can be purified and used as a medicine, which can be life saving. Along with this, *Āyurveda* also gives us knowledge about the diet, lifestyle and other substances in a systematic way that helps to increase the life-span, as well as guide us about the nature, soul and God beyond the cycle of life and death, to attain liberation. There is no doubt that this amazing knowledge of *Āyurveda* generated by our learned sages is beneficial for the lives of all human beings. Today's need is to spread this *Āyurvedic* medicinal science in the entire world. New experiments and research in this field are required so that the *Āyurvedic* treatments can be carried out effectively. Even today, there are *Āyurvedic* doctors who are working in a traditional way and are experienced and capable of treating chronic diseases, but due to lack of interaction, mutual contact, communication and coordination between them *Āyurveda* is out of the reach of millions of people and they are deprived of the world's safest and most effective health science.

We have established *Brahmakalpa* hospitals to serve millions of patients utilizing the knowledge of *Āyurveda* and succeeded in curing patients suffering from many fatal diseases. We believe that research in *Āyurveda* with modern technological updates is mandatory. This necessity has been understood in depth by Swami Ramdev, under whose leadership, the teachings of *Āyurveda* for the benefits of mankind has been publicized and propagated by *Divya Yog Mandir Trust* and *Patanjali Yogpeeth.*

Today man has moved far away from the nature and from his own intellect which deprives him of the natural state of health. *Āyurvedic* guidelines are necessary to retrieve a healthy body, pure mind and intellect because it is *Āyurveda* which links human beings with nature and with their own intellect. This book makes one aware of amazing, deep-seated and unrivalled mysteries of *Āyurveda.*

Sister Kanchan, a disciple of Vaidya Bhagwan Das, has given us important assistance in writing this book. After a deep and thorough study of several *Āyurvedic* scriptures, she has collected the gist. I express my heartfelt thanks to her. I also thank and bless all the doctors of the *āśrama* who gave their assistance in documenting this text. I extend my sincere thanks and blessings to Dr. Parul Saxena for her suggestions in revising and translating this book in English. I appreciate Mr. Pawan Sharma and his team for such wonderful sketches. May God give them sincere desire and interest in serving others.

At last, I bow and pay tribute to my elder brother, the revered Swami Ramdevji Maharaj, who has been the source of inspiration for me in carrying out the services at the *āśrama.* He has provided me strong help and support; it is owing to his blessings that I am able to perform my duties. All my successes and achievements are the result of his efforts. Swamiji is the representative of those learned sages of *Āyurveda* whose efforts and knowledge of *Āyurveda* has been propagated all over. I am grateful and bow down to all the learned sages who have protected, added to and expanded the *Āyurvedic* treatises. With homage to them, we should take an oath and move ahead to propagate, preserve and follow the path of spirituality, *Āyurveda, Yoga* and *Vedic* tradition. We have firm faith that we will be blessed and supported by everyone in this sacred task.

Acharya Balkrishna

Contents

Chapter 8
The Classification & Examination of Disease 200-230

Chapter 9
Therapeutic Methods **231-255**

Chapter 10
Yoga* Therapy and *Āyurveda **256-264**

Appendix **265-273**

Glossary **274-305**

List of Tables

List of Figures

List of Plates

Abbreviations

A.Hr.ci	:	*Aṣṭāṅga Hṛdaya cikitsāsthāna*
A.Hṛ.śā.	:	*Aṣṭāṅga Hṛdaya śārīrasthāna*
A.Hr.sū	:	*Aṣṭāṅga Hṛdaya sūtrasthāna*
A.Saṁ.sū.	:	*Aṣṭāṅga Saṁgraha sūtrasthāna*
Atharva.	:	*Atharva Veda*
Ā.Pra.	:	*Āyurveda Prakāśa*
Bhā.Pra.	:	*Bhāvaprakāśa*
Cakra.	:	*Cakrapāṇī*
Ca.ci.	:	*Caraka Saṁhitā cikitsāsthāna*
Ca.ka.	:	*Caraka Saṁhitā kalpasthāna*
Ca.ni.	:	*Caraka Saṁhitā nidānasthāna*
Ca.śa.	:	*Caraka Saṁhitā śarīrasthāna*
Ca.si.	:	*Caraka Saṁhita siddhisthāna*
Ca.sū.	:	*Caraka Saṁhitā sūtrasthāna*
Ca.vi.	:	*Caraka Saṁhitā vimānasthāna*
Chāndo.	:	*Chāndogyopaniṣada*
Dha.ni.	:	*Dhanvantari nighaṇṭu*
Kaṭho.	:	*Kaṭhopaniṣada*
Nyāya.da.	:	*Nyāyadarśana*
Praśno.	:	*Praśnopaniṣada*
Śā.Saṅ.pū.kha	:	*Śāraṅgadhara Saṁhitā pūrvakhaṇḍa*
Śā.Saṅ.ma.kha	:	*Śāraṅgadhara Saṁhitā madhyakhaṇḍa*
Śā.Saṅ.utt.kha	:	*Śāraṅgadhara Saṁhitā uttarakhaṇḍa*
Su.ci.	:	*Suśruta Saṁhitā cikitsāsthāna*
Su.ni.	:	*Suśruta Saṁhitā nidānasthāna*
Su.śā.	:	*Suśruta Saṁhitā śārirasthān*
Su.sū.	:	*Suśruta Saṁhitā sūtrasthāna*
Taitti	:	*Taittirīyopaniṣad*
Vai.da.	:	*Vaiśeṣikadarśana*
Yaju.	:	*Yajurveda*
Yo.da.	:	*Yogadarśana*
Yo.ra.	:	*Yogaratnākara*

Sanskrit and Allied Word Alphabets Scheme of Transliteration

VOWELS

अ	आ	इ	ई	उ	ऊ	ऋ	ॠ	ऌ	ॡ	ए	ऐ	ओ
a	ā	i	ī	u	ū	ṛ	r̄	ḷ	lṛ	e	ai	o
औ	अं		अः									
au	ṁ, aṁ		ḥ, aḥ									

CONSONANTS

क्	क	क़	ख्	ख	ख़	ग्	ग	ग़	घ्	घ	ङ्	ङ
K	Ka	q	kh	kha	kh	g	ga	g	gh	gha	ṅ	ṅa
च्	च	छ्	छ	ज्	ज	ज़	झ्	झ	ञ्	ञ		
c	ca	ch	cha	j	ja	z	jh	jha	ñ	ña		
ट्	ट	ठ्	ठ	ड्	ड	ड़	ढ्	ढ	ढ़	ण्	ण	
ṭ	ṭa	ṭh	ṭha	ḍ	ḍa	r̲	ḍh	ḍha	r̲h̲	ṇ	ṇa	
त्	त	थ्	थ	द्	द	ध्	ध	न्	न			
t	ta	th	tha	d	da	dh	dha	n	na			
प्	प	फ्	फ	फ़	ब्	ब	भ्	भ	म्	म		
p	pa	ph	pha	f	b	ba	bh	bha	m	ma		
य्	य	र्	र	ल्	ल	ळ	व्	व	श्	श	ष्	ष
y	ya	r	ra	l	la	ḻ	v	va	ś	śa	ṣ	ṣa
स्	स	ह्	ह	क्ष्	क्ष	त्र्	त्र	ज्ञ्	ज्ञ			
s	sa	h	ha	kṣ	kṣa	tr	tra	jñ	jña			

: (Visarga)=ḥ . (Anusvāra)=ṁ

ँ (Anunāsika)=m̐ X (Jihvāmūlīya= h̲

ᳶ (Upadhmānīya)=h̲ S (Avagraha)= '

(Udātta)= − (Anudātta)= ̲,

(Svarita)= Δ

All the English terms mentioned in the book to explain the *Āyurvedic* terminology based on the principles of *Āyurveda* does not described the exact sense of the *Sanskrit* words completely, still we have used those words in English as they are the most appropriate words to understand the nearest sense of *Āyurvedic* terminology for the better understanding for the readers. Consult the glossary of *Āyurvedic* terminology given at the end of the book to understand the correct sense of the basic principles of *Āyurveda*.

Chapter 1
An Introduction to *Āyurveda*

1. What *Āyurveda* Signifies

All of us have experienced at different times that not only human beings, even the smallest life-forms always struggle to survive; all beings strive to prevent pain caused by disease, loss, injury, indignity and ignorance, and try to remain happy always. Ever since human civilization began, we have been engaged in a continuous effort to fulfill our natural needs for food, water and sleep and to ward off disease and discomfort. The genesis of *Āyurveda* is embedded in our natural inclination towards health and happiness. Today, we use modern medicine, homeopathy, naturopathy and many other systems of medicine which improve our overall well-being. However, *Āyurveda* is closest to our hearts as it is a comprehensive science for holistic healing based upon the ancient and spiritual beliefs of India.

In daily life, we see that people suffering from simple problems, like stomach ache or digestive disorders are advised to use thymol seeds (*ajavāyana*) and asafoetida (*hīṅga*); they are advised to avoid drinking cold water in case of common cold, sore throat or cough; rather they are encouraged to use ginger (*ardraka*) and holy basil (*tulasī*) tea, black pepper, honey mixed with ginger juice and turmeric powder along with warm milk. In *Āyurveda*, each and every ingredient is either 'hot' or 'cold' in its nature and subsequently has corresponding usages. Such practices of *Āyurveda* have passed down through many generations and we have learned it from our ancestors. Most of the ingredients or simply remedies are available in our homes. We can find these in our kitchen or garden and these can be consumed with much ease. Thus, *Āyurveda* is an integral and inherent part of our daily life, rather than just another modality to treat disease.

Therefore, it is important for us to understand what *Āyurveda* actually is and how it is beneficial for us. First of all, it is of prime importance to know about the origin of the word '*Āyurveda*.' Etymologically, the word '*Āyurveda*' is a combination of two words: "*Āyuṣaḥ*" which means 'life' and "*Veda*" which means 'science.' Hence, "*Āyurveda*" means the 'Science of Life[1].' Yet, this science or *Veda* is not hypothetical or superficial knowledge about diseases and their remedies, but a profound understanding of the essence

1. *Āyuṣo vedaḥ āyurvedaḥ.* (*A.Hr.sū* 1.3)
Āyurasmina vidyate, nena vā,, yurvindatītyāyurvedaḥ, (*Su.sū.* 1/12)

or true nature of a substance. Simply stated, *Āyurveda* is the art of living in harmony with the science of life and is not just confined to diagnosis and treatment of various diseases. *Āyurveda* provides us wisdom to lead a productive and disease-free life. [PLATE 1]

Āyurveda is a science, a culture or practice which provides detailed and organized information about both health and ailments. *Āyurveda* is believed to be a comprehensive science that not only imparts physiological, but also psychological (mental) and spiritual well-being to all living beings. In *Caraka Saṁhitā*, one of the great classics of *Āyurvedic* thought, *Maharṣi Caraka* defined *Āyurveda* as follows: "The science that teaches us about the benefit or harm (favorable and unfavorable), the reasons for joy or sorrow, compatibility or incompatibility of substances, their properties and actions, as well as the duration and characteristics of life[(2)]." Thus, it specifies that *Āyurveda* is not restricted to certain individuals, caste, creed or a particular region, but it has a universal significance[(3)]. Just as life is a cosmic truth and has its own natural intelligence, so are *Āyurvedic* principles and philosophies, which are universal and reflect the wisdom of life. *Āyurvedic* practices are valid wherever there is life. These are eternal and rooted in enduring cosmic principles. The aim of these principles is to guide us towards complete well-being and lasting joy - ***"Sarve bhavantu sukhinaḥ, sarve santu nirāmayāḥ."*** In conclusion, *Āyurveda* is not only confined to medicine; rather, it is a complete lifestyle and spiritual practice. [PLATE 2]

2. Unique Features of *Āyurvedic* Treatment

While using the *Āyurvedic* system of medicine, some basic considerations should be kept in mind. This system of healing has certain unique features, rationales, logic, methodology and background as summarized below:

- **Comprehensive cure**

During diagnosis, an *Āyurvedic* practitioner does not confine his attention to the affected parts of the body or to the particular symptoms of the illness. In addition, he/she examines the patient's overall constitution, emotional state, spiritual orientation and other conditions responsible for the patient's physical and mental makeup. The practitioner also takes into consideration the condition of the *doṣas, dhātus* (body tissues) and *malas* (body waste or excreta). The overall diagnosis explains why different remedies are prescribed to various patients suffering from the same symptoms in *Āyurveda*.

2. *Hitāhitaṁ sukhaṁ duḥkhamāyustasya hitāhitam.*
   Mānaṁ ca tacca yatroktamāyurvedaḥ sa ucyate. (*Ca.sū.* 1/41)
3. *So, yamāyurvedaḥ śāśvato nirdiśyate anāditvāt,*
   svabhāvasaṁsiddhalakṣaṇatvāt, bhāvasvabhāvanityatvācca. (*Ca.sū.* 30/26)

- **Psycho-somatic nature of disease**

According to *Āyurveda*, no disease can be exclusively physical or psychological in nature. Physical ailments may affect the *psyche*, and mental disturbances affect physical health too. Therefore, the body and mind cannot be segregated and considered separately for treatment. This is the rationale why *Āyurveda* treats every disease as a psycho-somatic disorder. According to *Acārya Caraka*, all diseases, whether *Vātaja* (*Vāta* related), *Pittaja* (*Pitta* related), *Kaphaja* (*Kapha* related) or psychological have one underlying cause - mistakes committed due to ignorance and with wrong or distorted knowledge (*Prajñāparādha*). The root cause of all disease lies in ignorance of how life functions and can only be corrected by bringing us back in harmony. The background of *Āyurvedic* remedies is the insight of ancient sages of India and experiences they garnered over several millennia. Nature is the primary source of all *Āyurvedic* medicines. All medicines in *Āyurvedic* formulations are derived from the plant kingdom (herbs, extracts or juices), from the animal world (milk, clarified butter, cow's urine and so on) or from metals and minerals that are found in nature. No synthetic chemical is used in the preparation of these medicines, and hence their side-effects are minimal.

One reason why modern (allopathic) physicians have reservations and concerns regarding *Āyurvedic* medicines is the presence of heavy metals such as copper or iron in some of the formulations. This is a mere misconception, because in *Āyurveda*, metals present in these medicines and as well as poisonous plant products (such as snakewood, marking nut, swallow wort, and so on) are never used in their original form. They are subjected to numerous purification processes and made safe for the body before usage. However, it is very important to stick to all the necessary precautions during the production procedures and while using these metal-based medicines. Consequently, the use of these purified medicines in proper doses is absolutely harmless, and rather they prove to be extremely beneficial to the patients.

- **Every medicine is a tonic or a rejuvenator**

Every *Āyurvedic* medicine acts as a tonic or a rejuvenator, by virtue of providing improved nutrition to the body and triggering special restorative processes in the brain, which in turn lead to healing of the *psyche* and correcting mental, psychological and emotional imbalances. The unique restorative characteristics make these *Āyurvedic* medicines useful not only for patients, but also for people who are in good health by strengthening their overall vitality.Thus, *Āyurvedic* medicines are not only curative for specific disease, but also nourishing and prophylactic. Certain preparations such as *cyavanaprāśa*, *candraprabhāvaṭī* and other rejuvenators are examples of common restorative *Āyurvedic* tonics which have wide applications for disease prevention and promote longevity. *Āyurveda* is basically a multi-pronged science to attain health in terms of strength, purity and equilibrium.

- **Importance of developing the immune system and dietary control**

The *Āyurvedic* system of medicine emphasizes strengthening the immune system so that one may become less susceptible to diseases due to improved immunity and vitality. For the same reason, healthy food habits and nutritional guidelines (*āhāra saṁhitā*) along with good conduct and lifestyle (*ācāra saṁhitā*) are elaboratively explained in *Āyurvedic* texts along with the nature of food, food as per seasonal variations and food at different times of the day to support one's own body constitution. These factors help to sustain vitality, immunity and longevity, even if we are confronted with disease producing factors.

- **Role of dietary regimen and importance of compatible food**

In *Āyurveda*, great attention must be paid in prescribing a diet in accordance with the physical constitution and medical history of a patient. Such a supportive dietary regimen hastens the healing process. In contrast, a diet that doesn't suit a patient's constitution or which might aggravate the problem is not recommended. An *Āyurvedic* dietary regimen strengthens the immune system in healthy people, on one hand, and gives quick recovery for a person who is ill. *Āyurveda* has one of the most comprehensive dietary therapies in the world, that withstood a clear system of food adaptation with respect to individual's constitution and season, which makes *Āyurveda* unique among all medical sciences.

- **Simple and affordable remedies**

In modern age, treatment usually does not begin until several complicated tests have been conducted. This causes physical, mental and economic stress to the patient. On the contrary, a learned *Āyurvedic* practitioner can diagnose and treat the ailment by examining the patient's pulse and other bodily conditions or symptoms. This helps to avoid unnecessary stress, delay and expenditure. Along with this, several chronic and hard to cure diseases are also treated in *Āyurveda* after examining them with the latest and most accurate methods. Contemporary diagnostic tests detect diseases like diabetes, bronchial asthma, cardiac disease, hypertension, gout and others when pancreas, lungs, heart, nervous system and bones start getting impaired by 70 to 80 percent. Whereas in *Āyurveda*, through pulse examination and diagnostic processes prescribed in the book *'Mādhava Nidāna'*, we can examine, diagnose and alleviate at a very early stage, diseases which have become common nowadays.

- ***Āyurveda* is not a symptomatic treatment but a systemic one**

One of its unique features is that it targets the root of an ailment. The treatment methods aim at eliminating the actual cause of a disease and do not just suppress the symptoms. Elimination of the actual cause makes possible the permanent cure of a particular ailment, because *Āyurvedic* treatment is not only a symptomatic treatment but is also systemic. The advantage of modern medicine is that it can effectively control the complications of diseases; however it fails to cure the root disease. Whether the cause is electrophysiological, biochemical, hormonal, immunological or a cellular-level imbalance, most diseases can be diagnosed and appropriate medicine can be given. This is the reason, the terms 'control' or 'management' are frequently used in modern therapeutics to treat problems such as hypertension, diabetes or pain management.

In *Āyurveda* we not only control the disease; rather, we treat the underlying cause of the disease and hence complete management of the disease is possible. Here again, care is taken to prevent side-effects as much as possible. This is the uniqueness of *Āyurveda* and the basic difference between *Āyurveda* and modern medical science.

Āyurvedic treatments detoxify the body, provide strength and maintain complete equilibrium, right from embryonic stem cells to the development of tissues, systems and the whole body.

There is no conflict between *Āyurveda* and modern science. In fact, we consider that modern medicines may be needed to control the advanced stages of certain diseases, but for the complete relief from hypertension, cardiac disease, gout, arthritis and various other diseases, *yoga* and *Āyurveda* are the best possible options. There is scientific evidence which proves the effectiveness of *Āyurveda* and further research is going on in this field.

- ***Āyurveda,* in spite of being an ancient medical system, is completely relevant and scientific today**

It is an indisputable fact that *Āyurveda*, *yoga* and naturopathy are among the oldest medical systems in the world. These are gifts from the ancient Indian sages to the whole world in the form of the *Vedas* ***"Sā prathamā saṁskṛtoviśva vārā"*** (*Yajurveda* 7:14). Indian sages have contributed to the world in various fields among which the major ones are education, health, the judiciary and the ruling system. Our ancient sages held a very lofty philosophy of idealism, right from man and human development to the formation of an ideal family, society, nation and an ideal era. Therein, an ideal and completely scientific therapeutic system is also a contribution from Indian sages. Modern medical science is not as old as *Āyurveda* , which originated in the *Vedic* period. The founders of medicine are *Brahmā* and *Rājarṣi Dhanvantari*. When we try to assess the knowledge and reasoning level of our sages we become enthralled and even surprised to find that their knowledge, their lives and their moral sense were so profound. The actual cause of the diseases which are diagnosed by medical professionals today were already known at that time. Today mainly eight causative factors are considered for all diseases according to modern medical science. They are:

1. Hereditary causes
2. Infections
3. Environmental factors
4. Lifestyle and stress related factors
5. Addictions
6. Complications of diseases
7. Diseases generated due to side effects of medicines
8. Iatrogenic disorders

Prevention and treatment of all related diseases were well-known to our sages in the *Vedic* era. Today modern medical science works mainly in these areas:

1. Primary prevention
2. Secondary prevention
3. Control
4. Cure
5. Acute management
6. Rehabilitation
7. Palliation

If we go through a comparative analysis of the above-mentioned factors we come to the conclusion that ancient traditional medical systems (*Āyurveda* and natural medicine) have several advantages:

1. **Primary prevention:** The main goal is to prevent diseases. For this purpose immunization is used in modern medicine. Starting from childhood until a certain age, vaccinations and similar precautions have been adopted but these are useful only to a limited extent. There are specific vaccinations for diseases like polio, measles and hepatitis, but in some cases polio and measles occur even after the vaccination. As has been mentioned earlier, *Āyurveda*, *yoga* and natural medicine are not only a medicine system, but are the best and most scientifically examined system of living life in harmony with nature.

One who practices *yoga* regularly and takes Indian gooseberry (*āṁvalā*), Tinospora (*guḍūcī*), Holy basil (*tulasī*), Aloe vera and a group of vitality promoting herbs, *Aṣṭavarga* along with a natural lifestyle can stay free from disease almost entirely. This is a big achievement and eventually the whole universe will have to revert to this path. By following *yoga*, natural medicine and an *Āyurvedic* lifestyle, all the cells of the body get recharged and promote longevity; by means of meditation and self-control, one moves on the path of salvation as has been said by the great sages of India. By following *yoga*,

Āyurveda and natural medicine we prevent the degeneration of cells, tissues, internal organs and the complete body system and also provide strength, detoxification and equilibrium to the receptors of every cell from genes and chromosomes to life itself, in a natural way. In this way we protect the body from degenerative lifestyle disease and also make the body youthful, energetic, healthy and productive. It is the science that keeps away diseases, aging and death. *Āyurveda* quotes:

Prayojanaṁ cāsya svasthasya svāsthyarakṣaṇamāturasya vikārapraśamanaṁ ca.

(*Ca.su.*30:26)

The primary aim of *Āyurveda* is to safeguard the health of a person, emphasizing the approach of healthy living by adapting a lifestyle and diet that meet the demands of the season and following a disciplined daily regimen suggested by *Āyurveda*. When it comes to hereditary disorders we have successfully treated those who were suffering from various diseases like bronchial asthma right from birth. We have also protected people at risk of genetic abnormalities. In medical science, this is our great contribution and achievement which is really a boon for the entire world. If there is any system that can achieve primary prevention close to one hundred percent, then it is only *Āyurveda* which also encompasses *Yoga* and natural medicines.

2. **Secondary prevention:** The main aim of secondary prevention is that if a person had a history of myocardial infarction, hemorrhagic stroke or status asthmaticus and such conditions, medicines should be given which do not let the disease recur. To accomplish this goal *Āyurveda* is more effective. As in the case of myocardial infarction, there are seven main causes including hypertension, diabetes, high cholesterol, obesity, tobacco and use of narcotics, lack of physical activity and hereditary causes.To some extent these causes can be controlled by modern medicine, but *Āyurvedic* treatment guarantees long term success and is permanently effective.

3. **Control:** In this context, modern medicines are more effective than *Āyurveda* under certain conditions such as bacterial, viral and other infections. However, high cholesterol level, hypertension, diabetes and other such disorders can be controlled in both ways.

4. **Cure:** The number of diseases that can be completely cured by modern medicine are very few such as chronic infections like tuberculosis, injuries and those needing surgical intervention. *Āyurveda* can completely cure diseases including dengue, hepatitis, colitis, pancreatitis, chronic bronchitis, arthritis, psoriasis, migraine, cancer and many others. In the complete eradication of disease *Āyurveda* plays an important role.

5. Acute management: In myocardial infarction, hemorrhagic strokes or in case of any accident, traumatic and surgical condition, modern treatments are more effective. *Āyurveda* needs to focus more on research in these areas.

6-7. Rehabilitation and Palliation: In rehabilitation and palliation, both *Āyurvedic* and modern treatment methods are very effective. *Āyurvedic* treatment is thousands of years old, easy, simple, authentic, safe and stems from a scientific heritage of Indian saints. We can preserve our culture by making use of *Āyurvedic* treatment. By adopting *Āyurveda* in life one can achieve an easy, healthy, and natural life and also benefit from the culturally rich ancient philosophy and ideology.

- ***Āyurvedic* remedies: Naturally and easily available**

Procuring most *Āyurvedic* medicines is easy as numerous herbs are available in our kitchens and gardens. Another benefit of using *Āyurvedic* medicines is that, since one is using natural products, we remain close to nature. This helps to develop interest and love for nature, fields, trees, shrubs and herbs. This prevents a person from being fully dependent on modern technology and an artificial lifestyle. *Āyurveda* provides a way to conserve nature. [PLATE 3]

- ***Āyurveda* complementary to *yoga* and spirituality**

As mentioned before, *Āyurveda* provides scientific knowledge to lead a happy and healthy life, and it also helps one in spiritual progress with complete well-being of the body, mind and soul. It is not only intricately bound up with *dharma* (duty), but also with the soul. *Āyurveda* also recognizes all the main goals of human life: the attainment of *dharma* (duty or religious and ethical virtues), *artha* (wealth or material benefits and goals), *kāma* (desire or lust) and *mokṣa* (liberation or salvation). The principles and procedures of *Āyurveda* are powerful aids in practicing *yoga* properly.

These characteristics of the *Āyurvedic* healing system demonstrate that it is unique in itself and is in complete harmony with the natural rhythms of life. One cannot run away from it. It is our basic nature and proclivity.

3. *Āyurveda* and its Diversified Areas

Āyurveda is concerned with the welfare of all living beings including plants and animals, in addition to humans. Together with treatises that examine diseases afflicting human beings, there are *Āyurvedic* texts on plant and animal diseases and their management as well. These were written by different sages. Among the better known are *Aśva Āyurveda* (related to the horse), *Gaja Āyurveda* (to the elephant), *Gava Āyurveda* (to the cow) and *Vṛkṣa Āyurveda* (to plants).

The expertise, subject area and scope of *Āyurveda* are also vast. On one hand, it provides detailed information to treat difficult-to-cure and complex ailments including those usually regarded as incurable. On the other hand, it teaches a healthy person to remain fit and free from disease throughout his/her life. In this context, clear instructions are given in '*svasthavṛtta*'(health horizons - an approach to a healthy life) about what to eat and when, according to different seasons and times, what to avoid and how to live so as to lead a healthy and stress-free lifestyle. *Āyurveda* also enumerates elaborately healthy and beneficial ways of fullfilling biological needs such as hunger and thirst. It also describes how to protect oneself from infirmities, particularly those which may occur with aging. It is a remedy that can be adapted to the needs of every person, place, time and culture. It is a system that connects us back to the great healing powers of life.

4. *Aṣṭāṅga Āyurveda*: The Eight Branches of *Āyurveda*

The vast topics of *Āyurveda* have been divided into eight categories by the sages, which are known as '*Aṣṭāṅga Āyurveda*[4],' the eight branches of *Āyurveda*. They are as follows:

1. ***Kāya cikitsā***[5] **(Internal Medicine):** Here the word '*kāya*' means '*agni*.' *Kāya cikitsā* means 'treatment of *agni*.' In *Āyurveda,* we need to understand the interpretation and complete philosophy of the word '*agni*'.

   Every single cell of the body, in fact the whole body, is continuously undergoing a vital process. It is named *tridoṣa* in *Āyurveda* whereas in modern medicine it is referred to as metabolism. As long as the fundamental energy of the body, i.e. *agni*, is co-ordinating well with all physiological functions within the body, all three *doṣas* and seven tissues remain in harmony and excretory processes and other physiological actions in the body go on smoothly. With an exhilarated mind and soul, one utilizes or develops complete energy for well-being and to keep the body in order. This is the complete definition of good health and sanity. *Āyurveda* mainly targets this fundamental energy of the body - '*jaṭharāgni*.' When the fundamental energy is co-ordinating well, a person will not suffer from disease. Apart from balance in the body weight, all the chemicals, electrolytes and hormones are also maintained in a state of equilibrium in the body.

4. *Kāyabālagrahordhvāṅgaśalyadaṁṣṭrājarāvṛṣaiḥ.* (A.saṁ. sū. 1/10)
5. *Kāyacikitsā nāma sarvāṅgasaṁśritānāṁ vyādhīnāṁ jvara raktapittaśoṣonmādāpasmārakuṣṭhamehātisārādīnāmupaśamanārtham.*(Su.sū. 1/3)

There are a total of thirteen types of *agnis* - *saptadhātvāgni*, *pañcabūtāgni* and *jaṭharāgni*. *Agni* is the basic driving force (energy) of existence which operates the body and again is composed of seven tissues and five basic elements. The metabolic activity of the body depends on '*agni*.' The baseline of *Āyurvedic* treatment is *kāya cikitsā* or *agni cikitsā*. All procedures of *Āyurvedic* treatments, *yogic* activities and naturopathy treatments aim to activate, control and to maintain the continuous, co-ordinated flow of this energy.

Among the thirteen types of *agnis* present, '*jaṭharāgni*' is the fundamental *agni*. '*Jaṭharāgni*' is also known as the '*pācāka agni*' or the digestive fire. This is the base of all diseases. It is the result of irregularity in digestion and due to slow and sluggish digestive fire. The treatment of these diseases is called *kāya cikitsā* (the treatment through internal medicine). In this branch all diseases and their remedies are prescribed which affect the entire body. All diseases related to endocrine, respiratory, digestive systems, mental health disorders, dermatological and sexually transmitted diseases come under this category.

2. ***Kaumārabhṛtya tantra or Bāla roga***(6) **(Pediatrics):** This branch deals with all types of arrangements and treatments for a woman during pregnancy, of neonates, infants and children. Selection of a wet nurse for an infant, problems related to breast milk and their treatment, symptoms of various bacterial diseases such as puerperal infection and their treatment all come under the scope of pediatrics.

3. ***Bhūta vidhyā***(7) **(Psychiatry and Exorcism):** Holy offerings, sacrifices, chanting and other holy rituals used to counter the bad effects of demons, demigods, ghouls and evil (in *Āyurveda* all these names signify various infectious agents), which are causative factors for the generation of certain types of diseases, comes under '*bhūta vidhyā*.' This branch also deals with mental disorders, emotional disturbances and psychological problems. It includes ligation, punishment, intake of snuff or nasya, collyrium and medicated smoking which are carried out only by a skilled physician.

4. ***Śalya cikitsā***(8) **(Surgery):** This branch deals with incision, excision, treatments by surgical procedures and equipments. It also includes

6. *Kaumārabhṛtyaṁ nāma kumārabharaṇadhātrīkṣīradoṣasaṁśodhanārtha duṣṭastanyagrahasamutthānāṁ ca vyādhīnāmupaśamanārtham.* (*Su.sū.*1/5)
7. *Bhūtavidyānāmadevāsuragandharvayakṣarakṣaḥpitṛpiśācanāgagrahādyupasṛṣṭaceta sāṁ śāntikarmabaliharaṇādigrahopaśamanārtham.* (*Su.sū.* 1/4)
8. *Śalyaṁ nāma vividhatṛṇakāṣṭhapāṣāṇapāṁśulohaloṣṭāsthibālanakhapūyasrāvaduṣṭa vraṇāntargarbhaśalyoddharaṇārtha yantraśastrakṣārāgnipraṇidhāmvraṇana viniścayārthaṁ ca.* (*Su.sū.* 1/1)

trauma management due to injuries from weapons like arrows, shafts, spears, guns, swords and so on. This branch includes treatment with surgical equipments, instruments, heat, chemicals, weapons, medicines and wholesome sources. According to *Suśruta*, foreign particles, pieces of wood, bullets and diseases due to accumulation of waste matter are included under this branch.

5. ***Śālākya tantra***[9] **(Otolaryngology (E.N.T) and Ophthalmology):** This branch includes the diseases above the neck, especially the ear, nose, throat and eyes. Since these treatments are carried out with the help of probes or '*śalākā,*' this branch is also known as '*śālākya tantra.*' In modern science it can be defined as otolaryngology (ear, nose and throat) and ophthalmology branches.

6. ***Agada tantra***[10] **(Toxicology):** Toxicology includes identification of different types of poisons and their remedies. This treatment involves *sthāvara viṣa* (poisons obtained from trees, plants, vegetables, other edible substances and minerals), *jaṅgama viṣa* (poison of insects, reptiles and other animals) and *saṅyoga viṣa* (poison derived from the wrong combination of medicines or from the mixture of various medicines and other substances).

7. ***Rasāyana tantra***[11] **(The Treatment for Rejuvenation):** The word '*Rasāyana*' is derived from two words '*Rasa*' + '*Āyana,*' where '*rasa*' means 'lymph and other tissues (dhḍtus) of the body, which are necessary and supportive to restore life' and 'āyana' means 'special methods to obtain these things.' So the word '*Rasāyana*' means the resources and methodology by which we can nourish the lymph, blood and body tissues (*dhātus*) to restore life. On this basis, the complete treatment which provides strength to the body, sensory and motor organs and teeth, which minimizes the effect of consequences of old age (such as wrinkles, gray hair and baldness), which counters the aging process and promotes longevity, which sharpens the brain and intellect and which helps to maintain body's health, is known as the 'Science of Rejuvenation.'

8. ***Vājīkaraṇa tantra***[12] **(The Treatment for Infertility and Virility):** The word '*Vājīkaraṇa*' is derived from two words '*Vājī*' and '*Karaṇa*.' The

9. *Śālākyaṁnāmordhajatrugatānāṁ śravaṇanayanavadanaghrāṇādisaṁśritānāṁ vyādhināmupaśamanārtham.* (*Su.sū.*1/2)
10. *Agadatantraṁ nāma sarpakīṭalūtāmūṣikādidaṣṭaviṣavyañjanārthaṁ vividhaviṣasaṁyogopaśamanārthaṁ ca.* (*Su.sū.* 1/6)
11. *Rasāyanatantraṁ nāma vayaḥsthāpanamāyurmedhāvalakaraṁ rogāpaharaṇasarmathaṁ ca.* (*Su.sū.* 1/7)
12. *Vājīkaraṇatantraṁ nāmālpaduṣṭakṣīṇaviśuṣkaretasāmāpyāyanaprasādopacayajanananimittaṁ praharṣajananārthaṁ ca.* (*Su.sū.*1/8)

last tissue considered in *Āyurveda* to be nourished by food consumed is '*śukra*' (semen). Therefore, here '*vāji*' means 'semen or *śukra*' and '*karaṇa*' means 'that which enhances.' Hence, a treatment that increases the quality and quantity of semen is called virilization. Those drugs and sources which help in increasing, purifying, collecting, facilitating reproduction and nourishment for normal production of semen are called '*vājīkara* or aphrodisiac.' It is therefore a detailed treatment of debility and disorders of the reproductive system. [PLATE 4]

A number of comprehensive treatises on all these branches have been separately documented by different sages and *Āyurveda* experts over the centuries and all of these treatments were prevalent and profoundly practiced in ancient times and had widespread acclaim and appreciation. Pediatrics throve under the guidance of sage *Kaśyapa*, which is elaborated in *Kaśyapa Saṁhitā*. Sage *Suśruta* was a master surgeon. His *Suśruta Saṁhitā* is available even today. Surgery was common and highly evolved in ancient India. Detailed descriptions of Cesarean section and plastic surgery are available in ancient texts. *Suśruta* is considered to be the father of plastic surgery. Complex surgical procedures were performed at that time. However, they suffered a great loss under hostile conditions in the medieval era due to which the practices were disrupted and declined. Many important *Āyurvedic* texts were either destroyed or lost. Various branches of *Āyurveda* suffered over time.

Chapter 2
Fundamentals of *Āyurveda*

1. *Pañcamahābhūta* (The Five Basic Elements) and *Āyurveda*

The four *Vedas* - *Ṛga*, *Sāma*, *Yajura* and *Atharva* - are considered to be the oldest texts in the world dealing with all matters pertaining to individual and society. *Āyurveda* originated from the *Vedas* as an *upaveda* or supplementary *Vedic* science and is primarily considered to be a branch of the *Atharvaveda*, although all four *Vedas* highlight different aspects of healing and reflect *Āyurvedic* considerations. In addition to describing medicinal herbs and plants, the *Vedas* mention the basic principles of *Āyurveda*, like the three *doṣas* (*Vāta*, *Pitta* and *Kapha*), the seven *dhātus* or tissues (*rasa, rakta* and other *dhātus*), *prāṇa*, digestion, metabolism and rejuvenation. Similarly, other important principles of *Āyurveda* are also mentioned in the four *Vedas*.

The basic principles of *Āyurveda* are in accordance with the great philosophies of ancient India, in particular with *Sāṅkhya, Yoga* and *Vaiseśika* philosophies, which are three systems among the *Ṣad darśanas* or six *Vedic* schools of thought. Just as *Sāṅkhya* and *Yoga* texts hold that the five elements - *vāyu* (air), *jala* (water), *agni* (fire), *ākāśa* (space/ ether) and *pṛthvī* (earth) combine to create the entire living and non-living world, similarly *Āyurveda* is based on the same belief that the human body, its constituent factors and energy components - *doṣa*, *dhātu* and *mala* also are comprised of the five elements. Although, all the five elements are present in a particular substance, one of these elements works predominantly. On the basis of the predominance of one inherent element, substances are classified accordingly. When the element of space dominates in a substance, it is called *ākāśīya*. Substances that have qualities of air are termed *vāyavya*; the ones with fire as the main constituent are said to be *tejas*; those with water as the main constituent are *āpya*, and substances with a predominance of the earth element are termed *pārthiva*. To identify the category that a particular substance belongs to, we must look at the qualities inherent in its nature and in its effects.

- ***Ākāśīya dravya***: These substances are soft, light, minute, homogenous and vocal in their attributes. Intake of these items increases tenderness, lightness, kinetic energy (motility) and porosity in the body.

- ***Vāyavya dravya***: These are light, cool, rough, dry, minute and with a feel or touch. Intake of these items increases roughness, repulsion, motion and energy.
- ***Tejas dravya***: These are hot, pungent, light, dry, minute, non-sticky and are attractive in form. Use of such ingredients increase burning, digestive power, metabolism, brightness (shine), enhance complexion and lend a healthy glow to the body. They also cause sensation of heat.
- ***Apya* or *jalīya dravya***: These are liquid, cold, heavy, smooth, soft and moist. They lend moisture and softness to the body, increase determination and bring calmness and happiness to the mind and emotions.
- ***Pārthiva dravya***: These are heavy, hard, tough, gross, solid, non-sticky and have an odor. These substances cause obesity with an increase in body weight and fat, and build muscles which provide strength and support.

After examining the properties and nature of these elements and the constitution of the human body, it is clear that the two elements - earth and water predominate in the body and its tissues. The solid part of the body (such as the muscles) is formed from the element earth, and the liquid part (such as the plasma) is formed from water. The empty spaces and cavities in the body relate mainly to the element of space (ether) and partially to that of air. Apart from this, various physical and mental processes are carried out with the help of the element of air. The food we ingest is metabolized and converted into *rasa, rakta* (blood), *asthi* (bone) and other *dhātus* by the fire element.

The three *doṣas* (*Vāta, Pitta* and *Kapha*) present in the body, the *dhātus* (*rasa, rakta* and other *dhātus*) constituting the body and the *mala*s (waste products) are also formed by the combination of these five basic elements. In the same manner, different kinds of food materials and medicinal substances that nourish and treat our body are also constituted by these five elements.

To categorize food materials, elements are identified according to their *rasa* (taste), *guṇa* (attributes), *vīrya* (potency) and *vipāka* (post-digestive effect). It is sufficient to note that whenever there is an imbalance or disequilibrium in the body, a diet should be prescribed that will either increase or decrease the affected element in order to balance and restore harmony.

2. The Principle of *Tridoṣa*: The Three Biological Humors

When we consult an *Āyurvedic* physician, they usually correlate our ailments with an increase in one or more of the three *doṣas* - *Vāta, Pitta* or *Kapha*. This may leave us confused if we have no idea what they are referring to. It is important that we should understand these important terms in order to know more about our individual characteristics and inclinations.

- ***Tridoṣa* principle:** *Tridoṣa* is comprised of two words: '*tri+doṣa*.' Here '*tri*' means 'a group of three basic elements (biological energy forces) viz., *Vāta*, *Pitta* and *Kapha*' and '*doṣa*' means 'which is capable of vitiation.' When *Vāta, Pitta* and *Kapha* are vitiated they produce disease and when they are in equilibrium, or in their natural state, they maintain a perfect balance or harmony between the body and *saptadhātus* (seven fundamental tissues) thereby upholding and maintaining the body. Hence, here *doṣa* does not have an ordinary, literal meaning. *Tridoṣa* does not mean an impaired or vitiated condition of *Vāta*, *Pitta* and *Kapha*. Instead, it is a well-defined theory of upholding the body and its physiology by means of three biological energy pillars. This is the principle of *Tridoṣa*. Similarly, the three mental qualities (*sattva*, *rajas* and *tamas*), in a state of equilibrium, are called *mūla prakṛti* (the basic nature). Here *prakṛti* does not literally mean nature. In a similar fashion, *mūla prakṛti* (the basic nature) of the body is in the form of three biological energy pillars (*Vāta, Pitta* and *Kapha*) that maintain and uphold the body constituting *Tridoṣa*. [PLATE 5]

Body constituents - *doṣa, dhātu* and *mala*: The human body is made up of related factors of *doṣa*, *dhātu* and *mala*. All the constituent elements of our body are a part of these three; out of which *doṣas* are the most important as they are the most powerful forces in the body which create either health or disease. This is the energy source of the body.

There are three *doṣas*: 1. *Vāta*, 2. *Pitta* and 3. *Kapha*. Hence they are named *tri* (three) *doṣa*[1]. The three *doṣas* are considered to be the pillars or mainstay of the body, responsible for its creation, preservation and destruction. Although the union of sperm and ovum results in the conception of an embryo, but without the support of these *doṣas* formation of a body is not possible. After birth, nourishment of the body, maintenance of good health, prevention and cure of various ailments rests upon these *tridoṣa*. This is because all bodily processes, physical or chemical, are controlled by them. They act as basic constituents and protective barriers for the body in its normal physiological condition. When an imbalance occurs, they cause diseases. A healthy body is possible, as long as the *doṣas* are in equilibrium orbalanced. In a balanced state they are also known as *dhātus*. Any type of deformity or imbalance in the *doṣas* (increase or decrease) results in ill-health

1. *Vāyuḥ pittaṁ kaphaśceti trayo doṣāḥ samāsataḥ.* (*A.Hṛ sū.*1/6)

and the body becomes susceptible to disease. However, when the *doṣas* are out of balance, the others also get imbalanced, which results in poor health and ultimately disease. These *doṣas* change their natural state due to an increase, decrease or dominance. They also vitiate the balance of *dhātus* and *malas* and progress towards disease development. Therefore they are termed *doṣas,* as the term *doṣa* literally means a fault or a blemish.

There are two main causes for the vitiation of the *doṣas*: (i) *vṛddhi* - an undue increase above the normal level in the body and (ii) *kṣaya* - a decrease below the normal level. However, most diseases are caused by an increase in the *doṣas*, because with a decrease in any *doṣa* its power to induce an illness automatically gets reduced. It is true that with a reduction in the amount of a particular *doṣa* its properties also weaken and it cannot work effectively. However, when there is a decrease in any *doṣa*, the contrasting attributes gain strength and the *doṣa* with contrasting attributes gets aggravated as a result of disequilibrium, leading to diseases associated with the aggravated *doṣa* and not the pacified one.

It is clear that a balance between the three *doṣas* is absolutely essential for the uninterrupted physiological activities and upholding of the body. Just as the mind permeates the entire body, so do the *doṣas*. However the *doṣas* are present even in external body parts such as hair and nails where the mind may not permeate. A brief introduction to the three important *doṣas* is as follows. [PLATE 6]

(I) *Vāyu* or *Vāta Doṣa:* The energy of movement

Vāyu or *Vāta* is the most important of the three *doṣas*. The *Sanskrit* root for *Vāyu* or *Vāta* is ***'vā'-'vā gatigandhanayoḥ,'*** referring to breath, vibration, movement and that which causes motility (activity), excitement and vitality in the body. It is termed '*vāyu*' or '*vāta.*' Hence, it is the source of kinetic energy in the body. Generally the term *Vāyu* is used for the greater element and *Vāta* for its specific action as a biological force, but both are common in *Āyurvedic* literature. *Vāta* is connected to *prāṇa* or the life-force and is the prime manifestation of *prāṇa* in the body. According to the *Atharvaveda* - ***"Prāṇāya namo yasya sarvamidaṁ vaśe,"*** which means that 'the whole universe is governed by *prāṇa* (the life-force).' According to *Caraka, Vāyu* is the activator of the digestive fire and activator of all sensory functions, bestowing happiness and enthusiasm. It is *vāyu* that holds the entire body together and maintains tissues normally. This *prāṇa* resides in *pañcamahābhūta* (the five elements) present in the body in the form of

Vāyu, and in the form of *Vāta* it resides in *tridoṣa*. This *Vāyu* maintains the body in the form of breath (respiration) and energy and is known as '*prāṇa-vāyu*' or '*Vāta,*' which represents the life-force. The factors that generate motion and vitality in the body constitute *Vāta doṣa*. *Vāta* is the originator of all movements in the body. It governs all nervous functions, controls the mind, senses and motor organs. *Vāta* is also responsible for stimulation of digestive juices and enzymes that break down and digest food. The empty spaces in all channels (*srotas*) of the body are constituted by *Vāta*. Even the subtle and gross forms of every *dhātu* (tissue element) and the communication between various organs of the body are due to *Vāta*. The foetus is nourished and developed in the womb because of *Vāta*, and it controls the entire nervous system of the unborn. Without *Vāta*, the other two *doṣas*, *Pitta* and *Kapha* also remain inactive, as they are incapable to perform without it. *Vāta* is also responsible for the stability of other *doṣas* and *malas* at their specific locations, and when required, it eliminates them through urine, sweat and other wastes from the body. When the *Vāta doṣa* is in a state of equilibrium, it keeps all *doṣas*, *dhātus* and *malas* balanced. When it loses its balance and equilibrium, it disturbs other *doṣas*, *dhātus, malas* and *srotas* (channels). Being active and mobile, *Vāta doṣa* is capable of transporting other *doṣas* to different parts of the body where they are already present, thereby increasing their levels in those parts of the body and cause disease development.

Hence, it is clear that all ailments are ultimately due to an imbalance or corruption of *Vāta doṣa*. When it is in balance, it maintains harmony among other *doṣas*, *dhātus* and *malas*. When it is agitated, it causes an inappropriate mixing of these, which results in diseases and ill-health.

A very important characteristic of *Vāta doṣa* is "*yogavāhita.*" It combines with and takes on the attributes of other *doṣas*, and this is the cause of many diseases. When it interacts with *Pitta doṣa*, it takes on the characteristic of heating, burning and other properties of *Pitta doṣa,* and on interaction with *Kapha* it becomes cold, moist and sticky. *Vāta* has five divisions or sub-types according to its location and function. They are:

1. *Prāṇa* - the life-energy or the vital-force in the form of breath;
2. *Udāna* - the ascending or upward moving force (rising breath);
3. *Samāna* - the balancing air (circulating in the abdominal region);
4. *Apāna* - the descending or downward moving force (downward breath);
5. *Vyāna* - the expanding air, diffused throughout the body, governing the integrity of all vital processes.

It is essential to keep these five *Vāyus* in harmony to control *Vāta*. As mentioned before, *Vāta* contributes to the evolution of all types of ailments, but the disturbances in *Vāta* alone result in eighty different types of diseases, the most of any *doṣa*.

- **Natural attributes of *Vāta***

Vāta is dry, cold, light, subtle (minute), mobile, clear and rough in its qualities[(2)]. These are the natural attributes of *Vāta**. When *Vāta* is in balance, its attributes are not usually felt. They can only be experienced during erratic breathing or in a state of excitement. The qualities of *Vāta* such as dryness, etc. manifests only when it gets aggravated. [PLATE 7]

Table 1: Attributes of *Vāta* and their Effect on Physiology

Attributes	Physiological Manifestations
1. *Rūkṣatā* (Dryness)	Dryness, emaciation and stunted growth; poor development of bodily tissues; vocal unclarity, low, obstructed, dry, rough and hoarse voice; and lack of sleep.
2. *Śītalatā* (Coolness)	Inability to tolerate cold substances, disliking towards cold climate, afflicted with diseases related to cold; stiffness of limbs and shivering of the body, cold hands and feet.
3. *Laghutā* (Lightness)	Lightness in the body; inconsistent gait, action, food intake and movement (speed).
4. *Cañcalatā* (Motility)	Movements of joints, eyes, eyebrows, jaws, lips, tongue, head, shoulder, hands and legs; irregular heart rhythm, muscle spasms; changeable mind and emotions.
5. *Viśadatā* (Non-stickiness, clear)	Dry and cracked skin; crackling sound in limbs or joints, flickering of body parts.
6. *Kharatva* (Roughness)	Coarse-textured and rough hair, skin, nails, teeth, face, hands and feet.
7. *Bahulatā* (Abundance or Excessiveness)	Talkativeness; abundance and prominent visibility of tendons and veins.
8. *Śīghramitā* (Quickness/ Swiftness)	Quick in initiating actions, acting on impulse, restless activities, gets frightened quickly; rapid susceptibility to diseases and infections; mood swings, scattered thoughts, quickly deciding likes and dislikes; picks-up new information quickly, which is also quickly forgotten, poor long-term memory; fast speech.

2. *Rūkṣaḥ śīto laghuḥ sūkṣmaścalo, tha viśadaḥ kharaḥ.*
Viparītaguṇairdravyairmārutaḥ saṁpraśāmyati. (*Ca.sū.* 1/59)

* According to *Caraka*, the main attributes of all the three *doṣas* (*Vāta, Pitta, Kapha*) are mainly seven, but other *Āyurvedic* seers describe several other properties, besides the seven. Therefore, the main qualities of all the three *doṣas* are mentioned here.

- **Reasons for *Vāta* aggravation**

Being born with *Vāta*-type is certainly a strong predisposing factor for its aggravation. Another factor is old age, a time when *Vāta* increases in everyone. Aging can bring out the worst signs of *Vāta* aggravation. Grief, fatigue, fear and exhaustion are again the causes of *Vāta* imbalance. Among the most typical reasons are:

1. **Suppression of urges:** Suppressing the natural urges of the body such as defecation, urination, sneezing and so on.
2. **Dietetics:** Eating before the digestion of the previous meal, eating foods with too many dry, pungent, bitter and astringent tastes, excess intake of dry fruit, overeating, eating cold foods, fasting, skipping meals habitually, and ignoring the body's hunger signals.
3. **Stress:** Physical and mental stress, too much worry, anxiety and tension, overwork, working more than one's capacity, suffering emotionally from grief, fear and frightening experiences, unexpected shocks, long trips and uncomfortable rides in vehicles, strain and exhaustion.
4. **Habits:** Poor sleep, sleeping late at night, talking loudly and over indulgence in sexual activity.
5. **Season:** During monsoon, *Vāta* gets aggravated naturally without the onset of these conditions, as the weather become windy.

In people with *Vāta* dominance, even minor causes may lead to considerable *Vāta* aggravation.

- **Symptoms of aggravated *Vāta*** (3)

To diagnose *Vāta* imbalance, a physician has to look upon the symptoms of the following kind:

1. **Physical indications:** When *Vāta* gets aggravated, it leads to dryness, roughness, stiffness in the body and organs, pricking pain, loose joints, dislocation of the bones, brittle bones, hardness, weak and fragile organs, shivering and numbness in the limbs, feeling of coolness, debility, constipation, pain, discoloration and dull skin, lack of luster in the teeth and nails, losing sense of taste and astringent taste in the mouth.
2. **Mental indications:** Worry, anxiety, loss of mental focus, an over-active mind, impatience, short attention span and depression.
3. **Behavioral indications:** Insomnia, fatigue, inability to relax, restlessness, low appetite and impulsiveness.

It is important to remember that any *doṣa* can cause any symptom. These are just the common signs of *Vāta* imbalance.

The place of origin of *Vāta* is the intestine. When *Vāta* is aggravated it affects the intestines, particularly the colon. When waste matter (*mala*) reaches the intestine, *Vāta* is aggravated, particularly as undigested food and flatulence.

3. *Tatra, vātakṣaye mandaceṣṭātālpavāktvamapraharṣo mūḍhasaṁjñatā ca.* (*Su.sū.*15/11)

- **Remedies for balancing *Vāta*[4]**

To restore the balance of *Vāta*, the causes of its aggravation must be determined and corrected with an appropriate diet and medicine. The treatment should be performed keeping in mind the attributes of *Vāta doṣa* and what is needed to reduce them, i.e. to provide an opposing therapy such as emesis which acts against the attributes of *Vāta doṣa*. *Vāta* is the "King of the *doṣas*" and provides motility to *Pitta* and *Kapha*. Hence, to keep it balanced is the prime requirement for everyone. "Regularity" helps to balance *Vāta doṣa*. *Vāta* is so sensitive and quickly changeable that it easily falls prey to over-stimulation. Following are the common remedies for balacing *Vāta*:

1. Consumption of oily substances (clarified butter, oil, fats); bathing with warm water and taking enemas or *basti*.
2. Stay warm - fomentation or sudation to induce sweating with the help of decoctions prepared from *Vāta* reducing medicines, bathing with hot water or with these decoctions along with the ingestion of heat producing foods to induce sweating.
3. Mild purgation using medicines prepared from oily, hot, sweet, sour and salty substances to eliminate excretory wastes.
4. Tying the diseased area of the body with a cloth or poultice (healing through medicated cloth), pressing the diseased area with hands and feet, massaging and bathing with *Vāta* reducing substances or inhaling them nasally (*nasya*).
5. Pouring *Vāta* - controlling warm decoctions gently over the head (*śirodhārā* therapy).
6. Drinking medicated *āsava* (fermented medicated herbal decoctions) prepared from *Vāta*-reducing herbs and substances.
7. Using oil, clarified butter and other oily foods processed with *Vāta*-decreasing and purgative herbal medicines that elevate the digestive fire and act as an appetizer; these work as a stimulant to pacify *Vāta* and as a laxative to excrete the waste. These oils and medications can be used as eatables, and they may be drunk and used for massaging.
8. Eat a *Vāta* pacifying diet containing wheat, sesame, ginger, garlic and jaggery.
9. Various types of *bastis* (enemas) using herbal medicines made from hot and oily substances.
10. Psychological treatment according to the ailment and condition of the patient to promote calmness and to relieve fear and anxiety.
11. Get plenty of rest, avoid mental strain and stress.
12. Do not drink alcohol or take any form of stimulants including coffee, tea and nicotine. Give them up altogether.

4. *Vātakṣaye kaṭutiktakaṣāyarūkṣalaghuśītānām.* (*Ca.śa.*6.11)

Oil is the best among all *Vāta* pacifying greasy substances, both taken internally and applied externally. Sesame oil and *anuvāsana basti* (oil enema) are particularly beneficial for patients with vitiated *Vāta*. As the primary location of *Vāta* in the body is the colon (large intestine), therefore to pacify *Vāta, bastis* (*nirūha* and *anuvāsana basti*) are the best cure. Medicated substances are introduced through the anus for easy and fast expulsion of impurities and to restore the balance of *Vāta*, treating the source of the trouble.

- **Symptoms of low level of *Vāta* and its treatment**

When the level of *Vāta* drops, there is a corresponding slowing down of physiological functions, laxity in the body organs and reduction in perceptive power of sensory organs. Behavioral indications are weariness, sluggishness, dipping of spirit (unhappiness), disinterest in speech (vocal uneasiness), slowing down of normal *Vāta* functions and symptoms arising as that of *kaphaja* diseases like weak digestion, nausea and so on.

To provocate *Vāta*, one should adopt food habits and lifestyle that increase it. Light, rough, cold, bitter, pungent, astringent and spicy foods increase *Vāta*. In addition, food types listed under the reasons for *Vāta* aggravation must be consumed. In *yoga*, *vāyu* represents *prāṇa* (*prāṇa vāyu*), hence *prāṇāyāma* (regulated breathing exercises) are recommended, which not only help to alleviate many types of disorders, but also prevent diseases. By the efforts of Swami Ramdev and the hard work done by Patanjali Yogpeeth to spread awareness for *yoga* and *prāṇāyāma* among the masses, today, millions of people worldwide have transformed their lives and achieved a new disease-free life.*

- ***Sāma* and *Nirāma Vāta***

When *Vāta* mixes with *āma rasa* (accumulated undigested food residue in the body due to improper digestion) it is called *Sāma*. The following signs are manifested in case of *Sāma Vāta* formation.

- Constipation or obstruction in elimination of feces, urine and *apāna vāyu.*
- Weak digestive power
- Laziness, sleepiness and sluggishness
- Intestinal disturbance (gurgling sounds)
- Pricking pain
- Backache
- Inflammation or swelling of the joints leading to gout or arthritis

If *Sāma Vāta* is not treated in the initial stages, it gets vitiated and spreads throughout the body. When *āma* is absent from *Vāta*, it is called *Nirāma Vāta* which causes dryness of the skin and other organs, a dry mouth and tongue, no constipation, but mild discomfort. It should be treated with a diet having inverse properties like an oily diet.

*For more information consult *'Pranayam Rahasya'* of Swami Ramdev.

- ***Vāta* and its divisions**

Vāta has been previously classified into five types. Each of the five types of *Vāta* have different places of origin and different actions, which are responsible for different ailments. On this basis they are divided into five types. The following table lists their locations, functions and ailments.

Table 2: Types of *Vāta* - Locations and Functions

S. No.	Types	Locations	Functions	Ailments due to vitiation
1.	*Prāṇa*	Head, chest and brain	Perceptions and movements of all kinds, respiratory activity, swallowing of food, conversion of breath into life-force, spitting and sneezing.	Hiccoughs, cough, bronchial asthma, cold, sore throat and other respiratory complaints, giddiness, syncope and other neurological disorders.
2.	*Udāna*	Throat and lungs (diaphragm, chest)	Controls the process of speech and the voice, upward movement of breath, responsible for strength, enthusiasm and will to work.	ENT (Ear, Nose, Throat) and eye ailments, speech defects.
3.	*Samāna*	Stomach and intestinal tract	Stimulating gastric juices to break down food and categorizing them into *dhātus* (*rasa, rakta, māṁsa,* etc.) and *malas*, digestion, assimilation, controlling *svedavaha, jalavaha* and *doṣavaha srota* (channels).	Dyspepsia or low digestive fire, indigestion, diarrhea and defective assimilation linked to too slow or too rapid digestion.
4.	*Apāna*	Colon (large intestine), lower abdomen, organs of the pelvic region (kidneys, bladder, navel, rectum)	Elimination of waste, keeps foetus in place and helps during birth, responsible for sexual function (ejaculation of semen) and menstruation.	Renal calculi (stone), diseases of bladder, anus, testicles, uterus and obstinate urinary ailments including diabetes, *prameha* and dysuria.
5.	*Vyāna*	Permeates the entire body especially the heart	Responsible for sweating, bending, heart rhythm, blinking of eyelids, yawning, governs peripheral circulation, dilation and constriction of blood vessels, transport nourishing juices and blood throughout the body, elimination of waste and ejaculation of semen.	Sluggishness in the circulatory function of *srota*, fever, diarrhea, bleeding, tuberculosis and other diseases.

(II) *Pitta Doṣa*: The energy of biotransformation and heat generation

Pitta is responsible for all aspects of heat, light and color in the body. It is derived from the *Sanskrit* word ***'Tapa'*** from ***'Taptati iti pittam'*** means heat or energy. The one that generates heat in the body is called *Pitta*. *Pitta* is a source of thermal energy in the body. Sometimes *Pitta* is translated as bile, which is one important aspect of its functions.

Pitta doṣa regulates the enzymes and hormones in the body. It is responsible for digestion and metabolism. Whatever is ingested as food and the oxygen we breathe in are converted to body constituents (*doṣas*, *dhātus* and *malas*) by the action of *Pitta*. Although *Pitta* and *agni* (digestive enzymes) are slightly different factors, it is *Pitta* that represents *agni* (enzymes) in the body. In other words, like the *agni* (enzymes), *Pitta* maintains body temperature and digests food. It imparts color to the blood and skin, gives form, beauty and glow to the body, keeps the heart healthy, absorbs oily substances that are massaged into the skin and lends it luster. In addition, *Pitta* controls mental functions like intellect, wisdom, perception, judgement, valor, courage, confidence and joyousness.

When *Pitta* is out of balance, the digestion is adversely affected. Digestive energy levels go down leading to an increase in *Kapha* tendency and its concerned attributes, which further results in the loss of enthusiasm and accumulation of *Kapha* in the heart and lungs. There are five types of *Pitta* on the basis of location and function:

1. *Pācaka Pitta* - that which promotes digestion.
2. *Rañjaka Pitta* - that which increases the formation of *rakta dhātu* or blood, imparts color.
3. *Sādhaka Pitta* - that which is responsible for intellect and memory and allows us to accomplish things effectively and promotes contentment and enthusiasm.
4. *Alocaka Pitta* - that which promotes sight.
5. *Bhrājaka Pitta* - that which maintains body temperature and provides a glow to the skin.

These five forms of *Pitta* can also get disturbed by disease and must be kept in harmony for total well-being. Forty types of ailments are caused by irregularities in *Pitta doṣa*, fewer than the number for *Vāta* but more than that for *Kapha*. In the three *doṣas*, *Pitta* comes next to *Vāta* in sequential order of importance. Following is the description of its various aspects.

- **Natural attributes of *Pitta***

Pitta is slightly oily, hot, sharp, fluid, sour, tremulous and pungent[(5)]. It is digestive and causes burning, and smells fleshy. When it is in *nirāma* state, it is bitter in taste and yellow in color. In the *sāma* state, it is sour and blue in color. Like *Vāta*, *Pitta* also helps to build the body constitution and determine its nature. Its different attributes affect the physiology in different ways (Table 3).

Table 3: Attributes of *Pitta* and their Effect on Physiology

	Attributes	Physiological Manifestations
1.	*Uṣṇatā* (Heat)	Causes intolerance towards heat and hot things; having a red and hot face, warm, flushed skin; tender and clean body; freckles, spots, moles, warts, blemishes; quick advent of wrinkles, premature graying of hair and baldness, soft-brown facial and body hair; overactive metabolism, excessive hunger and thirst.
2.	*Tīkṣṇatā* (Sharpness or Acuteness)	Tendency to over exhibit body strength; sharp mind and sharpness of character; strong digestive power, intake of food and fluids in large quantity due to over secretion of stomach acids; flexibility; and inability to face difficult situations.
3.	*Dravatā* (Fluid, Moist or Oily)	Causes tenderness and laxity (looseness) in joints, bones and muscles; excessive sweating, urination and excretion.
4.	*Amlatā* and *Kaṭutā* (Sour and Pungent)	Results in low semen quantity, poor sexual desire and maternal ability.
5.	*Visragandnitā* (Sour Smelling or Pungent Odor)	Causes strong and pungent odor in underarms, mouth, head and other body parts.

When *Pitta doṣa* dominates in the body, one is said to have a *Pitta* constitution. The properties of *Pitta* result in moderate strength, life-span, material and spiritual knowledge, material assets (wealth), other abilities and endowments in life.

- **Reasons for *Pitta* aggravation**

By nature *Pitta* is inclined to "Moderation" and consequently excessive stress, overwork or sheer thoughtlessness are the reasons for imbalance. *Pitta* also aggravates naturally during young age. The following are the major reasons of imbalance:

5. *Sasnehamu ṣṇaṁ tīṣkṣṇaṁ ca dravamḍmlaṁ saraṁ kaṭu.*
Viparṣtaguṇaiṛ pittaṁ dravyairāśu praśāmyati. (*Ca.sū.* 1/60)

1. **Dietetics:** Consumption of large quantities of pungent, bitter, spicy, sour, hot, oily substances, fried foods and large amount of sour or fermented foods such as cheese, vinegar, sour cream, alcoholic beverages and fermented drinks. In addition, consuming dry vegetables and salty foods (alkaline substances); irregular food habits (not eating at a fixed time, not eating when hungry, eating without hunger) and indigestion; certain foods like sesame oil, mustard, horse gram, whey, certain green vegetables, citrus and acidic fruits, yogurt, buttermilk, cream of boiled milk, vinegar, intoxicating drinks, *Goha* and *Kaṭvara* fish and flesh of sheep and goat especially aggravate *Pitta*.
2. **Emotional disturbances and stress:** Anger, fear and depression, stress, constant pressure, heat and fatigue also affect *Pitta doṣa*.
3. **Habits:** Excessive sexual intercourse and too much exposure to heat and sun.
4. **Season:** It is also aggravated naturally in autumn, when the weather is in transition phase.

- **Symptoms of aggravated *Pitta***

  For the identification of *Pitta* imbalance, the following symptoms are to be looked upon:

1. **Physical indications:** Excessive *Pitta* in the body leads to lack of strength, excessive sweating, hunger and thirst, increased body temperature and burning sensation; skin inflammation, boils, rashes, acne, hot flashes, ulcers and heart burn; darkening of the complexion; unpleasant body odor, bad breath; oiliness/stickiness; sore throat (pharyngitis), dizziness and syncope; sunstroke, sunburn; yellowing of skin, fecal matter, urine, nails and eyes are special symptoms of aggravated *Pitta*.
2. **Mental indications:** Anger, hostility, impatience, resentment, irritability and self-criticism are the signs of *Pitta* imbalance.
3. **Behavioral indications:** Intolerance of delay, outburst of temper, criticism of others, argumentative nature, fatigue, lack of sleep, craving for cold foods and drinks, bitter and sour taste in the mouth, and intolerance to heat are results of elevated *Pitta* levels.

   These are the most common signs of *Pitta* imbalance.

- **Remedies for balancing *Pitta***

The key to balancing *Pitta* is 'Moderation,' so the very first thing is to stay away from the causes for aggravation of *Pitta*. The following methods help in balancing *Pitta*:

1. *Virecana* or therapeutic purgation is the best way to reduce excess *Pitta*. *Pitta* initially accumulates in the stomach and duodenum (small intestine) and purgatives reach these sites and eliminate the accumulated *Pitta*.
2. Meditation is very useful to regain inner calm and equilibrium, and coolness in any form helps to counteract the imbalanced *Pitta*.
3. Regular intake of *ghee* (clarified butter), which has *Pitta*-opposing qualities like sweetness, coldness and other moderate features is also very useful to keep *Pitta* in state of balance. Other such oily and smooth substances are also helpful. In fact chronic *Pitta* diseases can be treated in different ways with different types of medicated *ghees*.
4. Aloe vera juice, sprouted grains and porridge in the diet also pacify *Pitta* provocation.
5. Avoid strenous physical exertion or overheating in sunlight outside, as *Pitta* types are heat-sensitive. In addition, enjoy nature's beauty - look at the sunset, watch the full moon, walk beside lakes and running water, and walk in the cool breeze.

- **Symptoms of low level of *Pitta* and its treatment**

When the level of *Pitta* falls in the body, there is a corresponding reduction in the digestive power, low body temperature, color and luster in the skin, and also an increased sensitivity to cold. There is a slowing down of the body processes controlled by *Pitta*.

In this condition, regular intake of *Pitta* increasing foods and medicines are useful, especially those predominant in the fire element. Similarly, herbal preparations which increase the digestive fire should be administered. These are mainly items that are pungent, spicy, sour and salty in taste. In addition, such a lifestyle is recommended which helps to aggravate *Pitta doṣa*.

- ***Sāma* and *Nirāma Pitta***

When *pitta* mixes with *āma (sāma)*, it ferments and changes into a sour-smelling, heavy, blackish or greenish liquid, which does not easily mix with water and other liquids. In this condition, sour eructation (acidity), heart burn and burning in the throat and chest are experienced. On suffering from *Sāma Pitta*, foods with bitter taste should be consumed to remove the *āma*. When *Pitta* is without *āma (nirāma)* it is very pungent, hot, bitter in taste, red or yellow in color and mixes easily in water. It increases the interest in food, appetite and digestion. When suffering from *Nirāma Pitta*, sweet and astringent substances should be taken in order to pacify it.

- ***Pitta* and its divisions**

On the basis of locations and functions, *Pitta* is divided into five types. (Table 4)

Table 4: Types of *Pitta* - Locations and Functions				
S. No.	**Types**	**Locations**	**Functions**	**Ailments due to vitiation**
1.	*Pācaka*	Lower part of the stomach and central part of the small intestine	Digestion, separation of nutrients and wastes after digestion, nourishing other *Pittas* from its own location and regulates the heat of digestion, generates hunger and thirst.	Indigestion and irregular digestion.
2.	*Rañjaka*	Red blood cells, liver, spleen and stomach	Blood formation from digested food energy. Converting *rasa* into *rakta* (blood) and imparting color.	Anemia, jaundice, blood disorders, skin inflammation.
3.	*Sādhaka*	Heart	Removes dark thoughts and desires, increases intelligence, memory, wisdom and self-esteem.	Psychological disturbances, fear, anger and greed; heart diseases.
4.	*Ālocaka*	Eyes	Lends vision. It functions in the retina to make possible the perception of *rupa* (form) and color of an object.	Impaired vision and other ophthalmic ailments.
5.	*Bhrājaka*	Skin	Maintains a glowing complexion, lending color, brightness and luster to the skin; absorbing oily substances to nourish various body parts; maintains body temperature.	Leucoderma and other skin diseases.

(III) *Kapha Doṣa* or *Śleṣmā:* For stability and lubrication

Kapha is derived from *Sanskrit.* ***'Kena jalena phalati niṣpadhyate iti Kaphaḥ'*** means 'that which originates from water' while *śleṣmā* ***'sliṣhyati iti śleṣmā'*** means 'that which joins together and brings about cohesion.' Often *Kapha* is translated as mucus or phlegm, which is an important part of *Kapha*, particularly in disease, but *Kapha* is much more than that. It represents potential energy in the body.

Kapha doṣa provides nourishment to all parts of the body and regulates the other two *doṣas*, *Pitta* and *Vāta*. *Kapha* provides moistness, oiliness and smoothness to the body organs. It lubricates and connects joints and bones, increases libido, strength, enthusiasm, heals wounds, improves immunity, provides energy for mental and physical activities, and it is responsible for behavioral and psychological changes. *Kapha* is also the primary cause for sleep, lethargy and inertia (*tamas*). When there is an increase in heat due to *Pitta* or dryness due to *Vāta*, then *Kapha* increases the secretion of oily and smooth fluids and protects the tissues from damage.

There is a corresponding increase in opposing *doṣas*, *Pitta* and *Vāta*, if *Kapha* decreases. This results in damage to the *dhātus* (tissues) by the heat of *Pitta*, and accumulation of *Vāta* causes dryness and lightness in the *dhātus*, joints, heart and other parts of the body. However, in normal conditions when *Kapha* is in balance, it nourishes and strengthens all the cells, tissues and organs and does not provide space for the flow of *Vāta*. The five types of *Kapha* according to their locations and functions:

1. *Kledaka* - that which moistens the food in the stomach to break it up.
2. *Avalambaka* - that which maintains body fluids and physical stamina; protects and fortifies the heart.
3. *Bodhaka* - that which controls the taste and sharpens taste perception.
4. *Tarpaka* - that which ensures the stabilityof sense organs.
5. *Śleṣaka* - that which connects and lubricates the joints and improves their mobility.

It is important to manage the *Kapha doṣa* by keeping these five types of *Kapha* in sound state. There are twenty types of *Kapha* diseases, the fewest of all the *doṣas*. Following is the description of its various aspects.

- **Natural attributes of *Kapha***

Kapha is heavy, cold, soft, oily, sweet, firm and viscous in its natural attributes[(6)]. Besides, it is dull, stable, moist and white in appearance. People with dominant *Kapha doṣa* have a *Kapha*-type body makeup. People with *Kapha* constitution usually have an abundance of strength, material wealth, knowledge, power and peace. They usually have a long life-span. However, weight of an individual also plays a significant role in this regard. Obesity can neutralize all the good qualities of *Kapha doṣa* and makes one more susceptible to various diseases. Qualities of *Kapha*

6. *Guruśītamṛdusnigdhamadhurasthirapicchilāḥ.*
Śleṣmaṇaḥ praśamaṁ yānti viparītaguṇairguṇāḥ. (*Ca.sū.* 1/61)

are mentioned in Table 5.

Table 5: Attributes of *Kapha* and their Effect on Physiology

	Attributes	Physiological Manifestations
1.	*Gurutā* (Heaviness)	Firm and steady gait; heavy digestion.
2.	*Śītalatā* (Coolness)	Low appetite and reduced thirst, low perspiration and reduced feeling of heat.
3.	*Mṛdutā* (Softness)	Pleasing appearance, soft skin and hair, soft manners, soft look in the eyes; cheerful, beautiful; tenderness and clarity of complexion.
4.	*Snigdhatā* (Smoothness)	Smoothness in body organs and tissues.
5.	*Madhuratā* (Sweetness)	Increase in quantity of semen.
6.	*Sthiratā* (Stability or Steadiness)	Slow initiation of actions, slow manifestation of serious illnesses.
7.	*Picchilatā* (Viscousness or Stickiness)	Firmness, stability and lubrication in tissues and joints; well-built and beautiful.
8.	*Dṛḍhatā* (Firmness)	Compactness, strength and firmness in the body.
9.	*Ghanatā* (Denseness)	Plumpness and tendency towards obesity; well-built body and sturdy muscles.
10.	*Mandatā* (Dullness or Slowness)	Slow in action, lack of physical activities; deliberate thinking.
11.	*Ślakṣṇatā* (Oiliness)	Oiliness in body organs and tissues.

• Reasons for *Kapha* aggravation

Kapha is the slowest and steadiest of all the *doṣas*. In *Kapha* imbalance, following are the major reasons for its aggravation.

1. **Dietetics:** Excess consumption of sweet, sour (acidic), heavy, oily and fatty foods. Over intake of mutton, fish, salt, sesame, milk and watery substances such as carbonated drinks (soft drinks) and cold refrigerated water. Eating while the previous meal is yet to be digested and overeating also lead to *Kapha* aggravation.
2. **Habits:** Noon siesta, lethargy and laziness, lack of exercise and physical activity increase *Kapha doṣa* in the body.
3. **Season:** Siesta, lethargic attitude and lack of physical activity increase *Kapha doṣa* in the body.
4. **Natural tendency:** *Kapha* aggravates naturally in the morning, during first part of the night, after meals and during childhood.
5. **Heredity:** If diabetes, obesity or allergies run in your family you are more prone to aggravated *Kapha doṣa.*

• Symptoms of aggravated *Kapha*

With an increase in *Kapha doṣa* the following symptoms are manifested:

1. **Physical indications:** Laxity in the body organs, sweet taste in the

mouth, pale skin, coolness, smoothness, itching, heaviness, stickiness in the *malas* (body wastes - fecal matter, urine, sweat), a feeling of being wrapped in a wet cloth, to feel as if the affected part is being plastered with some substances, swelling, congestion, sinus, cold, increased mucus secretion from the nose and eyes, slow sensory responses, bronchial asthma, sore throat, cough, diabetes and fluid retention in the tissues.

2. **Mental indications:** Dullness, feeling of lifelessness, disinterest in any work, depression and over attachment.
3. **Behavioral indications:** Lethargy, over sleeping, drowsiness, possessiveness, slow movements, greed, inability to accept changes.

- **Remedies for balancing *Kapha***

Kapha is balanced by "Stimulation." With precautions and knowledge of the above-listed reasons one can pacify and keep *Kapha* in balance. The following remedies can be used to restore *Kapha* to its normal state.

1. Using pungent, astringent and hot herbal preparations to induce vomiting and increase laxity in the stool.
2. Intake of *Kapha* pacifying foods those are bitter, pungent, astringent, dry and hot because they can balance the characteristics of *Kapha doṣa*.
3. Intake of food that have *Kapha* reducing *vīrya* (potency), *ipāka* (post-digestive effect) and *prabhāva* (action).
4. Intake of old honey and old fermented substances like *Ayurvedic* herbal *āsava* and *ariṣṭa*.
5. Smoking of medicinal anti-*kapha* herbs and fasting to reduce weight.
6. Staying warm (dry heat is best), different kinds of fomentation therapies and sudation so as to induce sweating, sun bath, powder (dry) massage and *ubaṭana* (smearing herbal pastes on the body).
7. Rigorous exercise, brisk walking, running, sit-ups, high and long jumps, wrestling, swimming and so on.
8. Wearing warm clothes and staying awake till late in the night.
9. *Nasya* (inhalation of medicines administered nasally).
10. Staying active and keeping away from lethargy and laziness.
11. Anxiety, worry and grief reduce *Kapha*, but they lead to several other ailments and psychological disorders.

Therapeutic vomiting (*vamana*) is the best remedy to balance increased *Kapha* because it clears the vitiated *Kapha* from the stomach and the chest regions, the primary Kapha sites in the body. However, the medicines used for this process (*vamana*) must be prepared from pungent and hot substances.

- **Symptoms of low level of *Kapha* and its treatment**[7]

When the level of *Kapha* is low, the body displays the contrary symptoms of dryness, a persistent burning sensation, a feeling of lacuna (emptiness) in the

7. *Śleṣmakṣaye rūkṣatāntardāha āmāśayetaraśleṣmāśayaśūnyatā sandhiśaithilyaṁ tṛṣṇā daurbalyaṁ prajāgaraṇaṁ ca.* (*Su.sū.* 15/11)
Tatra śleṣmakṣaye svayonivardhanānyeva pratīkāraḥ. (*Su.sū.* 15/12)

Kapha locations (lungs, heart, joints and especially head), looseness and laxity in joints, excessive thirst, weakness and lack of sleep. Low *Kapha* affects the normal functioning of *Kapha doṣa* leading to a reduction in its actions and properties.

- ***Sāma* and *Nirāma Kapha***

When *Kapha* gets corrupted with *āma* (*Sāma Kapha*), it becomes turbid, dense, thick, sticky and unpleasant to smell. This prevents belching and reduces hunger. In contrast, *Nirāma Kapha* (without *āma*) is foamy, condensed, light, odorless and settled. It does not stick in the throat and keeps the mouth clean and fresh.

- ***Kapha* and its divisions**

The five types of *Kapha*, on the basis of location and function are listed in Table 6.

Table 6: Types of *Kapha* - Locations and Functions

S. No.	Types	Locations	Functions	Ailments due to vitiation
1.	*Kledaka*	Stomach	Moistens food and helps in digestion.	Weak and impaired digestion, feeling of heaviness, common cold, nauseous feeling.
2.	*Avalambaka*	Chest	Energizes limbs, lungs and heart.	Lethargy
3.	*Bodhaka*	Tongue and throat	Perception of taste.	Impaired taste buds and salivary glands.
4.	*Tarpaka*	Head	Protects and nourishes the sense organs.	Loss of memory and retardation of sensory activities, general dullness of senses.
5.	*Śleṣaka*	Bones and joints	Connect bones to joints and lubricate joints to protect, nourish and smoothen their movements.	Pain in the joints and slowing down of their functions.

- **Location of *Doṣas* in the body and their positive psychological traits**

Normally all three *doṣas* pervade the entire body, but they keep changing according to seasons, diet, digestive fire in the body and the strength of the alimentary canal, but any one of them is prominent in certain organs and parts of the body and this is known as the specific location (shelter) of that *doṣa*. [PLATE 8]

Doṣa	Location	Positive Psychological Traits
Vāta	Below the navel region; in the urinary bladder, small and large intestine, pelvic region, thighs, legs and bones.	Imaginative, sensitive, spontaneous, resilient, exhilarated.
Pitta	Between the navel and chest; in the abdomen, digestive organs and excretory organs; in sweat, lymph and blood.	Intellectual, confident, enterprising, joyous.
Kapha	Throat; parts above the throat, head and neck, chest, in the joints, upper portion of abdomen and fat of the body.	Calm, sympathetic, courageous, forgiving, loving.

• Relation between the three *doṣas* and the five elements

Āyurveda believes that the body has originated from the five elements as mentioned before. Like everything else, the *doṣas* are also made up of the five elements. The predominant elements in each *doṣa* are as follows. [PLATE 9]

Doṣa	**Predominant elements**
Vāta	Space (ether) and Air
Pitta	Fire and Water
Kapha	Water and Earth

3. *Prakṛti*: Know Your Constitution

The constitution of any body type is called '*prakṛti*' in *Sanskrit*, a term meaning 'nature.' Each individual is born with a unique body type determined by the dominance of one or more of the three *doṣas*. This is referred to as *Prakṛti* or the body constitution of an individual. According to *Āyurveda*, *prakṛti* plays a very important role in a person's health, well-being and to diagnose diseases in an individual. It helps to determine the most beneficial diet and lifestyle that an individual should follow. Diagnosis of disease and the type of treatment to be followed are also dictated by *prakṛti*. An individual's constitution is determined on the basis of body structure, nature, character, attributes and a wide variety of factors

The constitution of an individual is determined at the time of conception. It is a universal law that a child is conceived in the mother's womb from the union of the sperm and ovum, after which foetal development starts. The *doṣas* that are predominant at the time of conception determine the child's bodily constitution, build, character, nature and mental makeup. These attributes and characteristics are referred to as *prakṛti* in *Āyurveda*. If all three *doṣas* are in balance during conception, the new born will be healthy in every respect. On the contrary, if the *doṣas* are completely out of balance, conception will not take place or if it does, the embryo will not develop or be deformed. If one of the three *doṣas* dominate, the child's physiological and psychological characteristics will be governed by that dominating *doṣa*. If two *doṣas* are in dominance, a combination of their qualities will determine the *prakṛti* of a child. The sixteen customary rituals starting from conception, engendering a male issue, hair parting to birth ritual, naming ceremony, first feeding ceremony and so on also possess much influence on socio-cultural dimension. Accordingly, there are thus seven possible types of *prakṛtis*[8]:

1. *Vāta prakṛti* 2. *Pitta prakṛti*
3. *Kapha prakṛti* 4. *Vāta-Pitta prakṛti*
5. *Pitta-Kapha prakṛti* 6. *Vāta-Kapha prakṛti*
7. *Sāma prakṛti* (Equal effect of all the three *doṣas*)

Here, the fact that should be kept in mind is that although the balance of *doṣas* in an individual is constantly changing during the course of life owing to various internal and external factors, the basic birth *prakṛti* is rarely altered. This means that the predominant *doṣa* of an individual can be easily aggravated. For example, the slightest disturbance and unregulated regime in a *Vāta prakṛti* individual increases *Vāta* immediately. The same is true for all other *prakṛtis*. Besides *doṣas*, some other factors that chiefly help in the development of an individual's *prakṛti* are as follows:

1. Condition of an ovum and sperm at the time of conception.
2. Season and environmental condition within the uterus.
3. Food and lifestyle habits adopted by the mother, during pregnancy.
4. Attributes and action of the elements that bring about the fusion of sperm and ovum.

A person's *prakṛti* is also affected by genes, ancestry, ethnicity, race, family attributes (such as purity, piousness, wisdom, humility, bravery and so on), geographical location (belonging to hilly areas, plains or cooler places), time, season and its effect on parents, age of the parents (especially of the mother) and the child's own qualities (based on previous births). Yet, despite being influenced by many factors, *prakṛti* is determined primarily by the *doṣas*. Hence, its nomenclature is based on the *doṣa* type. The three *doṣas*, their attributes and effect on the body have been listed earlier. Here the characteristics of the three body-types (*Vāta prakṛti*, *Pitta prakṛti* and *Kapha prakṛti*) are mentioned. (Table 7)

People with mixed *prakṛti* (like *Vāta-Pitta, Vāta-Kapha* and so on) display the characteristics of both constituent *doṣas*. *Vāta prakṛti* people are susceptible to *Vāta* diseases, which easily and swiftly trap them. The same is true for other *prakṛti* as well. They tend towards diseases of their birth *doṣa*. Avoid dietary habits and lifestyle that aggravate the dominant *doṣa* and adopt habits that pacify them and keep them in balance.

It has been generally observed that life-span, strength, children, knowledge, luxuries, comfort in life and wealth are enjoyed most by *Kapha prakṛti* individuals. *Pitta prakṛti* individuals have these in moderation while *Vāta prakṛti* individuals tend to have them in limited amount, though there are many exceptions to this general rule.

8. *Sapta prakṛtayo bhavanti doṣaiḥ pṛthag dviśaiḥ samastaiśca.* (*Su.śā.* 4/61)

Table 7: Characteristics of Different *Prakṛtis**				
S.N.	**Characteristics**	***Vāta***	***Pitta***	***Kapha***
1.	Body frame	Short height; light and thin build; stiffness or shivering in the body; physically weak.	Medium frame, medium build with moderate strength and endurance; softness of muscles and bones.	Tall frame; symmetrical, beautiful and strong body; solid, powerful build or tendency to gain weight easily.
2.	Skin and external appearance	Dryness in the body, roughness on face, nails, teeth, sole of feet and palms; skin color brown or black.	Softness in the body; red hot face; fair or ruddy skin, often freckled with moles, warts and wrinkles.	Cool, smooth, thick, oily, pale white, glowing skin.
3.	Hair	Dry, split-ends,easily breakable hair; less dry and rough hair on body and beard.	Blond, light brown or reddish tone; normal to less hair, prematurely gray or bald.	Thick, curly, long, black and beautiful hair.
4.	Other body parts	Prominent veins; a crackling sound produced during walking, stretching of joints or limbs; cracked soles and palms.	Blackness (pigmentation) in body parts, nails, eyes, tongue, soles and palms.	Prominent (raised) forehead, chest and arms; due to obesity, unsymmetrical and fatty abdomen, thighs or buttocks.
5.	Eyes	Dry, dull or sleepy eyes.	Small or reddish eyes, less eye lashes.	Big and attractive eyes, reddish at outer corners; thick eye lashes.
6.	Sleep and dreams	Light, scanty, interruped sleep; fearful and insecure; fearful dreams.	Moderate sleep, little but sound; fiery, angry, violent dreams.	Heavy, prolonged, sound sleep; tranquil nature; pleasant, nature loving dreams.
7.	Food and digestive power	Variable and scanty appetite, irregular hunger and digestion, easily skips meals; aversion to cold weather and cold food.	Good, excessive and unbearable appetite, takes large amounts of food, strong digestive fire, sharp hunger and thirst, cannot skip meals, feels ravenously hungry; aversion to hot food and hot weather.	Slow but steady appetite, slowly takes food many times in a day in small quantity, slow digestion, mild hunger, scanty thirst; interested in oily, fatty foods, heavy meals and fast foods.

8.	Gait, temperament and memory	Walks quickly; changeable, unpredictable, very active; changing mood and liking towards others; excitability, fickle-minded, short-tempered, vivacious; quick to grasp, also quick to forget, makes quick decisions without thought; runs away from difficult situations; very talkative.	Intense, short-tempered, tendency to be angry, moderate activities; has a determined stride while walking; aggresive, lacks patience, irritable, adventurous, enterprising, likes challenges; good sharp memory and intellect.	Lethargic, slow to grasp but good long-term memory, slow decision making; careless, slow but sincere and graceful in action or works with steady energy; tolerant, patient; slow and steady walk; relaxed personality, slow to anger, calm, cool, tranquil, affectionate, forgiving, possessive.
9.	Mind and thoughts	Deformity in the mind and body, diseases occur quickly; poor mental state; mental and physical energy comes in bursts. Displays bursts of emotions that are short-lived and quickly forgotten; lack of knowledge, restless and impatient.	Excessive negativity in thoughts; moderate physical and mental state; diseases occur at normal pace but symptoms manifest quickly.	Calm mind, does not think much, but positive approach; even in severe diseases symptoms manifest slowly.
10.	Sex desire	Unstable sex desire (sometimes more or sometimes less).	Reduced sexual desire or low reproductive capability.	High sexual desire.
11.	General susceptibility to diseases	Bronchial asthma, cough, cold, sore throat; supraclavicular diseases (disease of eyes, ear, nose); loss of appetite, indigestion, chronic constipation; piles, prolapse of anus, rectum and urinary bladder diseases; mental disorders, loss of memory; tendon disorders (musculo-skeletal disorders), body edema and joints pain, muscle spasms or cramps.	Sour burps (acidity), bitter taste, indigestion, loss of appetite, peptic ulcers, anemia, jaundice; skin diseases (eczema, leucoderma, rashes, acne); eye diseases and poor eyesight; diseases due to heat stroke; mental imbalance (fear, anger, fascination, hostility and so on).	Loss of appetite, decreased digestive fire, nausea, tastelessness; heaviness, cough, cold, congested sinus, bronchial asthma, allergies; loss of memory; lethargy, unproportionate body and obesity, diabetes, high cholesterol, depression, chronic sluggishness.

Table 8: Method to Determine Your *Prakṛti* (Body-Type) Based on General Characteristics

S. No.	Characteristics	*Vāta*		*Pitta*		*Kapha*	
1	Body frame	Small frame or thin and weak body	☐	Medium frame	☐	Tall frame, powerful built (gain weight easily)	☐
2.	Types of hair	Dry	☐	Normal or less hair growth (reddish or brownish hair)	☐	Thick, curly, oily hair	☐
3.	Eyes	Dry, sleepy eyes	☐	Small and reddish eyes	☐	Big and attractive eyes	☐
4.	Skin	Dry and rough	☐	Soft or reddish	☐	Oily and tender	☐
5.	Mental activity	Impatient, restless	☐	Sharp intellect, perfectionist and aggressive	☐	Steady, stable, full of patience	☐
6.	Memory	Quick to grasp, quick to forget	☐	Sharp memory	☐	Good long-term memory	☐
7.	Gait	Fast and quick	☐	Moderate speed and determined walk	☐	Slow and steady gait	☐
8.	Reaction to stress	Anxious, worried and nervous	☐	Anger, easily irritated	☐	Not easily ruffled, stubborn	☐
9.	Sleep	Light-interruped sleep	☐	Moderate sleep, little but sound	☐	Heavy, prolonged, sound sleep	☐
10.	Effect of weather	Aversion to cold weather	☐	Aversion to hot weather	☐	Aversion to cool, damp weather	☐
11.	Temperament	Quickly changeable, fast speaking	☐	Slowly changeable	☐	Steady, stable and not changeable	☐
12.	Hunger	Irregular	☐	Sharp	☐	Slight, can easily skip meals	☐
13.	Body parts	Prominent veins, a crackling sound produced while walking	☐	Profusion of moles and black spots, freckles and wrinkles	☐	Fatty (obese), bulging abdomen, unproportionate body.	☐
	TOTAL	w	☐		☐		☐

Give an appropriate ☑ sign in the boxes next to what matches your

* These characteristic types must be further adjusted according to racial tendencies and cultural preference. Different races have natural proclivities for specific body and lifestyle characteristics, e.g., Africans have dark skin.

constitutional makeup in the above table according to the characteristics of *Vāta + Pitta + Kapha* best fitting in your body-type and add the total number of characteristics in each constitution types. Comparing these will determine your body-type. The maximum number of characteristics manifested represents the main *prakṛti* and the lowest number represents the subsidiary *prakṛti* for you. According to *Āyurveda* this chart is helpful in determining the *prakṛti* according to your physical, mental and behavioral characteristics.

The importance of knowing your body-type, *Vāta*, *Pitta* or *Kapha* is that it sharply focuses your diet, exercise, daily routine and other measures for preventing disease. By eating and adopting a lifestyle accordingly, one can have balance everywhere. This quiz will help you to find it yourself. Remember, however, that all the three *doṣas* are present in everyone, and all three need to be kept in balance. The knowledge of body-type obtained by solving the quiz is your key to total balance. It provides all important aspects for change - to change yourself as nature made you.

Knowledge of *prakṛti* is not only beneficial for an individual but absolutely essential for a physician. Medication, diet and lifestyle changes are prescribed keeping in mind the *prakṛti* of a patient because, even when the symptoms in two different individuals suffering from the same disease are the same, the medication and diet given to a *Pitta prakṛti* individual will be of a cool nature and potency (*vīrya*) whereas the medicine and diet prescribed for *Kapha prakṛti* individual will have hot attributes, potency (*vīrya*) and post-digestive effect (*vipāka*). Only those medicines and foods, which are chosen according to the *prakṛti* of an individual, are beneficial. Others are likely to aggravate the illness or cause further complications. For example, while black pepper is beneficial for *Kapha prakṛti* patients, it is not suitable for *Vāta prakṛti* patients, and can create complications in *Pitta prakṛti* individuals. This proves how essential the knowledge of *prakṛti* is in *Āyurvedic* practice. Hence, a complete knowledge of *prakṛti* is an intrinsic part of the *Āyurvedic* system of healing. In contrast with modern medical science it can be shown that different substances can cause varied reactions or allergies in different people due to an altered bodily constitution. It is even very essential for a dietician to have knowledge of suitability and unsuitability of diet and lifestyle according to *Āyurveda*.

One's basic *prakṛti* (constitution) is of two types: (1) Natural or basic *prakṛti,* and (2) *Prakṛti* governed by external factors.

1. **Natural or basic *prakṛti*:** Generally, the body constitution in terms of *tridoṣa (Vāta, Pitta* and *Kapha*) governed by the body at the time of

conception is called natural or basic *prakṛti*. It is the stable body-type of an individual. In general, the interests and working capacity of a person is governed by the condition of these *doṣas*.

2. ***Prakṛti* governed by external factors:** The second type of *prakṛti* depends upon our diet, lifestyle, nature, conduct, conditions, daily routine and seasonal fluctuations. This is changeable (increases and decreases) according to conditions and it is unstable, but when you recognize your basic *prakṛti* based on *doṣas* and when you try to alleviate your *doṣas*, then your *prakṛti* also transforms. As and when one brings the *doṣas* back into equilibrium, they acquire a *sāttvika* property and become free from diseases and deformities.

4. *Traiyopastambha*: Three Supporting Pillars of the Body

According to *Āyurveda*, the body is built up of three biological energy forces (*Vāta, Pitta* and *Kapha*) which are designed by the combination of five elements. To keep the body healthy and strong, *Āyurveda* recommends three supporting pillars of the body in the form of diet, sleep and celibacy[9]. Just as a building requires pillars for its foundation, similarly the three supporting pillars - diet, sleep and celibacy are important for body maintenance. On the foundation of these three pillars, equilibrium of the three *doṣas* (*Vāta, Pitta, Kapha*) depends, and this is the basic principle to keep the body balanced and healthy. [PLATE 10]

(a) ***Āhāra* (Diet):** Diet is the main factor to achieve good health. It is impossible to have good health without a proper diet. Our *Upaniṣads* and classical texts state that diet is essential for life - ***'Ánna ve prāṇa.'*** Virtually, diet is a medicine in itself. Food replenishes and supports the *doṣas, dhātus* and *malas*, and stabilizes life. By the knowledge of this science (food science) we can treat many diseases. Food not only affects body, but mind too functions accordingly. There is a famous saying that "the food you eat reflects your state of mind." Purity of food ensures purity of mind. Purity of mind ensures steady recollection. When recollection is secured there will

9. *Dehadhāraṇād dhātavaḥ* (*Ca.sū.* 28/4)
Dhātavo hi dehadhāraṇasāmarthyāt sarve doṣādaya uccyante. (*A.saṅ.sū.* 1)
Dhātvo rasaraktamāṁsamedosthimajjaśukrāṇi teṣāmapi śarīradhārakatvāt. (*Su.ci.* 5/21)
Rasāsṛṅmāṁsamedo, sthimajjāśukrāṇi dhātavaḥ, sapta dūṣyāḥ. (*A.hṛ.sū.* 1/13)

be liberation of all blockages. Food as a whole regulates the body functions and processes, thereby protecting the body from various diseases. It provides the body with fuel and energy. Inevitably, food strengthens the sensory and motor organs, promotes strength and vitality to the *prāṇa* (life-force) and nourishes the proclivity of mind. It provides the material needed for growth and upkeep of the body. Even after growth has ceased, the body continues to change throughout life and constantly worn out tissues need to be changed and repaired.

Actually diet can be beneficial for our health only when we eat for the sake of health rather than taste. Always remember that our life is not meant for food, but food is essential for our life. *Vāgbhaṭa*, a disciple of *Sage Caraka* being questioned by *Caraka* on the subject concerned with health, replied ***"Hitabhuk, mitabhuk, ṛtubhuk."*** This means 'eat food according to your own constitution, in an appropriate quantity and earned by right means or sources, which makes the food beneficial for health, otherwise there is a probability for several diseases to develop.' A person who can control his taste can keep good food habits. *Sage Caraka* had described eight important facts regarding food intake, which is known as a food directory (*Ahāra Saṁhitā*)*. Thus, food should be taken according to the prescribed method, keeping in mind these eight factors: the nature of the food, processing, combination, quantity, place, time, dietary rules and one's own constitution. By following these factors, this supporting pillar of diet becomes stable, but otherwise it gets disturbed and shattered.

Sage Caraka also stated that - 'food is vital for living beings that is why people rush to it.' Ones complexion, cheerfulness, life-span, voice, appearance, intelligence, contentment, desires, nourishment, corpulence, strength, power and intellect, all depend upon food.

(b) ***Nidrā* (Sleep):** The second important supporting pillar is sleep. After whole day's routine, when one's body and mind are completely tired, the sensory and motor organs become relaxed, then one goes to sleep. By means of sleep, the body and mind get rest which compensates the loss during activities. Sleep is invaluable. When one falls asleep, all the lax and inactive sensory and motor organs along with the mind get refreshed and energetic. To hasten the development of a child's physical and mental growth, God arranged the cycle of sleep for 18-20 hours in 24 hours among infants, while for a healthy adult 6-8 hours of sleep in 24 hours is essential and sufficient. A

* For detailed description on diet consult chapter 6 - Dietary Facts and Rules

sound sleep at a proper time brings cheerfulness, strength, vitality, longevity and wisdom. On the contrary, improper sleep results in debility, feebleness, infertility, a sluggish brain, sorrow and petulance.

To sleep early and to wake up early is beneficial for good health. This has been an eternal part of Indian culture. It has been quoted that: '***Brahme muhūrte budhyeta puruṣto rakṣārthamāyuṣḥ,***' and in English it is well said that "early to bed and early to rise makes a person healthy, wealthy and wise." Today, with a materialistic and pleasure-seeking lifestyle, this has changed a lot. Sleeping late at night and rising late in the morning has become a general trend. This is very harmful and can deteriorate the mind and the body.

In this context, one must also remember that while on the one hand insomnia or less sleep is harmful for health, and on the other hand excessive sleep also causes lethargy, indolence, *Kapha* vitiation, obesity, loss of appetite, indigestion and several other disorders.

(c) ***Brahmacarya*** **(Celibacy):** The third pillar of the body is celibacy (sexual restraint). Celibacy means 'to protect the semen' by keeping control over all the senses. The last *dhātu* (body tisssue) formed after the digestion of food substances we eat is the *śukra* (semen). According to *Āyurveda*, the strength of the body depends upon semen. This fact is proved by the following statement: "strength of the body depends upon digestive fire and vitality depends upon the semen." It is also quoted that: ***'Maraṇaṁ bindu pātena, Jīvanaṁ bindu dhāraṇāt'*** which means 'excessive discharge of semen may result in death while its retention provides life.' Here the word ***'bindu'*** represents ***'śukra'*** or semen. Opposite to celibacy, sexual indulgence and enjoyment results in loss of semen corresponding to loss of strength. By celibacy one becomes full of '*ojas,*' brightness, intellect, strength and majesty. Celibacy prevents diseases, preserves health and promotes strength. Therefore, it is considered an essential supporting pillar. At some places the word 'uncelibacy' is used in place of 'celibacy.' It concludes that even a married couple should undergo sexual intercourse within a limit, in a controlled manner and not freely and frequently. The term '*vīrya*' is considered as semen in males and it relates to an ovum in females. To follow celibacy has been set for both males and females.

It should be noted that to follow the rules of celibacy, one should avoid sexually stimulating drugs, pictures, photographs, diet, liquids and lifestyle. Pious conduct and simple food support celibacy. Only one who understands the importance of celibacy can adapt themself to such conduct. Its importance has been mentioned in our *Vedas* as - ***'Brahmacaryeṇatapasā devā mṛtyumapāghnata'*** (*Atharvaveda* 11.5.19) which means "by the penance of celibacy, deities have defeated death."

5. *Saptadhātu*: The Seven Fundamental Tissues

The most important elements that constitute our body are the *dhātus*. They are the basic tissues that play an important role in development, nourishment, sustaining the body and they support the formation of the basic body structure. Hence, they are termed as *'dhatus*[10]*'* as the Sanskrit word *'dhatu'* means "constructing element." There are seven types of *dhātus*. [PLATE 11]

1. *Rasa* or *Lasikā* (Plasma or Nutrient Fluid)
2. *Rakta* (Blood or the hemoglobin part of the blood*)*
3. *Māṁsa* (Muscular tissue)
4. *Meda* or *Vasā* (Adipose or fat tissue)
5. *Asthi* (Bone tissues: tendons and ligaments)
6. *Majjā* (Bone marrow)
7. *Śukra* (Reproductive or Generative tissues)

Like the *doṣas*, the seven *dhātus* are also composed of the five elements and one or two elements predominate in each *dhātu*.

Dhātu	**Dominant Element**
Rasa	Water
Rakta	Fire
Māṁsa	Earth
Meda	Earth
Asthi	Air and Space (ether)
Majjā	Fire
Śukra	Water

The *dhātus* are formed as a result of the action of *jaṭharāgni,* the digestive fire (enzymes) that breaks down food in the stomach and gastro-intestinal tract. Digestive enzymes break down food into two parts - *sāra* or nourishing essence and *kiṭṭa* (*mala*) or waste materials that require elimination. *Sāra* is carried to different parts of the body by *vyāna vāyu*, where it nourishes and replenishes *rasa, rakta* and other *dhātus*. Conversion of food into the building blocks of the body or *dhātus* takes place in a definite order. Food (nutritive part - *sāra*) is first converted into *rasa dhātu*, which then makes *rakta*, which is further transformed into *māṁsa*, *māṁsa* converts into *meda, meda* changes to *asthi, asthi* into *majjā* and *majjā* finally nourishes and develops into *śukra*.

10. *Rasastuṣṭiṁ prīṇanaṁ raktapuṣṭiṁ ca karoti.* (*Su.sū.* 15/7)

There are some special cells in the body and brain that never change or transform while other cells of the body, right from blood cells to sperms and ova, all undergo the process of construction, degeneration and regeneration in a cycle of origin, development and dissolution. Blood, muscles, adipose tissue, bone and all the tissues are continuously undergoing this cycle, which depends on *jaṭharāgni* (digestive fire). Thus for complete wellness, proper digestion and assimilation of nutrient rich food is necessary. Along with the digestive system, thirteen *agnis* including the *jaṭharāgni* (digestive fire) all should perform a balanced action, which is of utmost importance. Therefore, the *dhātus* are also part of the biological protective mechanism. With the help of *agni*, they are responsible for the immune mechanism. The post-digestion of food, called 'nutrient-plasma' (*āhāra rasa*), contains nutrition for all the *dhātus*. This *āhāra rasa* (nutrient-plasma) is transformed and nourished with the help of heat called *dhātvagni*, of each respective *dhātu*. In this sequence *rasa dhātu* is the first to get nourished. Hence, *rasa dhātu* (formed after digestion of ingested food) is the base element useful for every moment ongoing - functional, mental and sensual activities and transformation into *rakta* (blood), *māṁsa* (muscles), *meda* (adipose tissue), *asthi* (bone), *śukra* (sperm) and *raja* (ovum). The three *doṣas*, seven tissues, five elements, body, sense organs, mind and all their functions are govered by this *rasa dhātu.* Body development, co-ordination, conservation, immunity (protection), growth, repair and nourishment of the body are all directed by *rasa dhātu*. *Rasa dhātu* is produced in the digestive tract after digestion from where it is transported throughout the body. Some portion of this *dhātu* is involved in the formation of other *dhātus* (tissue) and elements like iron, fat, carbohydrates, protein, calcium, magnesium, vitamins, minerals, nutrients and micronutrients required for *dhātu* (tissue) formation are absorbed through the intestines and fat is absorbed by the lacteal ducts. When this *rasa dhātu* moves to the liver from the intestine it mixes with *rakta* (blood) and is circulated throughout the body thereafter.

Like the *doṣas*, the amount of *dhātus* in the body usually remains constant, but they can be easily vitiated by the *doṣas*, which in their increased state overflow into the *dhātus*. This imbalance in *dhātus* is a result of imbalance in *doṣas* and leads to many diseases in the body. Since it is the *doṣa* that affects and vitiates the *dhātus*; *dhātu* is also called a '*dūṣya*' (one which gets polluted or corrupted). The diseases so caused are named after the *dhātus* which have been corrupted. Hence, *rasaja roga* refers to an illness caused due to the vitiated condition of *rasa dhātu*. Similarly there is *raktaja roga*, *māṁsaja roga*, *medaja roga, asthija roga, majjāgata* roga and *śukraja roga*, emerging due to the vitiation of their respective *dhātus*. Below is a brief description of the natural characteristics and deformities caused by the seven *dhātus*.

(i) ***Rasa dhātu* (Plasma or Nutrient Fluid)**

Normal functions: It contains nutrients from digested food that nourish all the tissues, organs and systems of the body. It produces joy and satisfaction and helps in the production of the next *dhātu*, *rakta* (blood)[11].

Symptoms of increase: Symptoms similar to *Kapha* vitiation are observed. Specific symptoms are decrease in digestive power, excess salivation, nausea, vomiting, lethargy, heaviness, coolness, weakness or laxity in the limbs, bronchial asthma, cough and excessive sleep.

Symptoms of decrease: These include dryness in the mouth and other organs, roughness of the skin, fatigue, increased thirst, vocal senstivity to sound, increased heart beat, cardiac pain, feeling of lacuna in stomach and heart, languor and rapid breathing, and a decrease in the quantity of other *dhātus*.

***Rasaja roga* or diseases caused by vitiation of *rasa dhātu*:** It causes loss of appetite, general apathy (anorexia), bad taste in the mouth, loss of sense of taste (inability to judge and enjoy taste), pain, fever, syncope, blockage in the *srota* (body channels), impotence, yellow skin tone, weakness, emaciation, loss of body weight, reduction in digestive power, premature wrinkling and graying of the hair.

Treatment: Rejuvenating and strength-promoting medicines are useful in the medication of diseases caused due to defectiveness in *rasa dhātu*.

(ii) ***Rakta dhātu* (Blood)**

Normal functions: It is life promoting and sustains *prāṇa* (life-force) by governing oxygenation in all tissues and vital organs. It improves the skin glow and complexion[12] and makes it possible for sense organs to perceive (stimulus). *Rakta* nourishes and replenishes *māṁsa dhātu*. The nutritive elements of all the *dhātus* are engrossed in *rakta* (blood) *dhātu*.

11. *Raktaṁ varṇaprasādaṁ māṁsapuṣṭi jīvayati ca. Teṣāṁ kṣayavṛddhī*
śoṇitanimitte. Taddhi śuddhaṁ hi rudhiraṁ balavarṇa sukhāyuṣā. (*Su.sū.* 14/21)
Yunakti prāṇinaṁ pāṇaḥ śoṇitaṁ hyamuvartate. (*Ca.sū.* 24/4)
Dhātūnāṁ pūraṇaṁ varṇaṁ sparśajñāna saṁsayam.
Svāḥ śirāḥ saṁcaradraktaṁ kuryyāccānyān guṇānapi. (*Su.śā.* 7/14)
Dehasya rudhiraṁ mūlaṁ rudhirenaiva dhāryate.
Tasmād yatnena saṁrakṣyaṁ raktaṁ jīva iti sthitiḥ. (*Su.sū.* 14/45)

12. *Māṁsaṁ śarīrapuṣṭiṁ medasaśca* (*Su.sū.* 15/7 [1])

Symptoms of increase: Redness in the eyes and complexion, and high blood pressure are the most important symptoms.

Symptoms of decrease: Weakening of the blood vessels and veins, weakening of digestive fire and provocation of *Vāta*; rough, dry, dull and hard skin; craving for sour and cold foods.

***Rakṭaja roga* or diseases caused by vitiation of blood:** Leprosyand other dermatological diseases, leucoderma, itching, dermatitis, urticaria, eczema, blemishes, ringworm, moles, red spots on the skin, pimples, naevi, corns, exudating pustules, erysipelas, abscesses, pseudo tumors, blood cancer, intrinsic hemorrhage (bleeding), metrorrhagia, discharge from male and female genital organs, splenomegaly, stomatitis (mouth ulcers), gingivitis (oral disease), jaundice, gout and redness in the urine.

Treatment: The best therapies for *rakṭaja roga* are blood purification by means of blood-letting, nourishment and purgation.

(iii) *Māṁsa dhātu* (Muscular tissue)

Functions: *Māṁsa dhātu*, the muscular tissue, is the main cementing component of the body[13], holding the body, limbs and organs together. It is a covering of delicate vital organs. It performs the movements of the joints and maintains sturdiness and physical strength in the body. It is involved in the production of *meda dhātu* and provides protection to the complete skeleton system.

Symptoms of increase: Weight gain (obesity) and heaviness in the body as a result of accumulation of muscular tissues on the neck, hips, cheeks, lips, thighs, legs, calves, arms, stomach and chest.

In this condition adopt lightning therapies that will reduce the body musculature such as purification therapies, fasting, balanced diet, physical exercise and *yogāsanas*. Avoid foods made from clarified butter, oil, animal fats, sweets and sugar

Symptoms of decrease: Symptoms due to reduction in muscular tissues are opposite to those of an increase. Thinning of flesh is seen along with weakness of muscles. The patient loses weight and experiences fatigue, dryness, prickling pain and weakening of blood vessels.

To increase the muscles, take a fat and protein-rich diet like milk, milk

13. *Medaḥ snehasvedau dṛḍatvaṁ puṣṭimasthnāṁ ca.* (*Su.sū.* 15/7 [1])

products and other dairy products, sprouted green gram, sprouted grains and Bengal gram in large quantities. Non-vegetarians will be benefitted from an increased intake of mutton and meat broth.

Māṁsaja roga **or muscular disorders:** These include accumulation of fat on thighs, goiter, scrofula (enlarged cervical glands), cyst formation on the tongue, palate and neck, tumors, warts, enlargement of abdomen and glandular swellings.

Treatment: *Māṁsaja* diseases respond best to surgery, alkalis, cauterization and heat treatment, as they usually involve excess development or inflammation of the muscles.

(iv) ***Meda dhātu*** **(Adipose or fat tissue)**

Functions: *Meda dhātu*, the fat (adipose) tissues provide warmth, lubrication and oiliness to the body(14). Fat protects the body and lends strength, sturdiness and stability to the organs. It helps to nourish *asthi dhātu.*

Symptoms of increase: Excessive oiliness in the body, symptoms similar to increase in *māṁsa dhātu* (goiter, development of belly), cough, bronchitis, exhaustion, breathlessness, flabbiness and sagging of the buttocks, breasts and waist due to fat accumulation and increased body odor. All precautions recommended in increase of *māṁsa dhātu* should be adopted.

Symptoms of decrease: Pain and feeling of emptiness (lacuna) in the joints, dull and sleepy eyes, dryness in the skin and hair, blocking of ears, fatigue, thin and lean body and stomach, emaciation, lack of tactility on the back and enlargement of spleen. The patient craves for fat rich and oily foods. All therapies for increasing weight and eradicating emaciation are helpful.

Medaja **roga or diseases of the adipose (fat) tissue:** Sweet taste in the mouth, burning sensation in the limbs, tangling of hair, lethargy, excessive thirst, dry mouth, throat and palate; increased secretion of

14. *Ābhyantaragataiḥ sārairyathā tiṣṭhanti bhūruhāḥ.*
Asthisāraistathā dehā dhriyante dehinā dhruvam. (*Su.śā.* 15/23)
Yasmācciravinaṣṭeṣu tvaṅmāṁseṣu śarīṇām. Asthīni na vinaśyanti sārāṇyetāni dehinām. (*Su.śā.* 5/21)

body wastes like sweat, increased secretion from the skin pores, burning sensation and numbness in the body.

Treatment: An increase in *meda dhātu* can be treated in the same way as obesity, by means of lightning therapies such as fasting, a light diet, weight-reducing pungent and bitter herbs; physical exercise and *yogāsanas*. A decrease can be alleviated by the treatment meant to increase weight (stoutening therapies), with increased intake of fat, clarified butter, milk, oily foods, tonic and rejuvenating herbs.

(v) ***Asthi dhātu* (Bone tissue)**

Functions: Bones constitute the basic structure and skeleton on which the body is constructed and upheld, and provide shape and support to the body as a whole[15].

Symptoms of increase and diseases: Abnormally large and thick bones, bone enlargement, excess growth in the nails and hair mass, extra teeth, enlargement of teeth, pain in bones and teeth, distortion of the nails, diseases of the hair, beard and body hair. It includes all the main types of arthritis.

Symptoms of decrease: Osteopenia, osteoporosis, degradation of bone, pain in bones and joints, loss of sensation (numbness), roughness in the bones and joints, hair loss from the body and beard, looseness (laxity) in the joints, and dryness and wreckage of teeth and nails.

Treatment: An increase in bone tissue can be treated through enemas with bitter herbal medicines. Ailments caused by a decrease in bone tissue respond well to a calcium rich diet, milk, buttermilk, cottage cheese, diluted yogurt (*lassī*), dry fruits, Bengal gram, green gram and other pulses, fresh fruits, leafy vegetables, clarified butter and milk flavored with bitter herbs. Vitamin D and sunlight is also beneficial. Other substances such as *muktāśukti* and *śankha bhasma* are effective too.

(vi) ***Majjā dhātu* (Bone marrow)**

Functions: Bones are packed with marrow in their empty spaces. Its function is to fill the bony spaces with nourishing fat and provide

15. *Majjā snehaṁ balaṁ śukrapuṣṭiṁ pūraṇamasthnāṁ ca karoti.* (*Su.sū.* 15/7)

lubrication, oiliness and strength to the body[16]. It also carries motor and sensory impulses.

Symptoms of increase and diseases: Heaviness in the body especially in the eyes, tenacious boils on the joints, bone and blood cancer, pain and boils in finger joints, dizziness, syncope and blackouts.

Symptoms of decrease: Hollowness in the bones, osteopenia, osteoporosis, rheumatoid arthritis, brittle bones and joints, small body frame, weak and thin physique, dizziness, blackouts and deficiency of *śukra dhātu* (sperm and ovum).

Treatment: Intake of all sources of proteinaceous substances and bone marrow cures *majjā* decrease.

(vii) ***Śukra dhātu* (Reproductive or generative tissues)**

Functions: *Śukra* is the last *dhātu* and is considered to be the quintessential sap of all the preceding *dhātus*. It is strength promoting and the most powerful among all *dhātus*. Its main function is to help in procreation[17]. Patience, courage, fearlessness, attraction towards the opposite sex, enthusiasm, excitement, sturdiness, sexual impulse, easy secretion and ejaculation of seminal fluid during intercourse are governed by *śukra dhātu*.

Symptoms of increase: Secretion of excess semen, increased desire for sex, stones (calculi) in the urethra.

Symptoms of decrease: Weakness, lack of energy, dry mouth, anemia, fatigue, impotence, absence of semen and ejaculation during intercourse, extreme pain in the testes and burning sensation in the genital organs.

***Śukraja* roga or diseases related to reproductive system:** Impotence, low libido, cause for unhealthy and physically/mentally challenged offspring, impotent or short-lived offspring.

Treatment: Excess of *śukra dhātu* can be corrected by fasting, balanced diet and intake of semen-decreasing bitter and pungent substances, whereas decrease in *śukra dhātu* benefits from using aphrodisiac substances and medicines that are sweet in taste and nourishes the semen.

16. *Śukraṁ dhairyaṁ cyavanaṁ prītiṁ dehabalaṁ harṣa bījārthañca.* (*Su.sū.* 15/7)
17. *Bhramaraiḥ phalapuṣpebhyo yathā sambhriyate madhu*
Tadvadojaḥ svakarmabhyo guṇaiḥ sambhriyate nṛṇām. (*Ca.sū.* 17/75[1])

- **Increase and decrease in *dhātus***

The level of all seven *dhātus* in the body is controlled by special digestive powers and enzymes known as *agnis*. The body has thirteen *agnis* in all, of which seven are *dhātvagnis*. If these *dhātvagnis* are in balance, the *dhātus* will remain in balance. When the *dhātvagnis* become too active, then there is a decline in the *dhātus* due to excessive metabolism of food, which is the primary source for the regeneration of all seven *dhātus*. In contrast, weak *dhātvagnis* will lead to an increase in the *dhātus* and poor digestion. When one *dhātu* is defective, it affects the successive *dhātus*, as each *dhātu* receives its nourishment from the previous *dhātu* in sequential order. Therefore, to keep the *dhātus* in balance, it becomes imperative to keep the seven *dhātvagnis* in balance.

6. *Ojas*: The Vital Essence

In the transformation of food from *rasa* to *śukra dhātu*, *ojas* releases at every step. *Ojas* is an essence of all the *dhātus*, the substance of all hormonal secretions which support the auto-immune system. It means 'that which invigorates' and in medical terminology it is also referred to as *'bala'* or the inner strength (immunity), which resists diseases. Just as bees collect honey from the nectar of flowers, the digestive fire collects *ojas* from the essence of all *dhātus*. Like the *dhātus*, *ojas* is also nourished by *āhāra rasa* (nutrient plasma - the nutrient-rich product from the metabolic processing of food)[18]. *Ojas* is the seat of '*prāṇa*' (life-force). Even though it permeates the entire body, it is closely connected to the heart, the prime location of *ojas*, and from there the arteries carry and distribute it throughout the body. One other interpretation of *ojas* residing in the heart is that it brings *sāttvika* mental thoughts and expression, particularly on the forehead, piousness, a good and truthful character, positive attitude, devotion, faith, belief, trust and enthusiasm. The more we perform *prāṇāyāma* (regulated breathing), meditation and prayer, the more *ojas* and *tejas* we gain and thus become more knowledgeable and enlightened. Its absence decays the body parts, and eventually loss of *prāṇa* (life). *Ojas* is smooth, cool and oily, and has reddish, yellowish and whitish hues. It is of two types:

1. ***Para*:** Located in the heart, it has eight vital points. Its complete degradation leads to death.

18. *Tatra balena sthiropacitamāṁsatāsarvaceṣṭāsvapratighātaḥ.*
Svaravarṇaprasādo bāhyanāmābhyantarāṇāṁ.
Karaṇānāmātmakāryaṁpratipattirbhavati. (*Su.sū.* 15/25)

2. ***Apara*:** Permeates in the entire body; its normal quantity is about a handful. A decrease in the *apara ojas* leads to lifelessness, loss of enthusiasm, strength and reduced immunity; cause to manydiseases.

- **Functions of *ojas* and its importance:** *Ojas* lends strength and radiance to the body. Being the essence of all *dhātus*, its decline in the body leads to a corresponding decline in the ability of *dhātus* to support the body, in spite of being in balance[19]. It keeps all *dhātus* stable stable and nourished. All physical, mental, sensory and motor functions are made possible by the action of *ojas*. It is also the source of joy, sorrow, will power, intellect, determination, arrogance, patience and enthusiasm. It refines the speech and appearance and strengthens immunity. In brief, it is the fuel of life, health and happiness.

  Some experts consider *ojas* an *upadhātu* (minor *dhātu*) as it is an essence of all *dhātus* and thus it supports the body like all other *dhātus*, but due to its meagre quantity, it can't nourish and sustain any single *dhātu*.

- **Causes of decrease:** Repressed anger, worry, fear, sorrow and other emotions; decline in the amount of *dhātus*, *doṣas* or *malas*; excessive fasting or inadequate diet; intake of dry food; overexertion; insomnia; excessive secretion of *Kapha*, blood, semen and waste matter; emaciation due to illness and injury can also lead to declined *ojas*.

- **Symptoms of decrease[20]:** A timid and frightened personality, dry and lusterless appearance, emaciation, restlessness, general weakness of the mind and body, increased worry and tension, painful and fatigued organs and a loss of zest for the life. It weakens the immune system, along with a decrease in will-power, determination and motivation in life.

- **Treatment[21]:** The use of sweet, cold, smooth, oily, light and wholesome foods, milk, life-prolonging herbal preparations, wintercherry (*aśvagandhā*) and other rejuvenating medicines and aphrodisiacs help to increase the amount of *ojas* in the body. In addition, keeping one happy and adopting a healthy lifestyle also boost *ojas*. Keeping the *srota* (channels) of *malas* and *dhātus* clean is also important. An increase in *ojas* results in contentment, joy, physical and mental strength. A surplus of *ojas* is also beneficial and does not lead to any deformity or illness.

19. *Ojaḥ kṣīyate kopakṣuddhyānaśokaśramādibhiḥ.*
Vibheti durbalo, bhīksṇṁ dhyāyati vyathitendriyaḥ. (*A.hṛ.sū.* 11/39)
20. *Jīvanīyauṣadhakṣīrarasādyāstata bheṣajam.* (*A.hṛ.sū.* 11/41)
Tanmahat tā mahāmūlāstaccaujaḥ parirakṣtā.
Parihāryā viśeṣeṇa manaso duḥkhahetavah. (*Ca.sū.* 30/13)
21. *Rasāt stanyaṁ tato raktamasṛjaḥ kaṇḍarāḥ sirāḥ.*
Māṁsādvasā tvacaḥ ṣaṭ ca medasaḥ snāyusambhavaḥ. (*Ca.ci.* 15/17)

Children should be encouraged to adopt a diet and lifestyle that boosts *ojas*, so as they may become physically strong, intelligent, energetic, pious and achievers in every sphere of life.

7. *Upadhātus*: Sub-Tissues

Those components of the body that uphold the body and lend support and structure, despite being present in small quantities and do not participate in the production of other *dhātus,* are called *upadhātus* or sub-tissues. The major difference between *dhātu* and *upadhātu* is that *dhātus* not only supports the, body but also generates the next *dhātu*, whereas *upadhātus* only shares the task of lending support. They are termed *upadhātus* because they are produced from *dhātus.*

- **Nourishment of the *upadhātus* (sub-tissues)**

Just as the nutritive (*sāra*) part of *rasa dhātu* nourishes the subsequent *dhātu*, *rakta* (blood) and also produces milk and menstrual blood as an *upadhātu.* While blood is produced regularly, menstrual blood is produced only once a month, and being an *upadhātu* it is produced in a limited quantity. In the same way, nutritive (*sāra*) parts of *rasa dhātu* produces *māṁsa dhātu*, and nourishes the veins and arteries. Similarly, *māṁsa* is transformed into *meda dhātu* which produces *meda* and *asthi*, respectively, and nourishes the nerves, ligaments and joints. Breast milk, menstrual fluid, arteries, veins, fat, skin and nerves are the seven *upadhātus*[22]. Since they are directly derived from the *dhātus*, they are termed '*upadhātus.*' A brief description of the three main '*upadhātus* is given below:

➤ **Skin**

The skin covers the entire body. It helps to perceive stimuli such as heat, cold, light, heavy, hard, soft and so on. It provides protection to the whole body. Even though the skin contains all five elements, but air predominates. That's why it adapts the tactile quality of air and perceives all sensations (touch). Apart from tactile perception, the skin keeps the body temperature normal, absorbs energy obtained from the sun, absorbs nutrients and lends luster. Sweat glands are also embedded in the .

➤ **Breast milk**

The presence of this *upadhātu* finds relevance only in females. Breast milk is the best nutrition for infants as it provides maximum nourishment and

22. *Kiṭṭamannasya viṇmūtraṁ rasaya tu kapho, sṛjaḥ.*
Pittaṁ māṁsasya khamalā malaḥ svedastu medasaḥ. (*Ca.ci.* 15/18)

antibodies. Hence, it is termed as life-giving. It is the residue of the sweet part of the *āhāra rasa* and like *śukra* it is present in the entire body, it reaches the breast when required. Healthy and nourishing breast milk mixes easily with water, is sweet, yellowish and odorless. It is considered as the best milk, which keeps all *doṣas* in balance and the body disease-free. A decrease in this *upadhātu* can be corrected with increased intake of *kaphaja* diet. Cumin seeds and asparagus (*śatāvarī*) also help improve milk production. Excess of breast milk should be treated by purification (draining by suckling or use of a breast pump) and in such condition one should consume light food substances.

➤ **Menstrual fluid**

This is also a female-specific *upadhātu*. Menstrual fluid is discharged from the female genitalia once a month after attaining the age of puberty (above 12 years). Normally the menstrual period lasts for three to five days. Between 40 to 50 years of age this discharge ceases at menopause. The basic function of the menstrual fluid is to promote follicular development which supports conception. Its characteristics are similar to those of blood.

Menstrual fluid that is discharged once a month without pain or burning, is neither too much nor too little in quantity, which resembles the color of the red lotus or lac or *Abrus* seed, which easily washes off clothes, which is not very mucilaginous and that lasts for not more than five days, is considered to be healthy. An undue increase in the *upadhātu* results in excessive bleeding, bodyache and malodorous fluid discharge. It leads to debility and even uterine tumors. On the contrary, the decreased, delayed or reduced bleeding may cause pain in the pelvis.

8. *Mala*: Waste Matter or Excretory Products

Metabolic action of food results in two products - *sāra (prasāda)*, the essence from which the *dhātus* are nourished and regenerated, and *asāra (kiṭṭa)*, the inessential portion from which body wastes such as fecal matter, urine and sweat are produced[23]. These waste products are called *malas* (from *malina* which means befouling). Since these excretory products are toxic to the body, they are known as *malas*. If they are contaminated (*dūṣita*) by *Vāta* and other *doṣas*, they are also termed as *dūṣyas* (pollutants). Regular

23. *Sirāḥ srotāṁsi mārgāḥ khaṁ dhamanyo nāḍya āśayāḥ.* (*Su.śā.* 9/3-*Ḍalhaṇa* comm.)
Ākāśīyāvakāśānāṁ dehe nāmāni dehinām.
Srotāṁsi khalu pariṇāmamāpadyamānānāṁ
dhātūnāmabhivāhīni bhavantyayanārthena. (*Ca.vim.* 5/3)
Sravaṇāt srotāṁsi. (*Ca.sū.* 30.12)

elimination of these *malas* is of utmost importance for good health.

'Jāyante vividhā rogāḥ prāyaśo malasañcayāt.

Sarveṣāmeva rogāṇāṁ nidānaṁ kupitaḥ malaḥ.'

Means if the toxic wastes accumulate in the body in excess, it causes the genesis of different types of diseases.

Apart from the undigested part of ingested food, the *malas* also contain toxins produced by tissues during metabolic activity; undeveloped, dead and lifeless tissues produced during digestive activity; vitiated *Vāta*, *Pitta* and *Kapha doṣas*; other toxins, harmful and useless substances produced in the body.

Malas have the natural property, on accumulation they move to the rectum, bladder, sweat glands and other excretory orifices for evacuation. Fecal matter, urine, sweat, secretions from nails, hair, body hair, facial hair (beard and moustache), nose, ears, eyes and mouth (like mucus and ear wax) are all waste products.

Like everything else, the *malas* also have a correlation with the five elements. A brief description of the three main *malas* - fecal matter, urine and sweat is given below.

	***Mala* (Waste Matter)**	**Dominating Elements**
1.	Fecal matter (*Purīṣa*)	Earth
2.	Urine (*Mūtra*)	Water + Fire
3.	Sweat (*Sveda*)	Water + Fire

- **Fecal matter**

The feces consist of undigested parts of ingested food (*asāra*) along with the wastes produced by the tissue cells. This is the reason why a person who has not eaten for many days and even the foetus in the womb also produces feces. It is imperative that feces should be expelled regularly from the body in order to keep the tissue cells healthy. When they are not regularly and properly excreted from the body, diseases like lumbago (backache), rheumatism, sciatica, hemorrhagic strokes, paralysis, bronchitis and bronchial asthma are easily contracted. Therefore, in *Āyurveda*, the first medicine for all these ailments is a laxative. The accumulation of *mala* in the bowels encourages growth of intestinal worms and other harmful microbes and also prevents the colonization of other useful microbes, thus decreasing its benefits by disturbing the natural microbial interaction within the body. Therefore, it is essential for a healthy body to be cleansed regularly and for all waste products to be excreted properly.

➤ **Functions of the feces**

Feces not only acts as an excretory waste, but it also provides support and gives strength to the large intestine to maintain its tone and sustain *Vāta* and *agni* (fire). If a person has no feces, the intestine will collapse. The base of human life is feces. Though *malas* are considered bodily waste products, urine and feces are not strictly wastes. They are, in fact, to some extent essential for the physiological functioning of their respective organs. For example, feces supply nutrition through intestinal tissues; many nutrients remain in the feces after digestion. Later, when these are absorbed, the feces get eliminated. This is the reason why a patient of tuberculosis, who suffers from a decrease in all the *dhātus*, gets strength and nourishment from the energy provided by fecal matter and it should be ensured that such patients do not pass excess fecal waste. The slightest increase in fecal elimination results in severe debility in such patients.

Too much fecal matter in the intestine causes shooting pain, flatulence, bloating, unsettled bowels, distention, discomfort and a feeling of heaviness. Too much increase in the fecal matter is a result of overeating and indigestion. On the other hand, when there is deficient production of feces, *Vāta* causes spasm in the intestine and moves it upward. The deficiency in fecal matter occurs due to diarrhea, passing of excessive stool or excessive purgation, fasting and eating less than the required amounts of food or fiber. To increase the production of fecal matter, high fiber foods like black gram, green gram, barley, leafy vegetables, flour with husk and other fibrous foods should be taken in large quantities.

- **Urine**

Urine also aids in the evacuation of waste matter from the body. Urine is formed in the large intestine, particularly from the liquid portion of *asāra* (the undigested part of food). The urinary system removes excess water, salts and nitrogenous wastes present in the body and keeps the urinary bladder full and moist. Urine helps to maintain the normal concentration of water and electrolytes within the body fluids. The functioning of this *mala* depends upon the water intake, diet, environmental temperature, mental state and physical condition of an individual. It is emphasized to drink plenty of water (at least about 3-4 liters) both in summer and winter in order to maintain good health. It will help in passing urine at least six times a day and also expel toxins from the body. *Āyurvedic* texts states that human urine is a natural laxative that detoxifies poisons in the system and helps absorption in the large intestine as well as the elimination of feces.

However, passing excess urine is also abnormal. It causes pain in the bladder, a feeling of heaviness, restlessness and discomfort due to frequent urination. These symptoms also occur when the urge to pass urine is suppressed or water is taken while the urge to urinate is strong. If the body retains water, urine will be scanty and this water will accumulate in the tissues. This condition, in turn, will affect the blood and increase blood pressure. A decrease in urine production also causes prickling pain in the bladder, reduced urine elimination, obstructed urination, pain while urinating (dysuria), change in the color generally being yellow or sometimes red (blood mixed with urine); excessive thirst and dry mouth are experienced. Sugarcane juice, liquids and foods that are sweet, sour and salty increase the quantity of urine.

- **Sweat**

Sweat is another very important *mala* or waste material. Sweating is essential to keep the skin healthy and to eliminate waste products from the body. Sweat keeps the skin soft, maintains the flora of the skin pores and also maintains skin elasticity and tone. It also assists the skin in regulating body temperature, so that a constant body temperature is maintained during summer and winter.

Excessive heat, exercise and physical work causes increased sweating. When sweat comes in contact with air it evaporates, lowering the body temperature. In contrast, during winter, the body sweats less and maintains its temperature. Although the body sweats to some degree in every season, it is felt only when it is released in excess or under humid conditions.

Excessive sweating causes smell and itchy skin. It can cause fungal infection and reduces the natural resistance of the skin. Reduced sweating causes blockage in the pores; dry, scaly and cracked skin; loss of tactile perception and a reduction in body hair. Massage, exercise, staying away from windy places, induced sweating (*svedana*) or fomentation with hot substances, consuming substances that cause sweating (honey in water, hot water) and sweat-producing, hot medicinal preparations are helpful in increasing sweat.

It is clear that even though they are waste products, these three *malas* are essential to maintain a healthy body.

- **Other waste products**

The above statement is also true for all other waste materials secreted in the eyes, ears, mouth, nose and other body parts. Their secretion should be just enough to maintain the required moisture in these organs. On increased production, these body parts feel heavy and there is increased secretion. On the other hand, owing to a decrease in the level of these *malas* dryness, pain, lightness and lacuna (emptiness) is experienced. Increased secretion results from their accumulation and decreased due to too much evacuation.

Even though, abnormal increase or decrease both are harmful, but decrease is more harmful than an increase, because it does not support or help the organs to perform their normal functions. Though, all these *malas* are naturally malodorous, an unbearable smell indicates that something is out of balance and needs attention.

- **Relation between *doṣa*, *dhātu* and *mala***

These three factors - *Doṣas*, *Dhātus* and *Malas* in some way or the other, build the foundation of the human body, they are the building blocks and primary sustaining forces. Hence, their mutual coordination and interdependence is of great importance. *Vāta* is located in *asthi dhātu* (bone), *Pitta* resides in *rakta* (blood), sweat and *Kapha* predominates in the remaining *dhātus*. Therefore, the treatments prescribed for balancing of *doṣas* have a direct impact on the *dhātus* they reside in. The only exception to this is *Vāta doṣa* and the bone tissue where it resides. Normally, an increase in *doṣa* and *dhātu* is treated with lightning (*asantarpaṇa*) therapies and fasting, and a decrease with nourishing and stoutening therapies (*santarpaṇa*). The therapies recommended for *Vāta* imbalance are inverse to it, i.e., the increase requires nourishing and stoutening therapies, while its decrease requires fasting and lightning therapies.

9. Digestion and Metabolism

The food we ingest in the form of protein, carbohydrates, fat, minerals and vitamins, nourish the *dhātus* and provide strength, sturdiness, color, perception, comprehension, understanding, intellect and longevity to the body as a whole. However, this is possible only when the ingested nutrients are successfully converted into bodily tissues. This entire process is called digestion and metabolism and the elements that carry out these processes are referred to as '*agni*' or the biological fire; a catalytic agent in digestion and metabolism. Different enzymes are produced by these *agnis* in the stomach, liver and cells of the *dhātu* channels to carry out the different phases and aspects of digestion. These enzymes convert solid, semi-solid and liquid foods into an appropriate *dhātu* and *mala*. Although *vyāna vāyu*, which carries digested food material all over the body and the *srota* (channel) that transport and distribute nourishment are very important for the digestive process, the digestive fire, *jaṭharāgni* plays the most significant role. Without it, food can neither be digested nor can the *dhātus* be generated in the right manner. According to *Āyurveda*, if *agni* is destroyed, it becomes fatal for a person's life. If *agni* gets corrupted, it leads to many ailments. When *agni* is normal and balanced, it supports a long and disease-free life.

- **Types of *agnis***

Agni in particular is a group of various types of *agnis*. In all, thirteen types of *agnis* are prevalent.

1. *Jaṭharāgni*

2-8. *Dhātvāgnis* - 7 types

9-13. *Pañcabhūtāgnis* - 5 types

➤ ***Jaṭharāgni*: The digestive fire**

Jaṭharāgni is also known as *pācakāgni* (digestive fire) or *kāyāgni* (bodily fire). The importance of this *agni* in the groups of *agnis* has been previously described. It is located between the stomach and the intestines (the small and the large intestines) around the navel. Just as the sun uses its rays to absorb water from ponds, lakes and rivers, *jaṭharāgni*, located in the navel region begins to digest food with its energy as soon as it is consumed. All that we eat is broken down into smaller units and transformed into substances that are analogous to our body constituents by *jaṭharāgni*.

Hence, the main function of *jaṭharāgni* is to initiate the metabolic process and facilitate longevity, complexion, voice, strength, energy, physical growth, enthusiasm, *ojas*, body temperature and to keep the other *agnis* functional. To sustain its functional activities in a controlled manner, it is required to keep this *agni* in a balanced state. *Jaṭharāgni* can be classified in the following four states according to its level and intensity:

(a) *Viṣamāgni*: Unstable state of *agni* (abnormal digestive fire)

As its name suggests, this type of *jaṭharāgni* is never stable. It oscillates between high and low intensity and is rarely in balance. The digestion of food is thus fast, slow or normal according to its changing condition. This state of *jaṭharāgni* occurs mainly due to an increase in *Vāta doṣa*. It results in stomach ache, constipation, flatulence, heaviness in the stomach, unsettled bowels, upward movement of *Vāta*, ascites, dysentery and diarrhea.

(b) *Tīkṣṇāgni*: Intense state of *agni* (increased digestive fire)

This is an intense state of *jaṭharāgni* and causes quick and immediate digestion of food which leads to overeating. This state is also referred as *'atyagni'* or *'bhasmaka,'* when a person becomes a glutton, capable of digesting even large amount of food very quickly. It is a consequence of *Pitta doṣa* aggravation. The patient suffers from dryness in the throat, lips and palate. At the end of digestion, it produces heat, a burning sensation and dryness in the throat, lips and palate.

(c) *Mandāgni*: Low state of *agni* (decreased digestive fire)

In this state, the intensity of *jaṭharāgni* is low and becomes incapable of digesting even small quantity of food. This state of weak and slow digestion is a consequence of *Kapha doṣa* aggravation. The patient experiences discomfort, heaviness in the abdomen and head, cough, bronchial asthma, increased salivation, vomiting or eructation and general body weakness.

(d) *Samāgni*: Balanced state of *agni* (controlled digestive fire)

When all the three *doṣas* - *Vāta*, *Pitta* and *Kapha* are in balance, *jatharāgni* is also in balance, and food is consumed in the proper proportion and digested well in time. This state is called '*samāgni*' (balanced state of *agni*). There is no abnormality in the digestive process in this state. It is an ideal *agni* for health and normal digestion.

➤ ***Doṣas* and *Jaṭharāgni***

Agni or the digestive fire aids in digestion and assimilation. Here it is important to mention that due to *doṣas*, the intensity of *agni* is also affected.

Doṣa	**Level *of agni***
Vāta	Irregular (sometimes intense, sometimes slow)
Pitta	Intense (acute)
Kapha	Slow (sluggish)
Vāta, Pitta, Kapha in equilibrium	Stable *agni* (balanced state)

- ***Bhūtāgnis*: *Agnis* of the five elements**

This group of *agnis* is located in the liver. They are five in number according to the five elements they act upon: 1. *Bhaumāgni* (earth); 2. *Āpyāgni* (water); 3. *Āgniyāgni* (fire); 4. *Vāyavyāgni* (air); and 5. *Akāśāgni* (space or ether).

Each of these *agnis* transform the corresponding elements present in the food that has already been broken down by *jaṭharāgni* to match the state of the same element already in the body and its tissues. Thus, these *bhūtāgnis* located in the liver divide food into five parts which nourish the five elements found in different parts of the body.

- ***Dhātvāgnis*: *Agnis* of the *dhātus* (tissues)**

Dhātvāgnis is the third group of *agnis* found in the body. They help in normal metabolic transformation of tissues. When *anna rasa* (nutrient-plasma), which has been transformed into five elements by the action of *jaṭharāgni* and *bhūtāgnis*, reaches the channels of the *dhātus*, it is further digested by the *dhātvāgnis* located there. This nutrient-plasma (*anna rasa*) gets transformed into *rasa, rakta* and other *dhātus*. Since *dhātus* are seven in number, so are the seven *dhātvāgnis*. These *dhātvāgnis* are named after the tissue that they work on: 1. *Rasāgni*; 2. *Raktāgni*; 3. *Māṁsāgni*; 4. *Medāgni*; 5. *Asthiagni*; 6. *Majjāgni*; 7. *Śukrāgni* (in males) and *Rajogni* (in females).

The actions of these *agnis* regenerate the *dhātus* and also produce *malas* (waste products). When the *dhātvāgnis* are aggravated, it leads to a corresponding decrease in the *dhātus* and vice-versa. When *dhātvāgni* burns too high, *dhātus* cannot build up to the required normal quantity. Conversely, low intensity in the *dhātvāgnis* leads to an increased *dhātu* formation.When the *dhātvāgni* burns too low, more *dhātu* emerge, but of an inferior quality. The entire digestive process due to the action of the three types of *agnis* is briefly explained as follows:

When food reaches the mouth, it is mixed with saliva and its taste is perceived by the tongue. The food then moves into the stomach where solid food particles turn watery, foamy and soft due to the action of the gastric acids and digestive juices. In the first step of digestion, foamy *Kapha* and *madhura rasa* (sweet taste) are produced. The digestion of food in the stomach is normal at this time. This half-digested food essence (*ahāra rasa*) reaches the small intestine through the duodenum. Here *jaṭharāgni* acts on it together with *samāna-vāyu* and *pācaka piṭta*. *Pācaka Pitta* absorbs the liquid part of the *āhāra rasa*, converting it into a solid mass, which is referred to as '*piṇḍa*.' *Kaṭu rasa* (pungent taste) and *Vāta* are produced during this stage. Here food is segregated into two parts: 1. *sāra* or *prasād,* and 2. *asāra* or *kiṭṭa*.

The properly digested part of the food which is in liquid form is the *sāra* part. This forms the first of the seven *dhātus* - the *rasa dhātu* or plasma, which is sweet and smooth due to the action of *jaṭharāgni*. This *rasa dhātu* then nourishes and produces other *dhātus*. However, if *jaṭharāgni* is working at low intensity, the *rasa* or taste turns pungent and sour. This is called the *āma* or *āma rasa* (improperly digested food mass). This *āma* is toxic and the cause of many ailments. The part of food that is undigestible or normally not absorbed is called *asāra* or *kiṭṭa*. Its solid part changes to feces and liquid to urine and collects in the lower parts of the large intestine in the form of *malas*. At this stage, the five *bhūtāgnis* join the metabolic process. They convert their own elements present in the digested food essence to match the forms of the same elements found in the body. This serves to particularly nourish the earth element found in different parts of the body.

The fully digested food essence or nutrient-plasma (*āhāra rasa*) is then circulated around the body as *rasa dhātu* (plasma) through the *srota* (body channel) that carries the nutrient-plasma. This nourishing *rasa*, which is inherently the building block of all *dhātus*, thus reaches all the limbs and organs. Then the digestive action of the *dhātvāgnis* replenishes *dhātus* and produces *ojas* (the essence of all the seven *dhātus*), which has been previously explained. *Pitta* plays a vital role in the entire digestive process. Hence, several *Āyurveda* experts do not differentiate between *agni* and *Pitta*, but there is a subtle difference. It is true that the seven *dhātvāgnis* contain parts of *pācaka Pitta* that helps them to function. The *agnis* also contain factors other than *Pitta*, and it is their combined action that completes the digestive process.

The *rasa* that is circulated around the body is acted upon by the seven *dhātvāgnis* to create the seven *dhātus*. The *dhātus* are said to have three parts, 1. *sthūla* (gross) 2. *sūkṣma* or *aṇu* (subtle) and 3. *mala* (waste matter). The gross part nourishes the same *dhātu*, the subtle part creates the next *dhātu*, and the waste or *mala* part forms the by-product or waste material of that tissue. This way, the action of every *dhātvāgni* produces some by-products and *mala*. For example, the *sāra* (the nourishing part of food) is acted upon by the gross part of *rasa dhātvāgni* to create *rasa dhātu*. The subtle part of the same *dhātvāgni* creates *rakta dhātu* and the *mala* part is converted to *Kapha* (phlegm, saliva and similar secretions). The other *dhātvāgnis* also act in a similar manner, which is described in table 9.

Table 9: *Dhātu, Upadhātu, Dhātvagni* and their Action

S. No.	*Dhātvāgni/ Dhātu*	*Upadhātu*	*Poṣaṇa* (Nourishes)	*Nirmāṇa* (Creates)	*Mala* (*Dhātu*-waste generated)
1.	*Rasa*	Breast milk, menstrual fluid	*Rasa dhātu*	*Rakta dhātu*	*Kapha*
2.	*Rakta*	Tendons, veins	*Rakta dhātu*	*Māṁsa dhātu*	*Pitta*
3.	*Māṁsa*	Fat, skin	*Māṁsa dhātu*	*Meda dhātu*	Secretions of nose and ears
4.	*Meda*	Ligaments	*Meda dhātu*	*Asthi dhātu*	Sweat
5.	*Asthi*	-	*Asthi dhātu*	*Mājjā dhātu*	Hair, body hair and nails
6.	*Majjā*	-	*Majjā dhātu*	*Śukra dhātu*	Oiliness in the skin, eye secretions
7.	*Śukra*	-	*Śukra dhātu*	-	-

- ***Āma rasa***

When *āhāra rasa* (nutrient-plasma, the nutritive part of the ingested food) is not properly digested in the stomach and intestine due to decreased activity of *jaṭharāgni* or *dhātvāgnis*. This undigested food is called *āma* or *āma rasa*. Being toxic, the presence of *āma rasa* in the body causes various ailments, because the elements in this undigested *asāra* or *āma rasa* do not convert into substances acceptable to the body. Hence, the next step in the metabolic process of assimilation by *dhātus* and other body parts does not occur. Due to their inability to move easily in the various body channels (*srotas*), *āma* accumulates in different parts of the body like the lungs, heart and other organs. The four major cavities (brain, chest, abdomen and pelvis) usually attract *āma rasa*, and the abdomen is the most common site of *āma rasa* accumulation. This leads to dyspepsia (indigestion) and other disorders. *Āma rasa* combines with *doṣas*, attacks other organs and causes allergies, bronchial asthma and various other ailments. When the low potency of *dhātvāgni* causes the formation of *āma rasa* (undigested food), the next *dhātu*, i.e. the *rakta dhātu*, is further deprived of nourishment, again leading to various ailments. Since almost all ailments are in one way or the other connected with the formation of *āma rasa*, sometimes they are also referred to '*āmaya.*' The ill-effect of *āma rasa* affects the *pācaka agni* (digestive fire), weakening the metabolic process and leading to improper digestion. It also blocks the *srota* (body channels). *Āma doṣa* can occur in any part of the body. The weakest organs and those with elemental composition similar to *āma doṣa* are most susceptible to its accumulation.

- **Symptoms of *sāma* diseases**

Blockage in the sweat, urine and other *srotas* (channels), weakness, low strength, heaviness, improper circulation of *Vāta*, lethargy, increased salivation and phlegm formation, absence of or inadequate elimination of feces and other *malas*, apathy (anorexia) and fatigue are the symptoms of *sāma doṣa* (*sāma* diseases). When characteristics opposite to these symptoms are manifested, it is a sign of clean *srota* and *nirāma doṣa*.

As stated earlier, a weak digestive system causes the formation of *āma doṣa*. When a *srota* is blocked by accumulation of either *āma doṣa* or *mala*, the remedy is to increase the release of digestive juices or the fire in that *srota* in order to transform the *āma rasa* into the *dhātus* or clearing away the *mala*. Therefore, most *Āyurvedic* medicines contain substances that increase the digestive power at some level. Purifying therapies such as *vamana* (emesis or therapeutic vomiting) and *virecana* (purgation) flush the *āma rasa* and *malas* accumulated in the blocked *srotas*, clearing them and making the *agnis* more effective.

Though the intensity of *agni* is high during childhood, the quantity of food intake is less at this stage. The power of *agni* increases with age, resulting in strong and healthy digestive and metabolic activity. This nourishes the body and boosts physical strength and the growth. The intensity of this digestive fire rises up to the age of 40 and it remains steady between 40-65 years. After 65 years, it begins to decline, preventing the body from getting all the necessary nutrients. This causes poor formation of the *dhātus* and depletion in their shape, quantity and strength. The body weakens and the quantity of *malas* increases. A person also experiences weakening of mental faculties and a decline in sensory activities. This is the old age. Rejuvenation therapies attempt to slow down this process of aging and protect an individual from associated ailments by strengthening the activities of various *agnis* (the complete digestive system).

10. Physical Strength

For good health and various vital activities of life, body strength (energy) is very important. One needs strength and energy to perform general day-to-day activities in life. Without the required energy, one cannot face the difficult and complicated challenges of life nor can one perform routine activities properly. One cannot estimate strength merely on the basis of body structure. Before selecting the proper line of treatment for a patient, a physician should properly examine the intensity of a disease and body strength. Body strength is determined on the basis of activities or physical work done by a person without fatigue.

- **What is strength or energy?**

The end product or the main essence of all tissue elements in the body is strength or energy. This energy or strength is also known as '*ojas*' in *Āyurveda*. This strength nourishes all the muscles and makes them stable and strong so that one can perform all types of activities energetically and courageously. The quality of voice and the glow of skin are also determined by *ojas*. All external and internal parts of the body are able to perform their tasks well because of this strength/energy which is produced within the body. Actually, the strength of the body is associated with the factors, namely '*Ojas*' and '*Tejas*' present in the body.

- ***Tejas* strength**

Tejas is considered to be derived from *agni mahābhūta* (the element of fire). During metabolism, the liquified fat or *vasā* is derived from the accumulated fat in the abdomen. This is '*tejas*'. It is found in abundance in females. Due to this factor, tenderness, softness, reduced and soft body hair, cheerfullness, good eyesight, strong digestive and metabolic activities, stability, attraction and beauty are comparatively more in females.

- ***Ojas* strength**

Ojas as has been previously described is a very important vital constituent of the body dominated by the qualities of the water element. When *Kapha* is at its normal level in the body, i.e. in a balanced state, it builds and strengthens *ojas*. On the other hand, when there is a drop in the normal level of *Kapha*, it turns into *mala* (a waste, toxic product) and gives rise to several disorders. Originally, *ojas* is a vital essence of all seven *dhātus* present in the body.

"*Ojas* is a protective substance that provides immunity to the body. Hence *ojas* should always be maintained and nourished. It strengthens the immune system. Without it, external medication is of no use. On losing *ojas*, all treatments lose their efficacy."

The energy produced by *tejas* and *ojas* is divided into three parts - *uttama* (superior or of high strength), *madhyama* (average or of medium strength) and *adhama* (below average or of low strength).

According to another classification, the energy is also categorized as follows:

1. ***Sahaja bala*** **(natural energy)**: This is the naturally occurring energy in the body. It is produced by *rasa dhātu* and is the most superior kind.
2. ***Kālakṛta bala*** **(periodic energy)**: This is age specific energy gained during different stages of growth.
3. ***Yuktikṛta bala*** **(acquired energy)**: This is the energy acquired through external nourishment by proper diet, good conduct, physical exercise, *yogāsanas* and from the essence of medicines.

- ***Sattva parīkṣā*: Examination of *psyche***

Along with body strength, the *psyche* (mind or mental behavior) also holds a great importance. It is considered to be of two types: (1) *Bhīrutva* (fearing nature), and (2) *Sahiṣṇutva* (tolerant nature). Patients with a fearful nature are not able to tolerate a strong penetrating treatment, so the physician needs to select mild treatment for such patients. Such patients need to be counseled and assured before starting the treatment. A physician has to put extra- efforts into their treatment. On the other hand, patients with a tolerant nature do not panic soon and a physician may unhesitatingly use strong penetrating therapies in his treatment, which a patient can easily tolerate. Therefore, their treatment is comparatively easier.

- ***Sātmaya parīkṣā*: Examination of compatibility**

In *Āyurveda*, knowledge of compatibility is also important to maintain health and to eradicate disease. One drug is favorable for one person and unfavorable for another. In brief, the diet, drugs, conduct (physical and mental activities), country, time and other aspects and products which by birth or by experience are beneficial or favorable for the normal health, to maintain health and to eradicate the disease are compatible or wholesome. Compatibility is very important and it is of four types:

1) ***Deha sātmaya*** **(compatibility for the body)**: The diet and lifestyle which suits a person, proves beneficial and favorable for the body are compatible or wholesome. For example milk, yogurt and alcoholic substances are suitable for some people, but for others thin gruel, vegetable soup, rice, wheat and other grains are more suitable.
2) ***Deśa sātmaya*** **(compatibility according to a specific area or country)**: Some particular substances that are suitable in a particular area might not be suitable in others. For example, yogurt, milk and sweet substances are suitable for people in a particular area. Milk is wholesome for people in the east zone of our country. Fish is beneficial for people of the Sindhu region and rice is compatible for the people of Bengal, Madras, Kashmir and other areas.
3) ***Ṛtu sātmaya*** **(compatibility as per the season)**: Some substances are beneficial in a particular season. Oily, hot substances are suitable in early winter. Pungent, bitter and dry substances are favorable in late winter. Cold and sweet substances are useful in summer.

4) ***Roga sātmaya* (compatibility according to the disease)**: A certain diet may be compatible or wholesome for a particular disease. For example, gruel is useful in fever, fomentation therapy is favorable in emesis and vomiting, and errhine and medicated smoking is beneficial in chronic cold.

Along with the above-said factors, dose of a drug, nature of a drug, effect of a drug, time, constitution, location and stages of the disease-cycle are also important factors for a physician to choose the appropriate drug or line of treatment.

- **Characteristics of an energetic and strong person**

One who is actually free from disease or ailments; displays minimum or no signs of aging; completes all tasks efficiently; enjoys the work; who has gained both material and spiritual knowledge; has a well-built, powerful and sturdy body, energetic and healthy.

Now the question arises, what is a well-formed and strong body? Is it a fatty body or one that looks healthy and strong? Is it a lean body that looks relatively healthy, yet is not strong? There are several such questions to which *Āyurveda* replies that a person with a well-constructed body structure, whose bones are in good shape, at the right place and distributed evenly, whose joints are well-formed and stable, having uniform distribution of muscular tissues, whose BMI (body mass index) is normal and balanced, one who is physically strong and does work efficiently is considered to have a strong and healthy body. This is the best kind of body to have, with superior or high strength. A heavy body which is not as capable as the previous one is of average type and so its strength is medium or average, while a body that is not well-formed and lacks balance between its various components is an inferior body with low strength. On the contrary, a person who lacks mental strength (faints on seeing blood, death, accidents and other traumatic events or suffers from mental illnesses) and who easily contracts disease and becomes seriously ill, is not considered to be a strong person. Such persons are considered weak both physically and mentally, in spite of strong and healthy looks.

- **Infirmities related to physical strength**

Heaviness or laxity in the body, lack of energy, numbness, sleepiness, fatigue, lethargy, lack of efficiency, bloating, lack of muscular tissues in the body, syncope, self-pity, complexes, depression, stubbornness - all these are the signs of a decrease in physical power and energy.

A physician must go through the nature of the vitiated *doṣa*, before deciding a treatment for infirmities related to strength or to increase the physical strength of a person. Thereafter, treatment should be selected keeping in mind the patient's body strength. For immediate results, a patient must be guarded against mental infirmities such as greed, fear, anger, envy, depression, self-pity and so on, tiresome physical exercises, over exertion and sexual activities. Such a patient should not indulge in activities that require the display of physical strength. Therapies, medicines, treatments, food and lifestyle habits that work in the case of tuberculosis and chronic fever are also recommended for these patients. Rejuvenation therapy and the use of aphrodisiacs for virilization (increasing semen) must be undertaken along with the use of *Vāta*-reducing oils. Besides a regulated lifestyle and food habits, *yogāsanas* and physical exercises are the best sources to increase physical strength.

11. *Srotas*: Body Channels

The word *'srota'* has been used frequently in the preceding pages related to the channel systems of the body. Many of the *srota* systems are equivalent to the physiological systems of the body like the digestive, respiratory and nervous systems. It should be clear by now that a clean and healthy srota with the proper flow of energy is necessary for a healthy body. *Srota* systems are as important as the *doṣas*, *malas* and *dhātus*. *Srotas* and their functions are briefly described in Table 10.

All body parts that are hollow (dominated by the space element), which carry water, food, mala, *dhātu*, sound and nerve impulses are called '*srota*.' They also transport essential materials like the *dhātus* from one part of the body to another. Since they circulate various substances throughout the body, they are termed '*srotas*' or the channels[24]. These hollow body parts have different shapes and sizes. Some are tubes, others are long, thin and wide and others have a complex system of branches, much like creepers. Some *srotas* are visible to the naked eye, while many others are not. They are usually of the same color as the substances that they carry.

- **Functions of *srotas***

According to their physical structure, they transport food, plasma, blood and other *dhātus*, *doṣas*, *malas*, life-force and so on. Their main functions are as follows:

1. Transports food nutrients from the gastro-intestinal tract to theirrespective *dhātus* to nourish them and making it possible for them to regenerate.
2. Cleanses the body by transporting wastes such as feces, urine and sweat to their sites of elimination, thus keeping the body fit and healthy.
3. Supports life by sustaining the breath.
4. No chemical element in the body can be produced, nourishedor experience an increase or decrease without the help of the *srota*.
5. *Srotas* are central to all the functions of the body, being responsible

24. *Tritayaṁ cedamupaṣṭambhanamāhāraḥ svapno, brahacaryaṁ ca. Ebhiryuktairupaṣṭabdhamupastambhaiḥ śarīraṁ balavarṇopacayopacitamanuvartate yāvadāyuṣaḥ saṁskāraḥ.*(A.Saṁ.sū. 9:36)

for all movements like transport of *malas*, sensory or tactile feelings, emotions, desires and so on.

Hence, they help in performing all body activities. *Srota* are present in every part of the body from the smallest cell of the body, to all minor and major body organs.

- ***Srotas* and emergence of diseases**

The importance of *srotas* for the smooth functioning of bodily processes is evident. Consequently, it is of utmost importance that the *srotas* remain in their natural healthy state like the *doṣas* and the *dhātus*.

> Even one of an unhealthy or diseased srota affects the surrounding srotas which causes ailments related to both. If any of the srota, whether a cell or any minor or major body part, does not perform its function perfectly, then toxic elements accumulate in these srotas and these cells or body parts suffer from severe diseases like cancer. For example, if the srota of the skin cells and blood cells get corrupted, it results in skin cancer and blood cancer.

Healthy *srota* enhance the smooth circulation of *doṣas, dhātus* and *upadhātus* throughout the body and speed up the movement of *malas* to their excretory orifices. Diseased *srotas* pass on their state of imbalance to the *doṣas, dhātus* and *malas* they carry, which in turn further corrupt the *srotas* due to the circulation of vitiated *doṣas, dhātus* and *malas*. It becomes a vicious cycle. If *dhātus* or *malas* accumulates in the *srotas*, the metabolic process of that *dhātu* is hampered. The adjoining *dhātus* are also adversely affected, due to the obstruction in the circulatory process of the *dhātus*. This leads to *āma doṣa*, which travels to other parts of the body, blocking other *srotas* and causing ailments. The common cold and related diseases are a good example. The out-of-balance *doṣas* travels from the diseased nasal channel (*srota*) to the *srota* in the thoracic region causing cough. Through these channels, *doṣa* reaches the ear and it causes earache, heaviness and deafness. When it flows to the head, it causes sinusitis. It causes bronchitis on reaching the lungs and dysentery on reaching the bowels. Hence, it is necessarily required to keep all the *srotas* clean and in good health.

- **Types of *srotas***

Our body is a network of innumerable large and small channels (*srotas*). Some *srotas*, like the gastro-intestinal tract, arteries, veins, lymphatic, reproductive and urinary tracts, and so on, are visible to the naked eye. Others are so small that they can be seen only under a powerful microscope, like the minute cells. In a complete human body there are millions of *srotas*.

Table 10: *Srotas* - Causes of Vitiation, Symptoms and Treatment					
S. No.	Name and Function	Controlling Organs	Cause of vitiation	Symptoms	Treatment
1.	*Prāṇavaha srota* (carries breath and life-force)	Heart and alimentary canal	Wasting, suppression of natural urges, eating dry foods in excess, exercising while hungry.	Obstructed, shallow or rapid breathing. Bronchial asthma also relates to it.	Treatment for respiratory problems such as bronchial asthma.
2.	*Udakavaha srota* (carries water and other liquids like juices of liver and pancreas)	Palate, pancreas	Exposure to heat, heat stroke, indigestion, excessive intoxication, eating extremely dry foods and remaining thirsty.	Dry lips, tongue, palate and throat.	Treatment for excessive thirst.
3.	*Annavaha srota* (carries food ingested from the mouth)	Stomach, left portion	Irregular eating habits, over-eating, eating unhealthy food and low digestive power.	Loss of appetite, anorexia, vomiting, indigestion.	Remedies for *āma doṣa* and indigestion work well.
4.	*Rasavaha srota* (carries chyle, lymph, plasma)	Heart and the blood vessels connected with heart	Worry, diet comprising of excessively heavy, cold and greasy foods.	Anorexia, nausea, heaviness, drowsiness, syncope, anemia, impotency.	Fasting
5.	*Raktavaha srota* (carries blood, especially hemoglobin)	Liver, spleen	Pungent, hot and oily food, exposure to excessive sun and heat.	Chronic skin diseases, intrinsic hemorrhage (bleeding), abscesses, inflammation in anus and genital organs.	Blood-letting in diseased parts.
6.	*Māṁsavaha srota* (carries ingredients of muscular tissues)	Tendons, ligaments and skin	Sleeping immediately after meals, frequent intake of heavy and gross foods in bulk.	Severe skin diseases, palate inflamation, granuloma, myoma, piles, goiter, adenitis, tonsilitis, cancers and non-malignant growths.	Surgery, heat therapy and *kṣāra* therapy (local application of alkalis). *Prāṇāyama* to strengthen the life force, which can even cure cancer and other malignant growths.
7.	*Medovaha srota* (carries ingredients of adipose tissues)	Kidney, adipose (fat) tissue in the abdomen	Sleeping during the daytime, lack of exercise, excessive alcohol and oil-rich diet.	Severe urinary disorders, diabetes.	Weight reduction remedies or anti-obesity treatment, lightning therapy, fasting, *yoga* and exercise.

8.	*Asthivaha srota* (carries nutrients that nourish bones)	Hip bone, lumbar bone and tissues	Excessive exercise involving friction of bones, intake of food that causes *Vāta.*	Cracking or distortion of nails and teeth, pain in bones, bone cancer, change in hair texture (because hair is the waste product of bone).	*Pañcakarma basti* (enema) using bitter herbal medicines processed with milk and clarified butter.
9.	*Majjāvaha srota* (carries nutrients of bones, joints and bone marrow)	Bones and joints	Incompatible food (fish and milk, honey and hot foods), injury to bone marrow by crushing, compression.	Pain in joints, giddiness, fainting, loss of memory, blackouts, deep abscesses.	Using sweet and bitter substances, sexual activity, exercise, elimination of *doṣa* on time and in right amount.
10.	*Śukravaha srota* (carries sperm, ovum and their nutrients)	Testicles, ovary	Sex at improper time, unnatural sex, suppression or excess of sex.	Impotence, infertility, abortion, defective pregnancy.	Virility and *dhātu* restorative treatment. Use of aphrodisiacs.
11.	*Mūtravaha srota* (carries urine)	Kidneys, bladder	Food, drinks and sex during urge for urination, suppression of the urge for urination, specially by those suffering from tuberculosis.	Excessive or no urination. Frequent urination, viscous urine.	Same treatment as for dysuria (difficult urination).
12.	*Purīṣavaha srota* (carries fecal matter)	Colon, rectum	Suppression of urge to defecate, intake of food before digestion of previous meal, weak digestion.	Less or excessive excretion of fecal matter, hard stool.	Treatment similar to the one given in diarrhea, using laxatives and purgatives, balanced diet and *yogāsanas.*
13.	*Svedavaha srota* (carries sweat)	Adipose tissue, hair-follicles	Excessive exercise, anger, grief, fear, exposure to heat.	Absence of or excessive perspiration, dryness of skin. Horripilation (Hair erection). Burning sensation on the skin.	Treatment as for fever, balanced exercise, balanced diet and drinks. In excess perspiration drink juice of tinospora *(giloya),* leaves of Bengal quince (*bilva*) and Indian rosewood tree (*śīśama*).

Chapter 3
The Body and its Vital Forces

Āyurveda, yoga and other scriptures describe the human body in relation to its interaction with the inner self.

By the activation of energies present within the inner self, one can protect oneself from various diseases and can also get rid of the diseases one is already affected. This way it also describes various routes to explore God and attain complete bliss. Below is the description and modality of the vital forces mentioned in the ancient texts of *Āyurveda*:

1. *Tridaṇḍa* (The three dimensions of life - body mind (*psyche*) and soul)
2. *Pañca pañcaka* (The five pentads)
3. *Pañcakoṣa* (The five spiritual body sheaths)
4. Body physiology and *Aṣṭacakrā* (The eight *cakrās)*
5. *Aṣṭacakra* and its relation with various *yogic* practices and *kuṇḍalinī yoga*

1. *Tridaṇḍa*: The Three Dimensions of Life - Body, Mind (*Psyche*) and Soul

Body, Mind (*psyche*) and Soul (The True Self or Consciousness) together constitute *Tridaṇḍa* in *Āyurveda.* They remain intact in mutual association with each other. This makes possible the existence of a life. The combination of these three in one entity constitutes a body, and it is the body where everything exists(1). By acquiring the precise knowledge of this *Tridaṇḍa*, i.e. Body, Mind and Soul, an expert physician can diagnose the nature, etiology or cause and location of a disease, and accordingly can choose a suitable treatment including medication, food and lifestyle.

(i) *Śarīra*: Body

According to *Āyurveda* the entire world and all its microcosms and macrocosms are brought into existence with the composition and combination of '*pañcamahābhūta*' or the five basic elements. According to this, all living beings including human beings have originated from *pañcamahābhūta*. Since all these substances originate from *pañcamahābhūta*, they are known as

1. *Satvamātmā śarīraṁ ca trayametatridaṇḍavat. Lokastiṣṭhati saṁyogātatra sarvaṁ pratiṣṭhitam. Sa pumāṁścetanaṁ tacca taccādhikaraṁ smṛtaṇam. Vedasyāsya tadardhaṁ hi vedo, yaṁ samprakāśitaḥ.* (*Ca.sū.*1/46-47)

'pañcabhautika.' These *pañcamahābhūtas*, which are also known as the basic elements, includes 1. Space or ether, 2. Air, 3. Water, 4. Fire, and 5. Earth.

This concept of the five elements lies at the heart of *Āyurvedic* science. In context to the human body, it is important to know the five elements and what elements are responsible to uphold and provide matrix to the body. The five sensory and motor organs are the main supports for upholding the body. The body is nourished by the six *rasas* (tastes) - sweet, salty, sour, bitter, pungent and astringent and the food substances containing these tastes. Human body is constituted from the seven *dhātu*s (tissues) - *rasa* (plasma), *rakta* (blood), *māṁsa* (muscular tissue), *meda* (adipose or fat tissue), *asthi* (bone), *majjā* (bone marrow) and *śukra* (semen); three *doṣas* (*Vāta, Pitta* and *Kapha*) and *malas* (waste matter - feces, urine and sweat). All these upholding factors of the body, nutritive components and constituent factors have been created from these five elements. [PLATE 12]

The body is made up of five sense faculties - eyes (optic), ears (auditory), nose (olfactory), tongue (gustatory or taste) and skin (touch or tactile). Though all these sense organs are formed by the combination of these five elements, fire, space (ether), earth, water and air dominate them, respectively. The five elements manifest in the functioning of the five sensory organs. These sense organs perceive knowledge from their surroundings to uphold the body and provide nourishment with the help of their related subject of light, sound, smell, taste and touch.

Besides this, to understand the body structure *Āyurveda* describes different organs and sub-organs that constitute the body in much detail.

- **Body structure: In view of body parts**

According to *Āyurveda* treatises, the complete body is divided into the following eight parts - head, neck, hands, legs, lateral (on both sides of the thoracic region), dorsal, abdominal and thoracic regions. The element of earth dominates each of these eight parts.The nose, chin, lips, ears, fingers of hands and feet, wrist and ankle joints are considered sub-parts (subsidiary organs).

Some scriptures divide the body into six principal parts known as *'ṣaḍaṅga,'* consisting of the head including neck, the trunk (thoracic and abdominal region); both hands and both legs. Both hands and both legs are known as the limbs of the body (*śākhā*). The trunk is called the thoraco-abdominal region, whose middle region is the abdomen(2). These six parts of the body are further divided into sub-parts, where the eyes are sub-part of the head and the heart is a sub-part of the thorax.

2. *Tatrāyaṁ śarīrasyāṅgavibhāgaḥ tadyathā dvau bāhū, dve sakthinī śirogrīvam, antarādhiḥ, iti ṣaḍaṅgamaṅgam.* (*Ca.śā.*7:5)

- **Excretory passages**

Nine passages of excretion are mentioned in male's including both eyes, both ears, both nostrils, the mouth, the anal region and the urethra(3), and twelve in females. Apart from the above nine passages, the remaining three include the vagina and both nipples on the breasts.

In *Āyurveda*, a detailed study of the anatomical structures constituting the body, are widely considered including veins, arteries, lymph, channels, nerves, muscles, ligaments, tendons, hair follicles (body hair), membranes, vital points of the body and skull, along with the mind, brain, intellect, pride and their location site, place, number, functions and all other related aspects of body parts.

(ii) Mana (*sattva*): Mind *(psyche)*

All organs of the body work in conjunction with the mind(4). No sensory organ can perceive anything without the support of the mind. Therefore, the mind is one of the most important parts of the human body. It is considered as both a sensory and a motor organ, and is responsible for co-ordinating both perception and action. Hence, it is known as '*ubhayendriya*(5).' *Āyurveda*, *yogaśāstras* and related treatises and teachings refer to the mind as '*manas.*' It is made up of '*mana*' *dhātu*. It is '*manas*' that is primarily responsible for any action or thought. In spite of having different meanings, words like *citta*, *hṛdaya* (heart), *sattva* and *svāntaḥ* are all *Sanskrit* synonyms of *manas* or its functions.

Mind has its own importance, as it is a crucial link between the *ātmā* and the sense organs, whose interactions lead to acquisition of knowledge. However, mind in itself is an unconscious (lifeless) entity and lacks touch, color, feeling and perception, which can only occur owing to the mind's ability to reflect the light of the *ātmā* or higher Consciousness. The body experiences it due to an interaction between the *mana* and the *ātmā*. Every individual *ātmā* has a *mana* (mind), which is considered its internal assistant and companion. Therefore, in *Āyurveda* '*mana*' is also known as '*sattva.*' Just as the sensory organs are the external means of collecting knowledge, mind is an internal receiver of the knowledge. It is one of the four main organs of the conscience.

3. *Naya mahānti cchidrāṇi sapta śirasi, dve cādhaḥ.* (*Ca.śā.* 7:12)
4. *Manaḥ punaḥ sarāṇīndriyāṇyarthagrahaṇasamarthāni bhavanti.* (*Ca.sū.* 8/7)
5. *Atīndriyaṁ punarmanaḥ sattvasaṁjñakaṁ ceta ityāhureke, tadarthātmasaṁpattadāyattaceṣṭaṁ ceṣṭāpratyayabhūtamindriyāṇām.*(*Ca.sū.* 8/4)

According to the sages, the *ātmā* is a traveler, the body is a chariot, the intellect is a charioteer and the mind is its reins. The sensory organs are the horses, worldly affairs and subject matters are the different paths available, and the mind in conjunction with *ātmā* is considered as its controller (co-ordinating with both perception and action or thought). One who remains ignorant, who is unconscious and has an intemperate and unregulated mind, loses control over his sensory organs, which then tend to behave like wild horses without being controlled by a charioteer.

- **Location**

Manas is said to reside in the heart and the brain. Both these organs are related to each other and are interdependent. In *Āyurvedic* texts, the heart is considered to be the primary location of the *manas*, whereas *yoga* treatises consider both the heart and the brain as its locations. Generally, the heart is the seat of deeper aspects of the mind, while, the brain is the site of its external functions through the sense and motor organs. Yet, it is not simply these physical organs that are meant, but the perception and awareness induce them to act. In *Śivasankalpa mantras* of *Yajurveda, mana* (mind) has been said to be omnipresent.

Yasmścittaṁ savata prajānāṁ tanme manaḥ śivasaṅkalpam astu.

(*Yaju*: 345)

Supposed size and number

According to *Āyurveda*, *manas* is is atomic in size, is a single entity and is material in nature. Alike body, the mind can also be perceived.

- **Functions**

The main function of *manas* is to interpret sensory data collected by the sense organs and communicate it to the motor organs, brain and other sites of emotional and intellectual activity. As a result of this process the sense and motor organs are able to perceive outside information and react appropriately.

- **Characteristics and strengths**

The mind is the center of all the overall knowledge of three periods (past, present and future), the three objects or goals of life (virtue, wealth and lust), and it governs liberty and limitations. The mind has unlimited knowledge, strength and infinite capabilities. Alike three *doṣas*, there are three types of mental constitutions that are found in human beings; they are related to the three prime *guṇas* or qualities of mind.

1) *Sattva* (*psychic* quality representing purity,modesty, balance and harmony)
2) *Rajas* (*psychic* quality related to motion and instability)

3) *Tamas* (*psychic* quality related to inertia, inaction and ignorance)

Sattva, *Rajas* and *Tamas* are together known as the *triguṇa* or the three attributes of the mind.

The state of mind is a very important aspect of a persons individuality. Generally these three modes are applied to understand the mind, since the mind is more subtle in nature. The three modes are not permanent, though they are minute in size and very subtle, they are mutually dependent and changeable according to our associations and actions. The qualities of all the three modes can be found in every human being, but like the *doṣas* one type is usually predominant. *Sattva* quality denotes knowledge and the light. It is characterized by balance and harmony and generates happiness and well-being. It is the state of harmony, indiscrimination, stability of mind, efficiency of handling matters without partiality and selfishness, emotional stability and detachment. *Sattva* is the peaceful, calm state of the mind. *Rajas* causes agitation and action. It has the inherent tendency to be active. This is essential to get things done. When in excess, *rajas* results in hyperactivity, aggression, passion, strong attachment, agitation and regrettable actions. When unbalanced, *rajas* is considered to have a disturbing influence on the mind. *Tamas* represents inertia and inaction. Rest or sleep is impossible without this quality, it provides grounding and stability. Its increase causes laziness, apathy, ignorance and depression. In the nutshell, excessive *tamas* is darkness.

Based on the aforesaid qualities, mental strength (*psyche*) can be divided into *Sāttvika*, *Rājasika* and *Tāmasika*. These three are considered the *prakṛti* of *manas*. *Sāttvika manas* is spiritual, pure, modest, ethical and conscious; *Rājasika manas* is restless, unstable, desirous, easily distracted and prone to anger; and *Tāmasika manas* is predominantly ignorant and unconscious. Qualities of people with these states of mind (*manas*) are illustrated below.

A. ***Sāttvika* characteristic people**

In *sāttvika* people, *rājasika* and *tāmasika* characteristics are absent and the quality of *sattva* predominates in them. *Sāttvika* people tend to have an inherent instinct for cleanliness, purification and are disease-free. They possess an effortless wisdom reflected in their actions.They do not tend to worry, nor are anxious or prone to panic. They are free from confusion, greed, anger, envy and do things in a systematic, intelligent and peaceful way. They have a high degree of consciousness, patience, satisfaction, forgiveness, kindness, softness, shyness, simplicity, generosity, asceticism, serenity and honesty. They are pleasing and have a clear heart and mind.

B. ***Rājasika* characteristic people**

In such people *rājasika* nature dominates and other qualities are absent. *Rājasika* people tend to be power hungry, having a nature to acquire more, and are dissatisfied with what positions or possessions they obtain. They constantly strive for more, often at the cost of those around them. They have a brave yet envious disposition.They possess instable and unsatisfactory characteristics and are playful, wanton, capricious, jealous, arrogant, back-biters, covetous (greedy), have longing (thirst or desire), worry, anxiety, fear, grief, spitefulness and sensuousness, which produces unhappiness, misery, increases lust and restlessness. They are often plagued by the consequences of their actions, which are guided by these qualities.

C. ***Tāmasika* characteristic people**

Tāmasika qualities dominate when other qualities remain absent. *Tāmasika* people tend to avoid work, with a penchant for uncontrolled sense of gratification and wasting time. They avoid cleanliness and are not health conscious. They are ignorant, inactive, inert, lazy, lustful, obsessive, meek, deluded, unaesthetic and dull.

Decrease or increase in the quantity of these characteristics or the combination of these qualities in different ratios results in infinite conditions of the mind (*psyche*).

- ***Manas* and *Āyurveda***

It is an established fact that the qualities and conditions of the mind and body affect each other. Therefore, in the *Āyurvedic* system of medicine, both physical and mental conditions (*psyche*) of the patient are taken into consideration before any treatment is finalized. *Āyurveda* divides ailments into two categories: (1) physical, and (2) mental or psychological.

The causes of physical ailments may also lead to physiological disturbances, whereas mental ailments may cause physical problems in a person. *Āyurveda* realises that the mind contributes to the genesis of both types of ailments.Where on the one hand, bodily functions and physiological processes affect the mind, conversely, mental processes are affected by physiological conditions. Therefore, there is a deep relationship between the two. This is the rationale behind treating physical ailments using therapies for mental health and well-being and emphasis given in *Āyurveda* on overall wellbeing of mind, body and soul.

(iii) *Ātmā*: The Soul (The True Self or Consciousness)

The central principle of *Āyurveda* is to maintain the health and harmony of the body (*puruṣa*). However, in *Āyurveda*, body is not merely a physical structure built by a combination of five elements and certain chemical compounds. Body and consequently life (*puruṣa*), results from the union between the five elements, mind, intellect (brain) and *ātmā* (individual soul or self). Therefore, *puruṣa* is a miraculous combination of the conscious and the unconscious. The body is inanimate while *ātmā* is pure consciousness, and the union of these two give rise to a human being (*puruṣa* - an active person).

The five elements, the organs (eyes and other sensory organs) and the mind lay down the foundation of the body. The conscious part of this foundation is the *ātmā*. The *ātmā* is considered to be the originator of all actions, as well as the bearer of their consequences. When the *ātmā* leaves the body, the body becomes non-functional or dead, even if all its organs remain intact. In the absence of *ātmā*, the organs cannot function and nothing can be felt or experienced by the body or mind. Hence, the *Ātmā* is regarded as the basis of all consciousness.

Ātmā is indestructible and continues to exist even after the body has been destroyed. It is immortal and hence fundamentally different from the body that is mortal. At demise, the *ātmā* takes on another body according to the *karma* (deeds) of the deceased body. Even though it is a conscious entity, it needs to be connected with the intellect (brain), mind and sensory organs in order to acquire knowledge, feel and make contact, communicate, beautify and be manifest in the external world. Knowledge is gained only when the *ātmā* aligns with the mind and intellect, the intellect interacts with the sensory organs and they experience perceptions and impressions. The *ātmā* is immutable, which transcends mind, body and sense organs, but it is a prime source of consciousness along with these. It is eternal and witnesses all the activities. *Ātmā* is free from disorders and transmutation, whereas the body and mind are prone to these.

- **Characteristics of the *ātmā***

Joy, sorrow, desire, hatred, endeavor, breathing, blinking and opening of the eyes, thought processes, determination, memory, knowledge, inter-sensory communication (the subject communicated from left eye to right eye), sound and other perceptions, motivation, beliefs, dreams, patience and pride are all considered to be the qualities of the *ātmā* because these characteristics are manifested only as long as the *ātmā* resides in the body and a person is alive. In fact, it is only with the existence of the *ātmā* in the body that sensory organs, mind and *prāṇa* become functional. However, *ātmā* exists in its own form as the *draṣṭā* or as a witness. A body can be treated only as long as the *ātmā* resides in the body. No treatment works on a body that is without the *ātmā* and it is referred to as dead.

Modern medical science does not discuss the existence of the *ātmā*, but founders of traditional Indian medical science like *Dhanvantari, Caraka, Suśruta, Patañjali* and all other sages have scientifically proven through experience, the existence of *ātmā* with their intellect, evidences, reasons and scientific proofs. We do believe that modern medical science will soon realize this

2. *Pañca Pañcaka*: The Five Pentads (The five sensory organs and their groups that are five each in number)

The sensory and motor organs on whom human body gathers the knowledge of perception and action is known as *pañca pañcaka* (the five pentads). Verbally it is known as the knowledge of five groups, all are five in number. All twenty-five elements constitute 'The Five Pentads.'

1. **The five sense faculties(6):** These faculties provide knowledge of varied types. They are five in number including: (i) Visual faculty, (ii) Auditory faculty, (iii) Gustatory faculty, (iv) Tactile faculty, and (v) Olfactory faculty.
2. **The five sense objects(7):** The knowledge perceived by these sense faculties is called subject. Each sense faculty has its own subject matter. Therefore, there are five subjects:
   (i) Auditory faculty deals with hearing;
   (ii) Tactile faculty refers to the means of perception to touch;
   (iii) Visual faculty perceives color, shape and seeing in general;
   (iv) Gustatory sense faculty is responsible for the knowledge of taste; and
   (v) Olfactory sense faculty perceives smell.
3. **The five sense organs(8):** These are the organs of perception. The sense faculties do not have their own individual identity or their own shape. The place where these faculties reside is known as its location or the organs of sense (sense organs). We see many such examples where in spite of the sense organs being duly present, one is unable to sense. In such a case, the strength of the faculty gets damaged due to some specific cause. Since there are five sense faculties, there are five sense organs:
   (i) Eyes - For visual faculty;
   (ii) Skin - For tactile faculty, which covers the entire body;
   (iii) Ears - For auditory faculty;
   (iv) Tongue - For taste faculty; and
   (v) Nose - For olfactory faculty

6. *Tatra cakṣuḥ śrotraṁ ghrāṇaṁ rasanaṁ sparśanamiti pañcendriyāṇī.*(*Ca.sū.*8:8)
7. *Pañcandriyārthāḥ śabdasparśarūparasagandhāḥ.* (*Ca.sū.*8:11)
8. *Pañcendriyadravyāṇī khaṁ vāyurjyetirāpo bhūriti.* (*Ca.sū.* 8:9)

4. **The five sense materials[9]:** The five sense materials are the five basic elements - space (ether), air, fire, water and earth governing the five senses.

(i) Auditory faculty - governed by the element of space (ether);
(ii) Tactile faculty - governed by the element of air;
(iii) Visual faculty - governed by the element of fire or *tejas*;
(iv) Gustatory faculty - governed by the element of water; and
(v) Olfactory faculty - governed by the element of earth.

5. **The five sense perceptions[10]:** Sensory faculties alone cannot gather knowledge and information. Conjunction with the mind is essential for sensory organs to recognize the subject area. By their combined action only, these faculties can perform their individual actions well, that is, the proper ability to hear, see, touch, taste and smell by ears, eyes, skin, tongue and nose respectively. At this stage the brain perceives the actions and thoughts and decides the words to be spoken, the type of touch (hot, cold, tender, rough and so on), the shape and color, the type of taste (whether sweet, sour, salty, bitter, pungent or astringent), and the type of smell (pleasant or pungent). On this basis, the experience or knowledge derived by the brain by means of conjunctive action of the mind and the sense organs with their faculties is also divided into five parts: (i) Auditory brain, (ii) Tactile brain, (iii) Visionary brain, (iv) Gustatory brain, and (v) Olfactory brain.

Table 11 : Consolidated Table of the Five Pentads

Five Sense Faculties	Five Sense Objects	Five Sense Organs	Five Sense Materials	Five Sense Perceptions
Visual Faculty	Seeing (Shape)	Eyes	Fire (*Tejas*)	Visionary Brain
Auditory Faculty	Hearing (Sound)	Ears	Space (Ether)	Auditory Brain
Olfactory Faculty	Smell	Nose	Earth	Olfactory Brain
Gustatory Faculty	Taste	Tongue	Water	Gustatory Brain
Tactile Faculty	Touch	Skin	Air	Tactile Brain

These brain percieve the image of an object, draws a conclusion and derives a shape or appearance. It is through these perceptions that an accurate and visible knowledge is obtained in a fraction of second. They comprehend the true nature of things. These sense materials and their properties together with the mind, brain and *ātmā* are responsible for all actions of the body and spiritual qualities which become the cause of inclination or aversion towards

9. *Pañcendriyādhiṣṭhānāni akṣiṇī karṇau nāsike jihvā tvakceti.* (*Ca.sū.* 8:10)
10. *Pañcendriyabuddhayaḥ cakṣurbuddhyādikāḥ, tāḥ punarindriyendriyārtha satvātmasannikarṣajāḥ, kṣaṇikāḥ niścayātmikāśca.* (*Ca.sū.*8:12)

good and bad deeds. The interaction of these senses with their subject matter in excess or a diminished state along with the mind, destroys the intellect and produces disorders. When these sense organs interact with what is percieved in a correct manner, then proper knowledge is obtained and the body remains in order (health)[11].

Hence, these are twenty-five important elements belonging to five groups each having five knowledge factors, known as 'The Five Pentads' in *Āyurveda*. The sensation of these five pentads not only helps us to understand the human body, but also helps us in comprehending the minute elements that exist within it. This contributes in the diagnosis of a disease and its corresponding treatment.

3. *Pañcakoṣa*: The Five Spiritual Body Sheaths

According to *yoga* and *Āyurveda,* the human body is a unique creation of God. The *Upaniṣads* and other scriptures on Indian spiritual knowledge very precisely and minutely explain the human body, its various activities and the complete mystery behind the functioning of this complex body system beyond the realization of existence of *ātmā* in the form of *pañcakoṣa*. *Ātmā* is beyond these *pañcakoṣa* (the five sheaths) and is very subtle and immutable. To be free from the bondages of afflictions, attachment and ignorance, there is a provision of self-realization, enlightenment and eternal self bliss. To reach these stages of self-realization and enlightenment, one has to go beyond these sheaths. Ancient sages firmly believed that one can keep oneself fit and healthy only after attaining an appropriate knowledge of the gross body, its activities, *mana*, intellect or brain power, self-importance and *ātmā*. By acquiring this knowledge, one can keep himself free of diseases so as to carry out all worldly affairs efficiently and perform good deeds, which leads one on the path of eternal bliss and subsequently the way to reach the Supreme soul. *Āyurveda* and *yoga* scriptures authentically explain the gross body, the soul, Supreme soul and all the subtle mysteries behind it. There is no direct relationship between *pañcakosā* and *Āyurveda* but it holds a very important position in *yoga*, it is briefly described here because of its relationship with the body science. These *pañcakoṣa* are of following types:

First - *Annamaya koṣa* (The physical sheath; literally 'the food sheath')
Second - *Prāṇamaya koṣa* (The vital air sheath)
Third - *Manomaya koṣa* (The mind sheath, which is instinctive)
Forth - *Vijñānamaya koṣa* (The intellect sheath)
Fifth - *Ānandamaya koṣa* (The bliss or emotion sheath)

These *pañcakoṣas* have their own importance. By means of spiritual endeavor, meditation, right food and lifestyle habits, *yoga* and other activities,

11. *Mano mano, rtho buddhirātmā cetyadhyātmadravyaguṇasaṅgraḥ Śubhāśubhapravṛttihetuśca, dravyāśritaṁ ca karma, yaducyate driyeti.*(*Ca.sū.* 8:13)

a devotee progresses from the gross form to subtlety. [PLATE 13]

It is also quoted:

"Dehādabhyantaraḥ prāṇaḥ prāṇādabhyantaraṁ manaḥ.
Tataḥ kartā tato bhoktā guhā seyaṁ paramparā."

(*Pañcadaśī. pañcakoṣa viveka, śloka*-2)

'In the gross body, *prāṇamaya koṣa* is more subtle than *annamaya koṣa*, *manomaya koṣa* is more subtle than *prāṇamaya koṣa*, followed by *vijñānamaya koṣa* and *ānandamaya koṣa* respectively.' This group of traditional *koṣas* from *annamaya* to *ānandamaya* located in the body is called '*Guhā*.' It is believed that *ātmā* resides in these '*Guhās*.'

When one moves from the gross body in the *annamaya koṣa* to subtlety, by means of *yoga*, meditation and other spiritual practices, one becomes free from disease, and after passing through each level or *koṣa*, finally one reaches the state of complete bliss and joy which is named *ānandamaya koṣa*. To enter this *koṣa (guhā)* one should possess the knowledge of the gross body and its deeds (*karma*), which makes one free from somatic and psychological diseases and helps to attain the goal of life.

According to the *Upaniṣada*, the management of this cosmic world/ universe is governed by divine power and energy. One who understands and accepts this does not need to know anything more. This is '*satya*' (the truth) or the reality of life and is infinitesimal (*ananta*). This divine power of the ultimate truth or creator "Brahma" resulted in evolutionary stages from space (ether) to air, from air to fire, from fire to water, from water to earth, from earth to drugs, from drugs to food, from food to *vīrya* (semen) and from *vīrya* to *puruṣa*, i.e., the body. It means that this gross body itself is known as *annamaya koṣa* (the food sheath). By the knowledge of this gross body in the form of *annamaya koṣa* and keeping it disease-free, we can attain complete happiness and eternal bliss(12).

1. ***Annamaya koṣa* (The food or physical sheath)**: The gross body has been formed by '*anna*' (food), thereby named as '*annamaya koṣa*.' This *annamaya koṣa* is related to earth as '*anna*' (food) is derived from the earth and subsequently this food builds a gross body. Therefore, health of the body and diseases are mainly related to *annamaya koṣa*. By practicing right food habits and lifestyle, *ṣaṭkarma* (six *yogic* practices involving purification of the body), medicines, *āsanas* (body postures) and *mudrās* (subtle postures), the body can be made strong, elegant, symmetrical and proportionate.
2. ***Prāṇamaya koṣa* (The vital air sheath):** In the gross body, *prāṇamaya koṣa* is subtle to matter predominated body (*annamaya koṣa*). The flow of '*prāṇa*' (life-force) is invisible, but life (consciousness) in the gross body depends on this *prāṇa*. It is also true that physical health depends on the '*nāḍī*' based body, where the *prāṇa* (life-force) flows.

12. *Annād bhatāni jāyante. jātānyannena vardhante. Adyate, tti ca bhūtāni. Tasmādannaṁ taducyata iti.Tasmādvā etāsmādannarasamayāt.* (*Tatti.Brahmānandvallī, Dvitīya Anuvāka*)

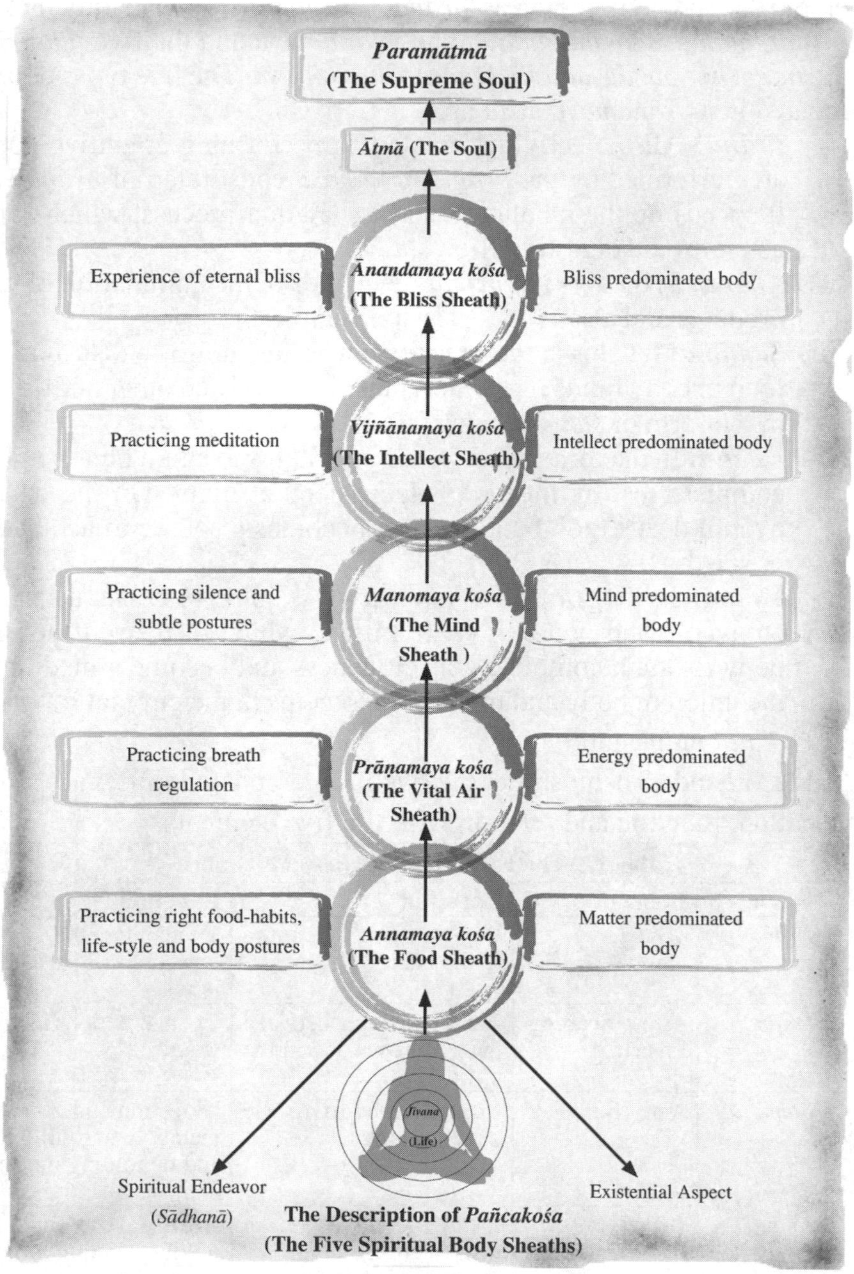
Paramātmā
(The Supreme Soul)
Ātmā (The Soul)
Experience of eternal bliss
Ānandamaya kośa
(The Bliss Sheath)
Bliss predominated body
Practicing meditation
Vijñānamaya kośa
(The Intellect Sheath)
Intellect predominated body
Practicing silence and subtle postures
Manomaya kośa
(The Mind Sheath)
Mind predominated body
Practicing breath regulation
Prāṇamaya kośa
(The Vital Air Sheath)
Energy predominated body
Practicing right food-habits, life-style and body postures
Annamaya kośa
(The Food Sheath)
Matter predominated body
Jivana
(Life)
Spiritual Endeavor (*Sādhanā*)
Existential Aspect

The Description of *Pañcakośa*
(The Five Spiritual Body Sheaths)

The source of power and vital energy in the body is *prāṇamaya koṣa*. The *vāyu* (element of air) present in the universe enters the body in the form of '*prāṇa*,' i.e., it is universally present everywhere, but when it enters the body it is known as '*prāṇa*.' *Prāṇamaya koṣa* mainly includes *prāṇa*, *apāna*, *samāna*, *udāna* and *vyāna vāyu* and the five *upaprāṇas* are *nāga*, *kūrma*, *devadatta*, *kṛkala*, *dhanañjaya*. The five types of *prāṇa* located in a *prāṇamaya koṣa* are:

(i) ***Prāṇa*:** All the activities related to performing cognitive actions are performed by the *prāṇamaya koṣa* constituted of *prāṇa vāyu*. It speeds up the inhalation and exhalation process, which further activates the digestive fire.

(ii) ***Apāna*:** In the form of *prāṇa vāyu*, aids in the elimination of waste products and also works as a spermatostatic.

(iii) ***Samāna*:** It helps in the transformation and uniform distribution of food in body fluids like water, plasma, blood and other body tissues in the form of *samāna vāyu*.

(iv) ***Udāna*:** In the form of *udāna vāyu*, it helps to attain bliss by giving complete rest by means of deep sleep at night. On the basis of overall deeds (good and bad), it becomes a source to achieve joy or sorrow.

(v) ***Vyāna*:** In the form of *vyāna vāyu*, it helps to consume various enjoyable and non-enjoyable things, which diffuse in the entire body to attain complete consciousness and become a medium for the union of body and mind. It also helps in the circulation of *rasa dhātu* in the entire body.

Tables 12 and 13 demostrates the five *prāṇas* and *upaprāṇas* at a glance, their location, function and relation with the five elements.

Table 12: The Five Main *Prāṇas* at a Glance

S. N.	Name	Element	Location	Function
1.	*Prāṇa*	*Vāyu* (Air)	Region from the mouth to the heart.	To maintain the working capacity of heart and lungs.
2.	*Udāna*	*Ākāśa* (Space/ Ether)	Throat, palate, between the eyebrows and in the brain.	Vocal functions in varied ways.
3.	*Samāna*	*Agni* (Fire)	From the heart to the navel region.	Digestion and metabolism; building and upholding the seven *dhātus*.
4.	*Apāna*	*Pṛthvī* (Earth)	From the navel to the lower abdomen up to the legs.	Elimination of waste products and mobility in the pelvis.
5.	*Vyāna*	*Jala* (Water)	Pervading the whole body.	Circulation of *rasa dhātu* in the entire body.

Table 13: The Five *Upaprāṇas*				
S. N.	**Name**	**Element**	**Location**	**Function**
1.	*Nāga*	*Vāyu* (Air)	Region from mouth to heart	Belching and hiccough.
2.	*Kṛkala*	*Agnī* (Fire)	Throat to mid brain, between the eye brows	Hunger and thirst.
3.	*Kūrma*	*Pṛthvī* (Earth)	In the eyelids	Blinking the eyelids.
4.	*Devadatta*	*Ākāśa* (Space/ Ether)	In the nose	Stretching, yawning and sneezing.
5.	*Dhanañjaya*	*Jala* (Water)	Pervading the whole body	To maintain glow on the body for sometime even after death or swelling on the body.

3. ***Manomaya koṣa* (The mind sheath):** The third *koṣa* is *manomaya koṣa* which is more instinct-based and includes five motor organs for action (mouth, hand, leg, anus and urethra) and sense of self or ego. By maintaining patience and control, one can know the potential of the motor organs.

   A beautiful example representing the relationship between the mind and *prāṇa* is found in the *Chāndogyopaniṣada*. As the kite being attached to its cord returns to its original place after having flown in several directions, in a similar manner, *mana* swings in different directions, but does not receive shelter at other sites and thereby takes the shelter of *'prāṇa.'* It is because the mind is bound with *'prāṇa.'* This is the reason why the scriptures emphasize to strengthen *prāṇa* by means of *yoga* and *prāṇāyāma*, because when *prāṇa* gets strengthened the mind also becomes stronger. As the '*prāṇa*' (breath) becomes steady, so the mind too becomes steady. Control over the unstable and motile mind prevents all sorts of psychological problems such as depression and stress. It is due to these disturbed emotions and distractions that one indulges in wrong deeds like addictions, intoxication, unhealthy desires, lust and so on. This instability of the mind is the cause of deviation from the right path and sorrow. This is the reason to bring *manomaya koṣa* under control making it disease-free by means of knowledge, meditation, *sādhanā*, concentration and by the use of other *sāttvika* remedies as suggested in the (*Chāndogyopaniṣada* 6.8.2).

4. ***Vijñānamaya koṣa* (The intellect sheath):** The fourth sheath is *vijñānamaya koṣa*. It includes the five sense organs (nose, ears, eyes, tongue and skin) along with intellect (brain) and mind. Its main components are the intellect empowered by knowledge and the sense

organs of perception. By keeping control on the intellect and reasoning one achieves self-control over the sense organs and their power or strength. The brain decides all the good and bad deeds that are performed by the sense organs, and therefore the power to decide is regarded as the *vijñānamaya koṣa*. By the control over the *vijñānamaya koṣa* one can escape from attachment, falsehood, illusions and delusions, and can also rectify the wrong speech.

5. ***Ānandamaya koṣa* (The bliss or emotion sheath):** The fifth sheath is *ānandamaya koṣa*. It is related to our inner self including affection, happiness, joy and pleasure. It is the residing place of life and bliss. Human life, the existence of the gross body and all worldly affairs depend on it. By meditation and self-control one reaches the stage of perpetual bliss and emancipates oneself from the bondage of worldly life. At this stage, one gains knowledge and realizes the true self (inner self).

   By knowing and controlling these five *koṣas* one can achieve the knowledge of body science and can get rid of psycho-somatic disorders. Moreover, one can achieve the path to reach the Supreme soul by attaining eternal bliss.

4. Body Physiology and *Aṣṭacakra*: The Eight *Cakras*

Yoga and *Āyurveda* are excellent, proven and scientific medicinal systems that provide an epitome of quality life and overall development. *Yoga* and *Āyurveda* are also the only ways for an individual to attain complete health, eternal bliss and a divine life by awakening the inner self and consciousness and by developing one's own intellect, internal strength and complete human energy.

Caraka Saṁhitā describes many divine medicines to be used as rejunevators for the complete health of an individual, achieving an inner glow (*teja*), longevity, youth, a pleasant voice, healthy complexion, development of the body, strength, intellect and all desirable attributes. In all the rejunevators, *ācāra* (healthy living habits) is considered to be the best *rasāyana* (rejuvenator). In reality all righteous deeds and healthy living habits are '*ācāra*.' This is also called '*sadācāra*.' There is no other way to achieve the best *sāttvika* nature (*sadācāra*) apart from *yoga*. The complete benefits of yoga can be achieved only by regular practice and detachment. Our ancient sages understood the subtle intricacies of physiology and described the body as a small model of the whole universe, a microcosm by saying "***Yathā piṇḍe, tathā brahmāṇḍe***." Our visual and non visual, gross and subtle personality is quite mysterious, adventurous and very scientific. To know this extensively, it is essential to understand the power centers located within the body, these power centers are called *cakras*. About these *cakras* the *Atharvaveda* states:

" Aṣṭācakrā navadvārā devānāṁ pūrayodhyā.
Tasyāṁ hiraṇyayaḥ kośaḥ svargo jyotiṣāvṛtaḥ."

(*Atharvaveda* 10.2.31)

It means that this body symbolises God's city, *Ayodhyā*, which has eight *cakras* (eight power centers) and nine gates (both eyes, both nostrils, both ears, the mouth, the anus and the urethra). In this city there is an illuminating golden treasure "*sahasrāra cakra,*" which is filled with infinite, eternal happiness, bliss, peace and divine light. Only *yoga* practitioners, worshippers and spiritual seekers can achieve this divine treasure. Though these *cakras* appear to be related to the physical body, they are actually associated with super power centers of the body. They cannot be seen by the physical senses as they are known only by means of extra-sensory or imperceptible knowledge and strength. These power centers help the body in obtaining the life-force. But, after death or assimilation of the body, this energy is diffused by itself. That is why in a post-mortem these *cakras* are not seen in the spinal cord. As they are not anatomically seen, these *cakras* are considered to be imaginary. We must remember that the soul or life-force cannot be seen in a post-mortem. Energy is experienced not by its visual existence but by its effect. These power centers distribute the life-force in each cell, each tissue and each nerve emerging from them. In these nerves the flow of *prāṇa* (life-force) is bidirectional. These *cakras* are situated from below the base of the spine, the *mūlādhāra* (filum terminale) to the *sahasrāra* (brain) throughout the spinal cord. This undoubtedly proves that the ancient sages had a more subtle and intense knowledge of physiology and anatomy and the body's invisible power centers than modern medical science has. They not only identified the main power centers of the body, but also discovered various techniques to awaken these invisible energy centers by vivid *yogic* activities, *sādhanā*, *prāṇāyāma*, *yoga* and meditation to get free from disease and to reach self-refinement. [PLATE 14]

- ***Aṣṭacakra* colors and their scientific approach**

The petals of the *cakras* imagined in the classics are the group of subtle nerve plexuses around that *cakra*. These nerves more than being a part of the nervous system is the medium for expansion of the Consciousness. Here '*nāḍis*' are not nerves rather they are channels for the flow of energy (Consciousness) in the subtle body. The literal meaning of *nāḍis* (nerve) is 'flow.' As negative and positive charges flow together in electric circuits, the *prāṇa* (life-force) and *manas* (mental-force) energies flow through all parts of our body via these *nāḍis*. These nerves (sources of subtle flow of Consciousness) are said to be from 72 thousand to 72 million in the *Upaniṣadas* and different classics[13]. These are distributed all over the body. These very subtle waves are white, blue, yellow and red. The color and subtlety of these nerves are also said to be like the color and subtlety of the sun's rays[14]. These nerves are said to dissolve in the Sun after death. *Iḍā*, *piṅgalā* and *suśumṇa* are important among these nerves. The energy of *iḍā nāḍī* flows through the *prāṇa vāyu* of the left nostril and *piṅgalā nāḍī* through the right nostril. They are also called *candra nāḍī* and *sūrya nāḍī* respectively. *Iḍā nāḍī* is cold and *piṅgalā nāḍī* is hot in nature. The origin of these *nāḍis* is called *mūlādhāra*. These two *nāḍis* form a circle (*cakra*) which combines with the *suśumṇa* at the base of the spinal cord. This is called the *mūlakendra* (origin) of energy. These *nāḍis* control the flow of *prāṇa* and Consciousness. From this supposed location the *suśumṇa* moves up vertically straight, *iḍā* moves up from the left and *piṅgalā* from the right side. These *nāḍis* meet each other at the locations of different energy centers (*cakras*) along the *suśumṇa* and they reach all the way up to the *sahasrāra cakra*.

One can know the deep and subtle aspects (secrets) of body physiology by understanding these *cakras* and can attain infinite powers and complete health by awakening the latent powers located in these energy centers. The energy when reaches the *sahasrāra* from the refining and awakening of these *cakras* through *yoga sādhanā*, brings immense happiness and eternal bliss. This is the main aim of all methods of *yoga sādhanā* (practices). These power centers or the centers of vital energy are known as '*Aṣṭacakra*' and the energy, extra-sensory or imperceptible knowledge or inner strength awakened by these *cakras* is known as '*Brahamavarcas*' (cosmic radiance or the radiance of the *brahamaṇa*) and '*Kuṇḍalinī Jagaraṇa*' (awakening of serpent power) in Modern *Tantra* Classics.

- **Description of the eight *cakras***

1. ***Mūlādhāra cakra* (The root *cakra*):** This *cakra* is associated with the lowest point of the spinal cord between the anus and genital organs (reproductive organs). It is connected with the instinctual behavior of human beings. Divine consciousness cultivates here leaving based thinking behind.
2. ***Svādhiṣṭhāna cakra* (The sacral *cakra*):** It is situated behind the sexual organs (reproductive organs) in the spinal cord. It is associated with the subconscious mind.

13. *Hṛdi hyeṣa ātmā Atraitadekaśataṁ nāḍīnāṁ tāsāṁ śataṁ. Śatamekaikasyāṁ dvāsaptatirdvāsaptatiḥ pratiśākhānāḍīsahasrāṇa bhantyāsu vyānaścarit.* (*Praśno.* 3.6)
Śataṁ caikā ca hṛdayasya nāḍyasyatāsāṁ mūrdhānamabhiniḥsṛtaikā. Tayordhva māyannamṛtatvameti viśvaṅnyā utkramṇe bhavanti. (*Kāṭho.* 6:16)
14. *Atha yā etā hṛdayasya nāḍyastāḥ piṅgalasyānimnastiṣṭhanti śuklasya nīlasya pītasya lohitasyetyasau vā ādityaḥ piṅgala eṣa śukla eṣa nīla eṣa pīta eṣa lahitaḥ.* (*Chāndo.* 8:6:1)

Table 14: *Aṣṭacakra* and their Anatomic Location

S. No.	*Cakras* (*Sanskrit* Name)	Gross form (English Name)	Location	Body parts and controlled functions	Diseases due to deactivation or non-awakening of *cakras*	Action on Endocrine gland	Physiological system concerned
1.	*Mūlādhāra cakra*	Root *cakra* or pelvic plexus or coccyx center	Base of spine	Rectum, urinary bladder; excretion and reproduction	Urinary diseases, kidney disorders, calculi, genital disorders	Adrenal gland	Excertory system, Urino-genital system
2.	*Svādhiṣṭhāna cakra*	Sacral *cakra* or sexual center	Below the navel	Genital organs; procreation	Infertility, tissue diseases, genital disorders	Adrenal gland	Reproductive system
3.	*Maṇipūra cakra*	Solar plexus *cakra* or lumbar center or epigastric sciar plexus	Below the chest	Stomach, intestine; digestion, assimilation, secretion	digestive system disorders, diabetes, low immunity	Islets of Langerhans (endocrine cells) in pancreatic gland	Digestive system
4.	*Anāhata or hṛdaya cakra*	Heart *cakra* or cardiac plexus or dorsal center	Center of the chest: Thoracic vertebra	Heart, lungs, diaphragm; circulation, immune regulation	Heart diseases, hypertension	Thymus gland	Circulatory system, Respiratory system, Auto-immune system
5.	*Viśuddha cakra*	Throat *cakra* or carotid plexus or cervical center	Thyroid and para thyroid	Neck, throat, vocal cords; all oral communications, growth in children, metabolism, temperature regulation	Bronchial asthma, lung disorders, thyroid, goiter	Thyroid gland	Respiratory system
6.	*Ājñā cakra*	Third eye or medul-lary plexus	Center of the forehead	Brain; all functions corresponding to the brain, concentration, will-power	Epilepsy, fainting, paralysis	Pineal gland	Nervous system
7.	*Mānas or Bindu cakra*	Mind *cakra* or lower mind plexus or point *cakra*	Below the thalamus	Brain and heart; regulation of all endocrine glands and autonomic nervous system, sleep, emotions, memory, overall homeostasis	Psycho-somatic and neurological disorders	Pituitary gland	Sensory and Motor system
8.	*Sahasrāra cakra*	Crown *cakra* or cerebral gland	Top of the skull, the vertex	Seat of the soul; synthesizes information, gathers all information from other sites	Hormonal imbalances, metabolic syndromes	Pituitary gland	Central Nervous System (CNS) via hypothalamus

3. ***Maṇipūra cakra* (The solar plexus *cakra*):** It is situated behind the navel in the spinal cord. It regulates the digestive system and *jaṭharāgni* or digestive fire. The whole physical (gross) body is regulated from here.
4. ***Anāhata cakra* (The heart or cardiac plexus *cakra*):** This is situated in the spinal cord behind the heart's right side, in the center of the chest (between the breasts). This regulates blood circulation, heart and lung functioning. It also regulates the nervous system and the immune systemm.
5. ***Viśuddhi cakra* (The throat *cakra*):** It is located in the throat (behind thyroid and parathyroid glands) in the spinal cord. It regulates the vocal cord and is responsible for the growth, development, hunger, thirst and temperature regulation.
6. ***Ājñā cakra* (The third eye or medullary plexus):** This is associated with the pineal gland behind the centre of the eyebrows above the spinal cord. This is associated with will-power and progressiveness. This is the center of materialistic knowledge and *Aṣṭavidya* on the intuitive level.
7. ***Manas cakra* (The mind *cakra* or the point *cakra*):** *Manas cakra* is situated in the hypothalamus. Its function is to develop thought processes, *saṁsakāras* (moral values) and brain secretions according to the emotions and mental processes by establishing the connection to the heart. We can also call it the center of mind and emotions.
8. ***Sahasrāra cakra* (The crown *cakra*):** All spiritual powers are achieved here. Its relation is with the brain and knowledge. This *cakra* is associated with the pituitary gland. It is the center of supreme knowledge and enlightenment.

These eight *cakras* (power centers) energize, balance and activate the vital energy in the whole body. *Yoga* is the name of the techniques for removing all physical-mental barriers and diseases and awakening the Consciousness. Many ancient and moderen *yoga* practices are described in various Indian classics and traditions [PLATE 15]

***Are the *cakras* six or eight? A resolution of contrary views**

The *Atharvaveda* describes eight *cakras*. Also in *Gorakha Bāṇī* eight *cakras* are described as: ***"E aṣṭa kamala kā jāṇau-bheṣa. Āpai karatā āpai deva. Iti aṣṭacakra kathanta jatī Gorașanāth sampurna."*** After awakening of the six *cakras* these two *cakras* in the brain, *manas cakra* and *sahasrāra cakra* are thought to be the two higher centers of Conscious illumination, to reach higher realms and the base source or termination centers of vital energy. Hence, it is definite that the main *cakras* are eight. It is beyond doubt that the knowledge of the awakening of these power centers by means of meditation and *sādhanā* (spiritual practices) helps a *sādhaka* (seeker) to reach from the *mūlādhāra* to the *sahasrāra cakra*, achieve a diseases-free life and experience eternal bliss.

• *Yoga* and *Aṣṭacakra*

For the knowledge of the eight cakras and the energy centers associated within them, it is very important to know what all *yoga* practices are required. *Yoga* reveals the true nature of *aṣṭacakra*, so here it is essential to know what is '*yoga.*'

The term '*yoga*' is derived from the verbal root of ***'Yujir' Yoge, na yuje samadhau,*** which means to unite, '*samādhi*' (deep transcendental meditation) and solution. If we comprehend this at spiritual level, it is union of '*jeevātmā*' (individual soul) with '*Paramātmā*' (Supreme soul) by means of a series of activities or methods. When one achieves the state of '*samādhi*' through the practice of *yoga*, in that sublime state the human soul gets engrossed into God, the Supreme soul. It is called '*yoga.*' It is through *yoga* that a person achieves cessation of mental suppression and acquires control on his mind. There are many more such practices which help us in restraining the inconsistencies of mind and elevating the spirit towards renunciation or sacrifice. All these are the integral parts of *yoga*.

One can achieve happiness and peace through the practice of *yoga*. Innovative power of inner self ignites and emits its glow elsewhere. Through the *yoga* practice and by means of meditation, this divine energy arises. It flows through the lower conscious centers to the higher ones. At this stage all power, be it mind power, resolution power or the power of self, work unitedly. Once the life-force awakens, these energies helps to elevate the incessant consciousness through the flow of life-force in *piṅgalā nāḍī,* through mind power in *iḍā nāḍī* and the power of self in *suśumṇa nāḍī*. This way, energy flows within the entire body. After the awakening of these energy centers, whenever the practitioner (*sādhaka*) settles himself in meditation, the power rouses once again. At this time, *sādhaka* experiences many miraculous effects which are unimaginary. Many new experiences, self realization and divine grace are attained by a *yoga* practitioner, while he dedicates himself in devotion (*bhakti*), practice (*sādhanā*), service (*sevā*) and penance (*tapa*). The body and mind also get transformed according to the need of the higher consciousness, which brings complete change in one's life.

▪ Relation of *Maharshi Patañjali's aṣṭāṅga yoga* with *aṣṭacakra*

Maharshi Patañjali has described eight limbs of *yoga* which are known as *yamas, niyamas, āsanas, prāṇāyāmas, pratyāhāra, dhāraṇā, dhyāna* and *samādhi*.

1. ***Yamas* (Moral restraints):** It is a series of rules for right living or ethical values. The *yamas* include *ahiṁsā* (non-violence), *satya* (benevolent truth), *asatya* (non-stealing), *brahmacarya* (celibacy and spiritual advancement) and *aparīgraha* (non-covetousness and absence of avarice). They are associated with the internal emotions of a person. A

person who does not follow the path of *satya, ahiṁsā* and other ethical values not only damages his own individual dignity, but also harms the society and nation. It happens due to the negative and disturbed emotions present in the body. Its association is with *mūlādhāra cakra*. Disturbed emotions like untruthfulness, violence, desire and other such disgraceful deeds end after the awakening of energy of *mūlādhāra cakra*.

2. ***Niyamas* (Observances):** The second limb of the eight limbs in *Patanjali's yogsūtra* is a set of prescribed actions codified as *niyamas* which are observances, requirements and obligations such as:

   ***Sauca*:** Cleanliness of thought, mind and body.

   ***Santoṣa*:** Satisfaction, contentment.

   ***Tapas*:** Penance, spiritual efforts, austerity.

   ***Svādhyāya*:** Study of the self for the awakening of the soul and God within.

   ***Īśvara-praṇidhāna*:** Surrender to God.

   These are associated with the character of a person. It is a loss to oneself if one does not adopt the *niyamas* in life, as a consequence of which society also has to suffer the loss. They are associated with the *svādhiṣṭhāna cakra*. By adopting *niyamas* in life, the *svādhiṣṭhāna cakra* gets awakened.

3. ***Āsanas* (Body postures):** *Āsana* are associated with the disease-free and healthy gross body. They are associated with the *maṇipūra* or *nābhi cakra*. After the awakening of *maṇipūra* or *nābhi cakra*, digestive and other physical disorders heal.

4. ***Prāṇāyāmas* (Breath extension):** It involves extension of the life-force by breath control. This is related to the *anāhata cakra,* which is situated in the lungs and the heart region. By the awakening of this *cakra*, the life-force can be strengthened by maintaining a perfect heart and respiratory system.

5. ***Pratyāhāra* (Sensory withdrawal):** *Pratyāhāra* is associated with the *viśuddhi cakra*. After the awakening of this *cakra*, attachment of the sense organs to external objects starts withdrawing and the practitioner can achieve control over the sense organs.

6. ***Dhāraṇā* (Concentration):** It involves concentration of the mind along with the retention of breath. *Dhāraṇā* is associated with the *ajñā cakra*. To stabilize the mind at a single focus after its withdrawal through the practice of *pratyāhāra* is called *dhāraṇā*.

7. ***Dhyāna* (Meditation):** *Dhyāna* is associated with the *manas cakra* or *bindu cakra*. The *manas cakra* awakens when the complete flow of Consciousness and life-force is controlled, stabilized and stored within the body through the practice of *dhāraṇā* (concentration).

8. ***Samādhi* (Deep transcendental meditation):** It is a state of total equilibrium of a detached intellect. *Sahasrāra cakra* awakens when the practitioner is free from all the disorders and desires and he is

established in the void, which is the true self or nature of the object through meditation. This state is also known as *samādhi* or blissful state.

- **Knowledge of *aṣṭacakra* and the ascension of power through the practice of *yoga***

The *cakras* present in our body are actually the centers of *prāṇa-śaktī*, the life-force. The awakening of these power centers enable the life-force to ascend. But this ascension depends upon the piousness, inner consciousness and on the practice of a practitioner. The more pure and pious the mind is, the higher the level of consciousness. In the form of *cakras*, we can precisely understand it as the person in his wretched state, whose mind is indulged in various kinds of desires, defects and disorders, and whose consciousness resides in *mūlādhāra cakra*, when progresses in the level of his consciousness, subsequently reaches from *svādhiṣṭhāna cakra* to *sahasrāra cakra*, through the ascension of power. Internal power inflames as the mind becomes pious and pure by means of *yoga* practice. Therefore, body is energized with the transformation of innovative power and vibration. These divine powers are called as different power centers (*aṣṭacakra*) in scriptures. When the power in these centers is aroused, the practitioner automatically switches to good intentions and ideas. His mind does not entertain any kind of negative feelings. His mind is always in the blissful state. Then many curable and incurable diseases starts healing even without any medication. One gets free of all kinds of mental and physical disorders like depression, delusion, anxiety and restlessness. When mind remains peaceful, favorable changes take place. Consequently, the power of determination and the will-power gets strengthened. In this state, ones priorities, interests and affections get changed. Hence, desired effect can be achieved in our body, mind and soul by awakening of these *cakras* which allows the *yogic* power to ascend through the regular practice of *yoga*.

5. *Aṣṭacakra* and its Relation with Various *Yogic* Practices and *Kuṇḍalinī Yoga*

In a debate on the practice of *yoga*, it is often assumed that the practice is related to awakening the power of *kuṇḍalinī*. However this is not true. The *cakras* are not confined to '*Kuṇḍalinī Jāgṛti*.' That is one of the most prominent practices of *yoga*, described in '*Tantra Yoga*.' In *Tantra Sādhanā*, the power of *aṣṭacakra* is depicted and *kuṇḍalinī* is explained as the perfect method to arouse power. In ancient times, many *yogis* attempted to arouse the power by connecting various *yogic* practices with *kuṇḍalinī* energy. However, the procedure of *aṣṭanga yoga* was not systematical in those days; hence their efforts were not fruitful. Some practitioners do not accept the theory of *aṣṭacakra*. But, one should not misunderstand the *aṣṭacakra*, which are latent power centers.

(A) *Aṣṭacakra* and different methods of *yogasādhanā*

Aṣṭacakra the names of various centers of subtle and invisible energy situated in the body. These *cakras* in our body are also centers of vital energy, the life-force. They are the center of *prāṇika* energy in the body. These energy centers are integral part of human physiology and they can be elevated and awakened by various sorts of *yoga sādhanā* (spiritual practices), *tāpas* (penance), *sañyama* (control), *sadācāra* (righteous and ethical conduct) and so on. The awakening of these power centers '*Aṣṭacakra*' and upliftment of energy depends on the piousness and mental status of the person. The more pious the mind of an individual, the higher the level of his consciousness. For the awakening of consciousness, along with *sevā* (services) and *sādhanā* (practices), various techniques of *yoga* and *prāṇāyāma* are suggested in *Patañjali's aṣṭāṇga yoga* which are very effective. Many *sādhanās* and *yogic* methods are in practice for the awakening of these power centers. Initially in *kuṇḍalinī yoga*, *kuṇḍalinī* energy awakens at random by the grace of a highly accomplished ascetic *gurū* (guide), but beyond this, to reach the higher realms a *sādhaka* (seeker) needs more practice (*sādhanā*) and much control, or otherwise this awakened *kuṇḍalinī* energy remains in the individual *cakra*.

In *aṣṭānga yoga*, initially a *sādhaka* (seeker) has to work hard to progress in *sādhanā* and for the awakening of the energies hidden in the eight *cakras*, but when he starts progressing, then effortlessly his mind becomes pious and he starts following the path of idealism and moral values in life, and at this stage his vital energy is enhanced. The same inner energy upswings and moves up through *maṇipūra*, *anāhata* and reaches the *viśuddha cakra*, and at this stage he experiences bliss, becomes energized and feels free from all stress. Inner excitement, energy and enthusiasm increases. Impurities in the form of mental infirmities and negativity starts cleansing, the mind becomes calm and a *sādhaka* starts experiencing *samādhi*. When the same energy of consciousness ascends from *ajñā cakra* to *manas cakra* and *sahasrāra cakra* and stabilizes there, then a *sādhaka* reaches *samprajñāta* (cognitive) and *asamprajñāta* (ultra-cognitive) *samādhi* and attains Supreme Bliss. This way the awakening of *cakras* is possible by *sāttvika sādhanā* (*aṣṭāṅga yoga*), *upāsanā* (service and worship), *vairāgya* (detachment from worldly pleasures) and *tyāga* (renunciation). Hence by *yoga sādhanā*, one's inner energy awakens and reaches the higher realms from *mūlādhāra* to *sahasrāra* through *svādhisthāna*, *maṇipūra* and other *cakras*. Whichever *cakra* this energy reaches, once it reaches the higher realms, it does not descend again from that center. With the awakening of energy, a *sādhaka* becomes unaffected by changes happening in the body and mind.

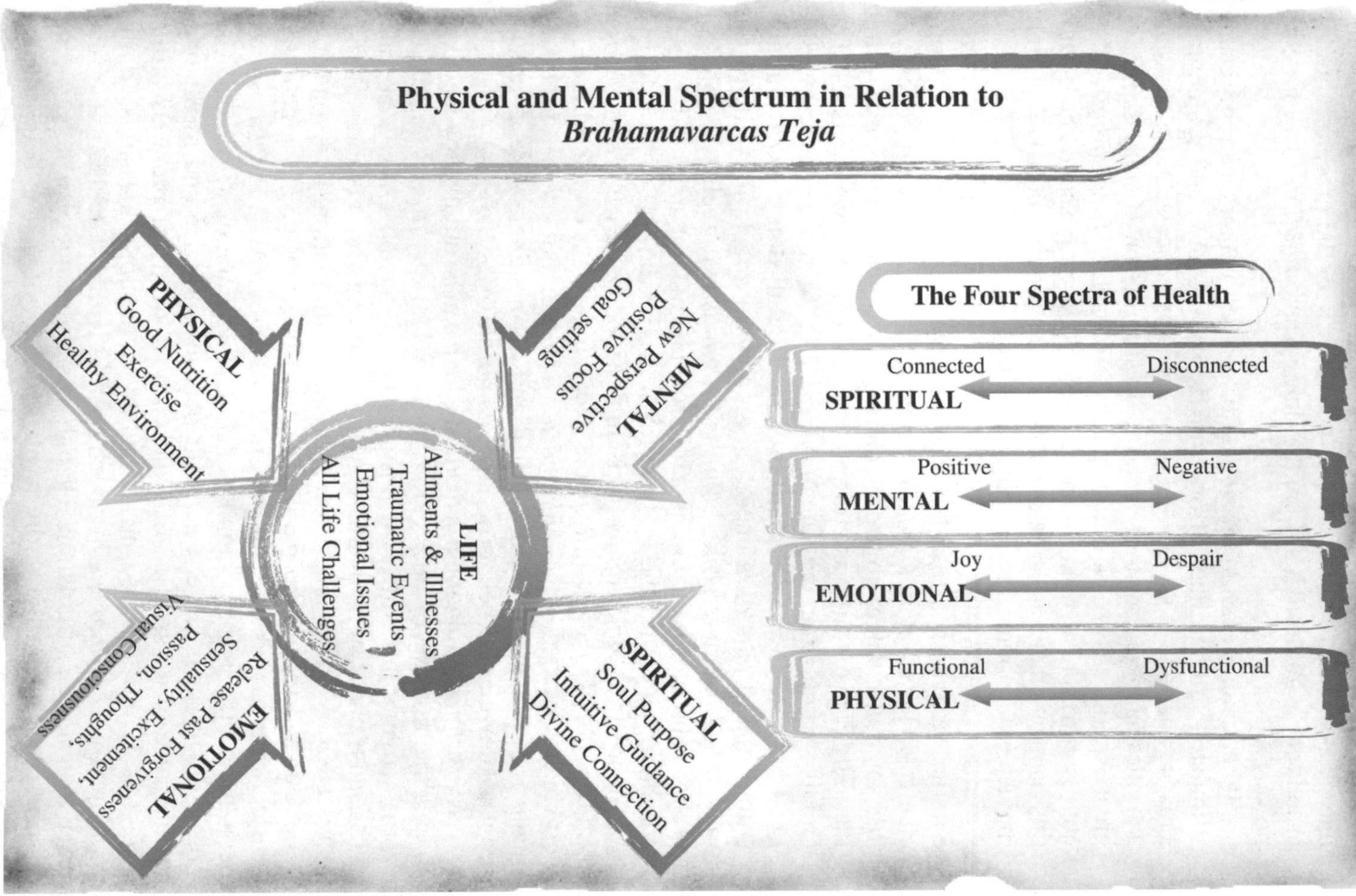
Physical and Mental Spectrum in Relation to
Brahamavarcas Teja
PHYSICAL
Good Nutrition
Exercise
Healthy Environment
MENTAL
New Perspective
Positive Focus
Goal setting
LIFE
Ailments & Illnesses
Traumatic Events
Emotional Issues
All Life Challenges
EMOTIONAL
Release Past Forgiveness
Sensuality, Excitement,
Passion, Thoughts,
Visual Consciousness
SPIRITUAL
Soul Purpose
Intuitive Guidance
Divine Connection
The Four Spectra of Health
Connected
Disconnected
SPIRITUAL
Positive
Negative
MENTAL
Joy
Despair
EMOTIONAL
Functional
Dysfunctional
PHYSICAL

(B) *Aṣṭacakra* and methods of *kuṇḍalinī yoga*

In *kuṇḍalinī yoga*, by small efforts of the practioner (*sādhaka*), the energy associated in *mūlādhāra* activates with the grace of a highly ascetic *gurū* (guide). This strength is known as *kuṇḍalinī śakti* (serpent's power).

By practicing *kuṇḍalinī yoga*, the power centers can be easily stimulated without much effort, with deep meditation and self control. This is experienced by the feel of energy waves, jerks and many such activities happening within the body. In stimulation of *kuṇḍalinī* many great experiences are naturally attained. However, if the *sādhaka* does not resort to self-restraint, then this power does not ascend and even if this happens, there are greater chances of its moving downward. Here movement is not used in the physical sense.

On stimulation of power by the method of *aṣṭāṅga yoga sādhanā*, external activities are reduced leading to an increase in internal changes. However, in *kuṇḍalinī yoga* by *kuṇḍalinī* energy, one feels less internal changes in the beginning but physical changes are felt intensely. This is the basic difference between the two methods. The aim for stimulating the *kuṇḍalinī śakti* is 'to realize' the almighty Lord Shiva (*Parama Brahma*) by targetting all other *cakras* through stimulation of *kuṇḍalinī* energy in an upward direction. Actually, the main target for undergoing both the *sādhanas* is to realize the bliss of feeling supreme and attaining a blissful state of soul and mind.

- ***Kuṇḍalinī yoga* and the method for its activation**

At present, *kuṇḍalinī yoga* is understood as a well-known *yoga* method for *aṣṭacakra* awakening. Here, *kuṇḍalinī* means coiled miraculous power which is located in the *mūlādhāra cakra* (the root *cakra*). It remains dormant here. Since it lives in a coiled and dormant state like a serpent, hence it is known as 'serpent power' or '*kuṇḍalinī śakti*.'

Kuṇḍalinī stimulation is a method which can be attained by means of following traditions set by ones *gurū* (guide). When *kuṇḍalinī* is stimulated, different activities like different postures of the hands, *prāṇāyāmas* and certain *āsanas* occur spontaneously. Many melodious sounds and waves of energy are felt. All these are signs of *kuṇḍalinī* stimulation. Everyone does not feel this and those who realize it, feel it differently. These activities arouse curiosity and interest in the minds of *sādhakas*. *Sādhakas* should understand that this is the beginning of *sādhanā* and not the final goal. This is possible without much efforts, with penance, practice and meditation, with the grace of an ascetic *gurū* and virtuous deeds of previous births. Hence, this is the knowledge attained by a mentor's blessings. If the *sādhaka* performs *prāṇāyāma* for a long period with full dedication, he can succeed in *kuṇḍalinī* stimulation. Though by self practice also the *kuṇḍalinī* gets stimulated, but in the tradition of *kuṇḍalinī yoga* it is believed that the *kuṇḍalinī* which has now stimulated, has been pre-activated by the blessings of a *gurū* gained in the previous birth. Here, a lot of caution is required. Even in the *gurū*-disciple tradition, the main method of *kuṇḍalinī* awakening (*jāgraṇa*) involves many kinds of *prāṇāyāmas* to be performed. In *Haṭha Yoga Pradīpikā*, it has been said, that the way a serpent straightens his body after being beaten repeatedly, similarly one should perform *jālandhara bandha* and take the air upward and practice *kumbhaka*. Then the air should be released slowly. It is advised not to perform it forcefully. This method has been suggested by experienced gurūs, by which serpent's power (*kuṇḍalinī śakti*) automatically gets straightened.

According to *Tantra Granthas* and *Haṭha Yoga*, the simplest way for *kuṇḍalinī* activation is to get the blessings of the *gurū* and follow the *gurūs* instructions.

After activation of *kuṇḍalinī*, if it is to reach the *sahasrāra cakra* or it is required to attain *samādhi*, then the *sādhaka* has to get rid of flaws. For this, after the activation of *kuṇḍalinī*, the *sādhaka* has to practice it regularly which helps to get rid of flaws. If this is not done, then it is most likely that the attainments go in vain. Therefore, regular meditation, *prāṇāyāma*, self control and positive thinking help us to reach the *sahasrāra cakra via svādhiṣṭhāna, maṇipūra* and other *cakras*, and also to experience eternal bliss and connection with Supreme Soul.

- **Qualities in a *yoga sādhaka* (practitioner)**

A *sādhaka* has to shun sensual inclinations, anger, greed, attachment, and continue *yoga* practice without any 'bad' habits.Therefore, a *sādhaka* has to be self-restrained, well-mannered, soft-spoken, disciplined and compassionate. He should have perseverance, strong will power and immense patience. A *sādhaka* has to be fully dedicated to the *gurū*. He/ she should not hide anything from the *gurū*. It is required to abide by the guidance of the *gurū*.

- **People unfit for *yoga sādhanā***

Those who indulge in sensual activities and are arrogant, dishonest and wicked. Those who are not reliable. Those who feel pleasure in disrespecting people and are cruel, have indisciplined eating habits, or are sensually weak, do not deserve to practice spirituality. Such people may practice *āsanas, prāṇāyāmas*, meditation and other *yoga* techniques, but it will be only for physical gain and will not help to attain the utmost success of *sādhanā* or spirituality. Such a person cannot attain enlightenment, strength, courage, power or eternal bliss.

In summary the path to ultimate Bliss involves a radical change in thinking, beliefs as well as constant *yoga* practice.

> "There are so many misconcepts about *kuṇḍalinī* stimulation and other *sādhanās* because there is no clarity in views, in ancient and modern texts. Here we have clarified things in this regard in the best ways."

Chapter 4
The Nature of Material Substances

The previous chapter dealt with the various components and elements that constitute the body. Whenever there is an abnormal increase in the quantity of *doṣas*, *dhātus*, *malas* and *srotas*, the balance can be restored by the consumption of right food, medicines or other curative substances having inverse qualities of the respective *doṣa*. Whenever there is a decrease in the quantity of these factors, the consumption of substances having similar qualities restores balance. Now the question arises, how does one determine what substances share the same or opposing qualities of a particular *doṣa* or *dhātu* to correct their vitiation? This is possible only when the practioner of *Āyurveda* has indepth knowledge about different types of substances.

All things in the universe are made up of five elements. Like the *doṣas* or *dhātus*, all substances are created by the combination of five elements in differing quantities. The shape and color does not necessarily indicate the predominant element of any substance. Only the *rasa* (taste), *vipāka* (post-digestive effect), *vīrya* (potency) and *guṇa* (properties) will help to identify the chief element of any substance. Based on this knowledge, a physician chooses the most appropriate food and medicinal substances to treat a particular patient, according to his/her constitution. All medicinal substances can be chiefly divided into three main categories:

a. ***Pārthiva dravya*:** Substances on and in the earth are known as *pārthiva* substances. Soil, sand, clay, red ochre (*gerū*), metals, minerals (like iron, copper, gold, silver, etc.), mercury, salt, stone, limestone, gems and precious stones, alkaline substances and collyrium fall under this category.

b. ***Jāṅgama dravya*:** These include all medicinal substances obtained from the animal kingdom such as honey, milk, milk products, leather, flesh (meat), animal fat, blood, bones, bone marrow, semen, blood, hair, nails, fur, horns, hooves, teeth, feathers, sinew, tendons, ligaments, muscles, nerves, urine, bile etc.

c. ***Audbhida dravya*:** This category includes substances that emerge from the earth such as plants and substances derived from them. Different kinds of flora, herbs, climbers, vegetables, fruits, flowers, roots, tubers, seeds, leaves, branches, bark, plant exudates, gums etc., are all categorized under *audbhida dravya*.

Based on their constituent elements, substances are also divided into five categories. It is important to remember that all substances contain traces of all five elements. Most substances are dependent on earth and water, which play a role in their formation. The three remaining elements - fire, air and space - complete the process of creation by their energy and add to the uniqueness of each substance. However, every substance has one or the other dominant element that decides its properties and makes it unique. On the basis of this fact, the five types of substances are:

1. ***Pārthiva dravya*** - dominated by the element of earth
2. ***Jalīya dravya*** - dominated by the element of water
3. ***Vāyavya dravya*** - dominated by the element of air
4. ***Tejas dravya*** - dominated by the element of fire
5. ***Ākāśīya dravya*** - dominated by the element of space (ether)

The characteristics of each of the above have been elaborated in the previous chapter.

In *Āyurveda*, a balanced diet does not revolve around fats, carbohydrates, proteins, vitamins and minerals. For the most part, conventional nutrition comes from laboratory analysis. *Āyurvedic* nutrition comes directly from nature. *Āyurveda* allows us to eat a balanced diet, guided by our own instincts. When taste buds receive any food, all useful information is delivered to the *doṣas*. When food communicates with the *doṣas*, it says many things because of different *guṇas* present in it. In *Āyurveda,* a substance is classified on the basis of *rasa, guṇa, vīrya* and *vipāka*, as per its different conditions and characteristics for medicinal purposes. The primary information lies in its taste. In *Āyurveda*, a balanced diet is one which contains all six *rasas*. Here, all these characteristics are described respectively.

1. *Rasa*: Taste

Rasa or taste is the main property that helps to determine the dominant element of any substance. To identify the type of *rasa* (taste) in any substance, one required great practice, though some items have stronger tastes than others, which anyone can recognize. Just as a touch felt on the skin helps us to understand the texture, similarly the tongue perceives the taste and helps us to understand its essence(1). The effect of a particular substance on a person also helps to determine the *rasa* (taste) of a substance. [PLATE 16]

There are six basic *rasas* (tastes): *madhura* (sweet), *amla* (sour), *lavaṇa* (salty), *kaṭu* (pungent), *tikta* (bitter) and *kaṣāya* (astringent)(2). The first *rasa,*

1. *Rasanārtho rasastasya dravyamāṇaḥ kṣitistathā.* (*Ca.sū.* 1/64)
2. *Svāduramlo, tha lavaṇaḥ kaṭukastikta eva ca.*
   Kaṣāyaśceti ṣaṭko, yaṁ rasānāṁ saṅgraḥ smṛtaḥ. (*Ca.sū.* 1/65)

madhura (sweet) provides the highest amount of energy. All other *rasas* are comparatively less energizing and low in potency. The astringent taste provides least amount of energy.

- ***Rasa* (taste) and the five elements**

Rasa or taste is the natural attribute of *jala* (water), interestingly, in *jala, rasa* (taste) is produced only after an interaction with other basic elements. Similarly, each *rasa* has some or the other predominant elements. [PLATE 17]

Indian sages have analyzed the properties of the substances on the basis of their *rasa* (taste) and the elements possessed by them. *Rasa* plays the most important role in characterizing the *pārthiva, jaṅgama* and *audbhida* substances and their medicinal properties - *guṇa*, *vīrya* (potency), *vipāka* (post-digestive effect) and *prabhāva* (action).

Types of *Rasas* and their Dominant Elements

Rasa (Taste) →	*Madhura* (Sweet)	*Amla* (Sour)	*Lavaṇa* (Salty)	*Tikta* (Bitter)	*Kaṭu* (Pungent)	*Kaṣāya* (Astringent)
Elemen →	Earth Water	Earth Fire	Water Fire	Air Space	Air Fire	Air Earth

The effect of any substance on *dhātu* and *doṣas* present in an individual's body depends on the main elements of the *rasa*. Though there are six primary tastes, they combine in several ways, in different ratios, to form innumerable taste variations. Apart from these, there are some other tastes too which are known as '*anurasa*' or '*uparasa*' and these are not immediately prominent on the tongue, but can be manifested faintly after a while.

- ***Rasa* and *Doṣa***

Depending on its dominant elements, a particular *rasa* will increase or decrease the intensity of some or the other *doṣa*. Therefore *rasa* (taste) can also be used to balance an aggravated *doṣa* and can even cause vitiation in *doṣa* as follows:

Rasa	**Increase in *doṣa***	**Decrease in *doṣa***
Madhura (Sweet)	*Kapha*	*Vāta, Pitta*
Amla (Sour)	*Kapha, Pitta*	*Vāta*
Lavaṇa (Salty)	*Pitta, Kapha*	*Vāta*
Kaṭu (Pungent)	*Pitta, Vāta*	*Kapha*
Tikta (Bitter)	*Vāta*	*Pitta, Kapha*
Kaṣāya (Astringent)	*Vāta*	*Pitta, Kapha*

It indicates that: *Vāta* is balanced by sweet, sour and salty tastes; *Pitta* is balanced by bitter, sweet and astringent tastes; and *Kapha* is balanced by pungent, bitter and astringent tastes.

Similarly sweet, salty and sour tastes aggravate *Kapha*; salty, sour and bitter tastes aggravate *Pitta*; pungent, bitter and astringent tastes aggravate *Vāta*.

- ***Rasa* and *Dhātu***

The six *rasas* (tastes) and seven *dhātus* are also intimately related. Usually:

Sweet, Sour, Salty	-	Responsible for an increase in the quantity of *dhātus*
Bitter, Pungent, Astringent	-	Responsible for decrease in the quantity of *dhātus*
Bitter	-	Responsible for decrease in *meda* (adipose tissue), *majjā* (bone marrow) and *lasikā* (lymphatics)
Sour	-	Responsible for decrease in *śukra dhātu* (semen)

- ***Rasa* and *Mala***

Sweet, Sour, Saline	-	Helps in excretion of waste products (hence very effective and useful in constipation and other abdominal disorders)
Bitter, Pungent, Astringent	-	Helps retain waste products (hence beneficial in diarrhea, colitis and dysentery, especially the astringent taste)

- **Categorization of *rasa* in *Āyurvedic* texts**

Based on the digestive pattern, *rasas* are categorized into two types - *vidāhī* (causing excessive thirst, acidity, heartburn) and *avidāhī* (causing no burning sensation during digestion and helps to recover from syncope).

Vidāhī: It includes pungent, sour and salty tastes.

Avidāhī: It includes sweet, bitter and astringent tastes.

- **Identifying *rasa* and their *guṇa-karma* (properties and actions)**

(i) *Madhura rasa* (Sweet taste)

That which is pleasant in taste, produces a certain amount of stickiness on chewing, nourishes the body and is enjoyable to the sense organs, i.e., increases *sāttvikatā* and exhilarates the mind, is sweet taste(3). Substances (medicinal and food substances) that contain *madhura rasa* (sweet taste) are most favorable by nature. They increase the quantity as well as strength of all the *dhātus* (from *rasa* to *śukra dhātu*) and thereby enhance the overall life-span. They improve the complexion and increase vitality. Intake of substances rich in *madhura rasa* (sweet taste) pacifies aggravated *Pitta* and

3. *Tatra yaḥ paritoṣamutpādamati, prahlādayati, tarpayati jīvayati, mukhopalepaṁ janayati, śleṣmāṇaṁ cābhivardhayati sa madhuraḥ.* (*Su.sū.* 42:11)

Vāta doṣa and neutralizes the adverse effects of toxins. Sweet substances lend strength, vigor, flexibility, stability and liveliness to the body. They make the nose, throat, mouth, tongue and lips smooth, soft and supple. Sweet substances are smooth, cool and heavy. They are good for the hair, sensory organs and *ojas*. They help to increase milk production and promote fusion of sperm and ovum. Therefore, feeble and emaciated people, children, aged persons and patients recovering from disease should increase their intake of foods with *madhura rasa*.

***Madhura Rasa* (Sweet Taste)**
Increases - *Kapha* (except honey)
Decreases - *Pitta* and *Vāta*

Yet, despite its beneficial and favorable qualities, an excess of sweet taste causes an increase in the *Kapha doṣa*. As a result *Kapha* dominant problems such as obesity, drowsiness, lethargy, excessive sleep, heaviness, lack of appetite, weak digestion, accumulation of fat around the neck and face, sweetish taste in the mouth, lack of sensation, weak voice and ailments such as diabetes, urinary disorders, dysuria, cough, cold, influenza, goiter, scrofula (enlarged cervical glands), swelling and stickiness in the throat and conjunctivitis can be easily contracted. Therefore, obese and overweight people, diabetics and those having abdominal worm infestation must refrain from consuming sweet products.

- **Sweet substances:** *Ghee* (clarified butter), milk, sugarcane, jaggery, honey, grapes, walnuts, bananas, coconuts, phalsa, jack fruit, asparagus (*śatāvarī*), roscoea's lily (*kākolī*), country mallow (*balā*), Indian mallow (*atibalā*), veronicalolia (*nāgabalā*), King Solomon's seal (*mahāmedā*), whorled Solomon's seal (*medā*), ticktree (*śālaparṇī*), dabra (*pṛśniparṇī*), African gram (*mudgaparṇī*), blue wiss (*māṣaparṇī*), leptadave (*jīvantī*), malaxis (*jīvaka*), honey tree (*mahuvā*), liquorice root (*muleṭhī*), Indian kudzu (*vidārī*), bamboo (*vaṁśalocana*), coomb teak (*gambhārī*), caltrope (*gokharū*) and gold are all sweet substances.
- **Exceptions:** Old unpolished rice, old barley, wheat, green gram and honey though sweet, do not cause *Kapha* vitiation. Hence it is prescribed in *Āyurveda* to consume old grains and new (fresh) *ghee*.

(ii) *Amla rasa* (Sour taste)

The taste that causes salivation, the eyes and eyebrows to pucker and the teeth and gums to tingle is the sour taste[4]. It adds taste to the food and makes food interesting. It stimulates appetite and is cool to feel. Sour foods nourish the body, strengthen and make it sturdy, make the brain more active, fortify and strengthen the heart, strengthen the sensory organs and energize

4. *Yo dantaharṣamutpādayati, mukhāsrāvāṁ janayati, śradhāṁ cotpādayati so, mlaḥ* (Su.sū. 42/11)

the body. The juices of sour food substances boost digestion by chymification, helps one to swallow food, soften it and hasten the downward movement towards the intestine for further assimilation. Sour foods are smooth, hot in potency, refreshing, light (easy to digest), helps in cleaning the bladder and colon and hastens waste elimination. Unripe fruits generally have a sour taste.

***Amla Rasa* (Sour Taste)**
Increases - *Pitta* and *Kapha*
Decreases - *Vāta*

The excess consumption of *amla rasa* (sour taste) increases *Pitta* in the body with symptoms like excessive thirst, horripilation, sensitivity in teeth, loosening of *Kapha*, damaged muscles, body-swelling in weak persons, weakness, feebleness, emaciation, laxity, itching, darkness before the eyes (blackouts), dizziness (vertigo), fever, burning sensation in the throat, heart and chest. It also results in dermatological diseases (erysipelas, eruptions and such other diseases), pus formation in cuts and wounds, trauma and fractures or dislocation of bones and other related disorders. Therefore, people suffering from skin diseases, trauma, bronchial asthma, cough, sore throat (pharyngitis) and joint pain should avoid sour foods. Feeble and emaciated persons and those whose diet lacks oil should also consume sour foods in restricted amounts.

- **Substances with a sour taste:** Indian gooseberry, vinegar, tamarind, lemon, star fruit (carambola), cranberry, mango, pomegranate, yogurt, buttermilk, wood apple, garcinia, Indian hog plum and silver.
- **Exceptions:** Pomegranate or dried pomegranate seeds and Indian gooseberry though sour, are not harmful.

(iii) *Lavaṇa rasa* (Salty taste)

The taste that causes salivation and a burning sensation in the throat and cheeks is the salty taste. Saline foods are carminative (carry *Vāta* downward), digestive, enhances taste, causes stickiness, helps to develop an interest in food, are pungent and scarifying. They reduce stiffness in the organs, accumulation of fat and excreta and blockages in the *srota*. Saline foods are neither very oily nor very hot or heavy. Salty taste dominates other tastes and tends to overpower them.

***Lavaṇa Rasa* (Salty Taste)**
Increases - *Pitta* and *Kapha*
Decreases - *Vāta*

Excessive salinity or overuse of this *rasa* vitiates both *Pitta doṣa* and the blood, leading to increased thirst and heat sensitivity. It also causes a burning sensation, syncope, decrease in *rakta* and other *dhātus*, suppuration of the eyes, edema, discoloration of the skin, hemorrhage (bleeding) from different parts of the body, weakening of gums and loosening of teeth, increased toxicity, decreased virility, baldness, graying of hair, wrinkles, hyperacidity, delayed wound healing and reduction of strength and *ojas*. It may also cause stomatitis (mouth ulcers), gout, erysipelas, ringworm and diseases of infected skin (leprosy and other severe dermatological diseases). Salt is considered incompatible for the eyes. Salt should not be taken by hypertensive patients and one suffering from skin diseases.

- **Salty substances:** Rock salt (sea salt), common salt (table salt), *sancala* salt, *sauvarcala* salt (black salt), *audbhida* salt (salt derived from the earth), *pāṁsu* salt, *biḍa* salt, lead salt (*śīśa*), *romaka* salt and other alkalies.
- **Exception:** Rock salt does not cause much harm.

(iv) *Kaṭu rasa* (Pungent taste)

This taste causes a stinging pain in the mouth, stimulates the front of the tongue, causes burning in the cheeks and watering of the eyes, nose and mouth. Pungent substances cleanse the mouth, aid absorption of food, boost hunger and promote digestion. They clean and improve the efficiency of sense organs, dispose of sticky waste products from the eyes, nose and *srota* more effectively and promote sweating. Hence, pungent foods and herbs help to keep the *srotas* of *anna, rasa* and blood vessels clear and open.

***Kaṭu Rasa* (Pungent Taste)**
Increases - *Vāta* and *Pitta*
Decreases - *Kapha*

The pungent taste helps to manage obesity, urticaria, hives, conjunctivitis, eye fatigue, itching, wounds, sores, abdominal worm infestation, *alasaka* (retention of undigested food in the abdomen), stiffness in joints, throat infection, dermatitis and bronchial asthma. It dries and putrefies oil, fat, muscles and moisture. It pacifies *Kapha* and helps circulate sluggish (viscous) blood. It improves the taste of food.

Excess of such substances with pungent taste leads to dizziness, anxiety, syncope, dryness of lips, fatigue, debility, reduced virility, decrease in sperm count and strength. Being dominated by air and fire elements, excessive intake leads to burning in limbs and back, increased body temperature, body aches, stinging and smarting pain, shivering and other debilities.

- **Substances with a pungent taste:** Asafoetida, black pepper, false pepper, *Pañcakola* (mixture of long pepper and its root, Java long pepper, white leadwort and dry ginger), green leafy vegetables, marking nut, all kinds of bile and urine as prescribed in *Āyurveda.*
- **Exceptions:** Dry ginger, long pepper and garlic are safe foods with pungent taste and do not cause much harm.

(v) *Tikta rasa* (Bitter taste)

This is the taste that removes feeling of slime from the mouth and numbs the tongue. Despite tasting unpleasant, the bitter essence enhances the taste of other substances, makes it more interesting and thus helps to develop an interest in food. Bitter substances detoxify and help to manage obesity, diabetes, intestinal worms, syncope, burning sensations, thirst, fever, itching, dermatitis and severe dermatological diseases. They help in carmination (downward circulation) of *Vāta* and bring dryness in the body. Consequently they help in drying up moisture, fat, cellulite, bone marrow, lymph, pus, sweat, urine and feces. They purify the throat and the liver and increase efficiency. Fever and toxins caused by accumulation of *āma* are effectively purged. They purify breast milk and pacify *Pitta* and *Kapha doṣa*. This taste's essence is light, dry, cool, smooth and is excellent in promoting intelligence.

***Tikta Rasa* (Bitter Taste)**
Increases - *Vāta*
Decreases - *Pitta* and *Kapha*

Excessive intake of bitter substances causes reduction in the tissues, plasma, blood, fat, bone marrow and sperm count. It leads to roughening of the walls of the *srotas*, dryness in the mouth, reduction in strength, feebleness, fatigue, dizziness, syncope and *Vātaja* ailments such as nerve palsies, headache, prickling pain and so on. It can increase many *Vāta* problems.

- **Substances with a bitter taste:** Pointed gourd, bitter gourd, sandalwood, vetiver, chiretta, margosa, sesban (*jayantī*), fragrant swamp mallow (*sugandhabālā*), colocynth (*indrāyaṇa*), tinospora (*guḍūcī*), sweet-flag (*vacā*), khorsan thorn (*dhamāsā*), *mahā pañcamūla* (five grass roots, an *Āyurvedic* medicine), yellow berried night shade (*kaṇṭakārī*), Indian night shade (*baṟī kaṭerī*) and aconitum (*ativiṣā*).
- **Exceptions:** Tinospora (*guḍūcī*) and pointed gourd though bitter are not harmful.

(vi) *Kaṣāya rasa* (Astringent taste)

Astringent is the taste that puckers the mouth, leads to numbness of the tongue and constriction in the throat and the *srota*. It reduces *Pitta* and *Kapha doṣas*, controls blood pressure and intrinsic hemorrhage (bleeding), helps in healing wounds, aids healing of injured bones, and dries *medā dhātu,* liquid *dhātus*, urine and other fluids. It also binds loose feces during dysentery and dissolves fat. Intake of astringent foods causes constipation and firmness in the body. They make the skin excessively tender or soft, causes pressure on wounds, boils and increases inflammation of diseased parts.They absorb the fluids present in the body. Astringent foods are dry, cool and heavy.

***Kaṣāya Rasa* (Astringent Taste)**
Increases - *Vāta*
Decreases - *Pitta* and *Kapha*

Excessive intake of astringent foods leads to dryness in the mouth, chest pain which may relate to the heart, flatulence, difficulty in speaking, blockage and shrinkage in the *srota*, darkening of complexion, reduced virility, excessive thirst, weakness, fatigue, firmness and downward movement of *Vāta* (*adhovāyu*), obstruction in the smooth elimination of urine, feces, other waste products and sperm. Being heavy in property, their digestion takes a longer time. Since the astringent tastes aggravate *Vāta*, their excessive intake in some cases may lead to an attack of palsy, strokes (paralysis), stiffness and convulsions.

- **Astringent Substances:** Myrobalan *(harar̲a)*, belleric myrobalan (*baher̲ā*), lebbeck (*śirīṣa*), white cinchona (*kadamba*), Indian fig (*gūlara*), catechu, honey, raw sugar, lotus, lotus stem, and all other substances belonging to the lotus family. Pearls, coral (*pravāla*), collyrium and red ochre (*gerū*) are also astringent substances.
- **Exceptions:** Even though myrobalan (*harar̲a*) is astringent, it is neither cool nor a binding agent and thus does not prevent fecal elimination like other astringent substances.

Qualities of all food substances depend on their *rasa* (taste). In medicinal preparations *vīrya* (potency) is more important, but it is also determined on the basis of *rasa* (taste). For example, medicines with sweet taste essence are cold (*śīta vīrya*) and sour or bitter medicines are hot in potency (*uṣṇa vīrya*).

2. *Guṇa*: Attributes

All substances have some attributes that cause various effects in the body. *Āyurveda* texts describe these attributes in different substances. There are 20 such prime attributes in 10 opposing pairs. These pairs become the cause of mutual conflict, because each of them has one opposing property. They are as follows[(5), (6)]:

1(a). ***Guru* (heavy)**: Increases *Kapha*, decreases *Vāta* and *Pitta*. Increases heaviness, stoutening and restorative, creates dullness and lethargy. For example, black gram, muscle (*mūsalī*), etc.

1(b). ***Laghu* (light)**: Increases *Vāta*, *Pitta* and *agni,* decreases *Kapha*. Helps in digestion, increases lightness in the body, creates freshness and alertness. For example, green gram, *lājā* (Parched rice flakes), etc.

5. *Gurumandahimasnigdhaślakṣṇasāndramṛdusthirāḥ.*
Guṇāḥ sasūkṣmaviśadā viṁśatiḥ saviparyayāḥ. (*A.Hr̥.sū.* 1:18)
6. ....*kriyate yena yā kriyā.* (*Ca.sū.* 26:65)

2(a). ***Manda* (dull or slow)**: Increases *Kapha*, decreases *Vāta* and *Pitta*. Creates sluggishness, slow action, relaxation and dullness. For example, pumpkin, etc.

2(b). ***Tīkṣṇa* (sharp or pungent)**: Increases *Vāta* and *Pitta*, decreases *Kapha*. They have an immediate effect on the body. Promotes sharpness and quick understanding. For example, marking nut *(bhilāvā)*, red chilly, etc.

3(a). ***Snigdha* (oily or greasy)**: Increases *Pitta* and *Kapha*, decreases *Vāta* and *agni*. Creates smoothness, moisture, lubrication and vigor, and promotes compassion and love. Its main action is oleation. For example, almond, sesame, etc.

3(b). ***Rūkṣa* (dry)**: Increases *Vāta* and *agni*, decreases *Pitta* and *Kapha*. Increases dryness and absorption; results in constipation and nervousness. For example, barley, guggula, etc.

4(a). ***Śīta* (cold)**: Increases *Vāta* and *Kapha*, decreases *Pitta*. Acts as a styptic, creates coolness, numbness, unconsciousness, fear and insensitivity. For example, sandal, couch grass, etc.

4(b). ***Uṣṇa* (hot)**: Increases *Pitta* and *agni*, decreases *Vāta* and *Kapha*. It acts as a sudative, promotes heat, digestion, cleansing, expansion, inflammation, anger and hatred. For example, white leadwort *(citraka)*, asafoetida, etc.

5(a). ***Ślakṣṇa* (smooth)**: Increases *Pitta* and *Kapha*, decreases *Vāta* and *agni*. It acts as a vulnerary, increases smoothness, love and care, and decreases roughness. For example, milk, etc.

5(b). ***Khara* or *khuradarā* (rough)**: Increases *Vāta* and *agni*, decreases *Pitta* and *Kapha*. It acts as a cautery, causes cracking of skin and bones, and creates carelessness and rigidity. For example, barley, gram, etc.

6(a). ***Sāndra* or *ṭhosa* (solid or dense)**: Increases *Kapha*, decreases *Vāta, Pitta* and *agni*. It nourishes, promotes solidity, density and strength. For example, butter, yogurt, etc.

6(b). ***Drava* (liquid)**: Increases *Pitta* and *Kapha*, decreases *Vāta* and *agni*. Promotes salivation, compassion and cohesiveness; dissolves and liquifies. For example, buttermilk, sugarcane juice, etc.

7(a). ***Mṛdu* or *komala* (soft)**: Increases *Pitta* and *Kapha*, decreases *Vāta* and *agni*. It causes loosening, creates softness, delicacy, relaxation, tenderness, love and care. For example, grapes, *ghee*, etc.

7(b). ***Kaṭhina* or *kaṭhora* (hard)**: Increases *Vāta* and *Kapha*, decreases *Pitta* and *agni*. Increases strength and rigidity; brings selfishness, callousness and insensitivity. For example, coral, pearl, etc.

8(a). ***Sūkṣma* (subtle or minute)**: Increases *Vāta, Pitta* and *agni*, decreases

Kapha. It quickly diffuses, pierces and penetrates subtle capillaries, increases emotions and feelings. For example, alcohol, poison, etc.

8(b). ***Sthūla* (bulky or gross)**: Increases *Kapha*, decreases *Vāta, Pitta* and *agni*. Causes obstruction and obesity, bring firmness. For example, semi-solid substances, *modaka* (sweet meat), etc.

9(a). ***Sthira* (stable or static)**: Increases *Kapha*, decreases *Vāta*, *Pitta* and *agni*. Promotes stability and faith; causes obstruction and constipation. For example, rejuvenating herbs.

9(b). ***Cala* or *sara* (tremulous or mobile)**: Increases *Vāta*, *Pitta* and *agni*, decreases *Kapha*. Promotes motion, shakiness and restlessness; reduces faith. For example, non-satiating substances.

10(a). ***Viśada* or *acipacipā* (non-mucilaginous or non-slimy or clear)**: Increases *Vāta, Pitta* and *agni*, decreases *Kapha*. It acts as a depurative or a purifier. Causes isolation and diversion. For example, margosa (*nīma*), alkali, etc.

10(b). ***Picchila* or *cipacipā* (mucilaginous or slimy or cloudy)**: Increases *Kapha,* decreases *Vāta, Pitta* and *agni*. Heals fractures and causes adhesion, vitality, unclearness and lack of perception. It is heavy to digest. For example, glue cherry (*lisoṟā*), resins of plants, etc.

These attributes in substances are not merely physical but medicinal. They are determined by the effect of different substances on the body. Just because a substance feels heavy does not mean that it necessarily has heavy attributes. Heaviness and lightness depend on the time taken to digest it, easily digested is light and that which takes time to digest is heavy. Similarly, mustard seeds which appear cold are actually hot, because they increase the temperature of the blood.

These attributes reflect the proportion of the five elements that substances contain. For example, if earth is the dominant element, it is heavy; if space dominates, it is light. As stated earlier, taste alone cannot determine the attribute of a substance. Attributes can be judged on the basis of both taste and effects of a substance on the body constitution.

3. *Vīrya*: Potency

All medicines have a combination of many attributes, out of which one or two dominate and are the most powerful and active, and thus are chiefly capable of curing ailments. These attributes determine the potency of a medicine. *Vīrya* (potency) is more powerful than *rasa* (taste), thus medicines are divided into two types based on their potency, cold and hot. This is popularly known as the hot or cold quality of a substance. Hot or cold medicines are prescribed according to the patient's body constitution. It is the potency that cures ailments and improves health. The physical, elemental and curative chemical composition of the medicine changes during digestion and metabolism. This brings about a reaction on the *doṣas* and the *dhātus*. As a result of these reactions sweet, pungent and astringent substances produce a cold effect, thus known as '*śīta vīrya,*' while sour, salty and bitter substances produce a hot effect, thus known as '*uṣṇa vīrya.*'

- **Effects on the body**

Śīta vīrya (cold potency) substances are anabolic (they create potential energy), cool in action, causing cheerfulness, exhilarating the mind and increasing moisture in the body. They increase sleep and urine, make the feces smooth and easy to eliminate and decrease appetite. These substances increases *dhātu* formation (especially *śukra dhātu*) and imparts life strength, sturdiness and steadiness, hence they act as a tonic. They cleanse the blood, calm *Pitta* and vitiate *Vāta* and *Kapha*.

Uṣṇa vīrya (hot potency) substances are catabolic (they create kinetic energy) and increase heat in the body. They increase the digestive power, sweat, thirst, exhaustion, fatigue and emaciation (feebleness). They produce giddiness and inflammation; promote dilation of blood vessels, relaxation of muscles, hard and difficult fecal elimination, decreased urine and sleep. They calm *Vāta* and *Kapha* and aggravate *Pitta*.

Some experts consider six other properties in addition to these two while deciding the attributes of any medicine. They are:1. *Snigdha* (oily or smooth), 2. *Rūkṣa* (dry), 3. *Guru* (heavy), 4. *Laghu* (light), 5. *Manda* (dull or slow), and 6. *Tīkṣaṇa* (sharp or pungent). It can be said that there are eight potencies including hot and cold, but the two main acceptable ones are the hot and the cold potencies.

When these two potencies are not expressed and are weak, they are referred to as merely an attribute (*guṇa)* and not a potency (*vīrya*). On this basis, there are some medicines which do not have potency. While food materials have prominant tastes, medicines are more potent.

4. *Vipāka*: Post-Digestive Effect

The taste essence produced after the digestion of a substance with the help of *jaṭharāgni* (digestive fire) is called *vipāka*[7]. The taste developed during the last stages of digestion of a substance is '*vipāka.*' During digestion, a substance interacts with several digestive juices that influence its properties and bring about several changes. During this process food

7. *Jāṭhareṇāgninā yogādyadudeti rasāntaram.*
Rasānāṁ pariṇāmānte sa vipāka iti smṛtaḥ. (A.Hr.sū.9:20)
Rasānāṁ pariṇāmānte jaraṇaniṣṭhākāle,
yadrasāntaraṁ rasaviśeṣaḥ udeti utpadyate sa vipākaḥ. (A.Hr.sū.9:20 Du.)

passes through three phases. In the first phase, its taste essence is sweet, in the second it is sour and in the third it becomes pungent. In the last phase of digestion the nutritive and the residual (waste) parts of a substance are separated. After the separation of undigested food, the digested portion of a substance remains only in the form of *rasa* (taste essence). It is a new form of *rasa* (taste), different from the original taste and is called the '*vipāka*' (post-digestive effect).

- **Types of *vipāka***

On the basis of *rasa* (taste essence), there are three kinds of *vipāka* (post-digestive effect), sweet, sour and pungent. Sweet and salty substances generally have a sweet *vipāka*, sour substances have a sour *vipāka*, and pungent, bitter and astringent substances have pungent *vipāka*[8]. Some exceptions are seen to the above stated types, for example:

Substances (*Dravya*)	**Taste (*Rasa*)**	**Post-Digestive Effect (*Vipāka*)**
Oil	sweet	pungent
A type of salt *(sauvarcala)*	salty	pungent
Indian gooseberry (*ām̐valā*)	sour	sweet
Dry ginger *(śuṇṭhī),* long pepper (*pippalī*)	pungent	sweet
Myrobalan *(harar̠a)*	astringent	sweet
Pointed gourd *(paṭola)*	bitter	sweet

- **Specific action of *vipāka***: The action of *vipāka* depends on the taste.

  Madhura vipāka (sweet): It is heavy in attribute, promotes smooth discharge of urine and feces and induces secretion of *Kapha* and semen.

  Amla vipāka (sour): It is light in its attributes, promotes excretory functions, destroys semen (*śukra*) and increases *Pitta*.

  Kaṭu vipāka (pungent): It causes constipation, destroys semen (*śukra*) and increases *Vāta*.

8. *Kaṭutiktakaṣāyāṇāṁ vipākaḥ prāyaśaḥ kaṭuḥ.*
Amlo, mlaṁ pacyate svādurmadhuraṁ lavaṇastathā. (*Ca.sū.* 26/58)

5. *Prabhāva*: Specific Action

Medicines usually act according to their *rasa* (taste), *vīrya* (potency) and *vipāka* (post-digestive effect), but there are many notable exceptions. Some substances have specific effect on the body which can aggravate or pacify the ailment. The property that determines this effect is called *'prabhāva'* (specific action)[9]. In other words, the different and unique effects produced by two substances on the body even those having the same *rasa, vīrya* and *vipāka* is termed as its *'prabhāva.'* Therefore, despite having similar *rasa, vīrya* and *vipāka*, one medicine might cure a particular ailment while another might aggravate it. For example, both purging cotton (*dantī*) or croton oil seed (*jamālagoṭā*) and white leadwort *(citraka)* have pungent *rasa* and *vipāka* and are *uṣṇa vīrya* (hot in potency), yet purging cotton and croton oil seed are strong purgatives, while leadwort is not. Both liquorice root (*muleṭhī*) and grapes (*drākṣā*) have the same *rasa,vīrya* and *vipāka* yet liquorice root is emetic (promotes vomiting) while grapes do not. Similarly, clarified butter (*ghee*) and milk also have the same properties but *ghee* is digestion promoting, not milk.

There are also some medicines that need not be ingested, merely tying or wearing them cures ailments such as fever, insomnia and so on. For example, tying the root of ash-colored fleabane (*sahadevī*) on the head cures fever. The trend of wearing charms, gems and precious stones, also relieve the disorder due to the *prabhāva* in them.

Substances are divided into three categories based on their *prabhāva*:

1. ***Śamana dravya* (Pacifying substances):** those that calm the *doṣas*.
2. ***Kopana dravya* (Provoking substances):** those that vitiate the *doṣas* and corrupt the *dhātus*.
3. ***Svāsthyahitakārī dravya* (Nourishing substances):** those that provide nourishment, promote well-being and sustain health.

Therefore, to understand the nature of a substance and its physiological effects on the body, one must be able to understand its *rasa* (taste), *virya* (potency), *vipāka* (post-digestive effect) and *prabhāva* (specific action) because these substances act accordingly on the body. The strongest trait among these dominates and weakens others. Hence, *vipāka* is stronger than *rasa* because it overshadows it, but *vīrya* is more powerful than both *rasa* and *vipāka* because it negates both of them. Thus, sequentially in a substance, *rasa* is the weakest and *prabhāva* the strongest. In order of power they can be arranged as ***rasa < vipāka < vīrya < prabhāva***.

9. *Rasavīryavipākānāṁ sāmānyaṁ yatra lakṣyate.*
Viśeṣaḥ karmaṇāṁ caiva prabhāvastasya sa smṛtaḥ. (*Ca.sū.* 26/67)
Rasādisāmye yat karma viśiṣṭaṁ tat prabhāvajam.
Dantī rasādyaistulyā, pi citrakasya virecanī. (*A.Hṛ.sū.* 9/26)

6. Types of Substances According to their Actions

Guided by their *rasa*, *vipāka*, *vīrya* and *prabhāva*, substances affect the body in various ways, which is known as '*karma*' (action). These actions or effects are of various types. On the basis of the effects, substances can be classified as:

SUBSTANCES	**ACTIONS**
Vamana (Emetic substances)	Induce vomiting and help to eliminate *Kapha* and *Pitta* through the mouth, e.g., vomiting nut (*madana phal*).
Virecana (Purgative substances)	Increases excretion of feces, eliminates both *pakva* (digested) and *apakva* (undigested) excreta through the downward tract (the anus), e.g., Indian jalap (*trivṛt*), Indian gooseberry (*āmalakī*), myrobalan (*harara̱*).
Saṅgrāhī (Absorbant/ Bowel binding substances)	Absorbs excess liquid from the intestines and binds and controls feces or causes constipation, e.g., cumin seeds.
Bṛṁhaṇa (Restorative substances)	Provides nourishment, e.g., new gum guggula.
Lekhana (Scarifying substances)	Helps to reduce obesity, dries up and eliminates unwanted *dhātus* and *malas,* e.g., old gum guggula.
Pācana (Digestive substances)	Digests undigested food, helps in metabolic transformation of *āma* (without stimulating the digestive fire), e.g., cobras saffron (*nāgakesara*).
Śamana (Palliative substances)	Pacifies aggravated *doṣas.* They mitigate the *doṣas* but do not expel them, e.g., tinospora (*guḍūcī*).
Anulomana (Carminative substances)	Promotes downward movement of *Vāta,* e.g., myrobalan (*harara̱*).
Sraṁsana (Bulk laxative)	Helps to eliminate hard excreta by dissolving the solid state, and hence relieves constipation, e.g., Indian laburnum (*amalatāsa*).

Bhedana (Emmolient laxative)	Helps eliminate both hard (solid) and loose (liquid) feces from the anal passage, e.g., gentian (*kuṭakī*).
Chedana (Expulsive substances)	Eliminates hard and tough accumulated *doṣas* and *malas,* toxins from the channels, e.g., alkali, black pepper, black bitumen (*śilājīta*).
Grāhī (Anti-diarrheal or Solidifying substances)	Strengthens appetite and digestion, binds the fecal matter and relieves diarrhea, e.g., dry ginger.
Stambhana (Styptic substances)	Stops bleeding, oozing and discharges; bein astringent they prevent the expulsion and flow of fluids (blood, *pus*) and *malas* and cause constipation, easily digestible, e.g., chenopodium (*vatsaka*).
Rasāyana (Rejuvenating substances)	Alliviates old-age ailments, increases life-span, e.g., Indian gooseberry (*ām̐valā*), gum guggula.
Vājīkara (Aphrodisiac substances)	Increases sexual desire and pleasure, e.g., milk, black gram, asparagus (*śatāvarī*), box myrtle (*tālamakhānā*).
Śukrala (Spermatic substances)	Increases the quantity of semen, e.g., wintercherry (*aśvagandhā*), muscle (*mūsalī*), sugar, asparagus (*śatāvarī*).
Sūkṣma (Minute substances)	Those that can enter the body through the pores, minute channels and thin capillaries, e.g., rock salt, honey.
Vyavāyī (Quickly Absorbed substances)	Those that diffuses throughout the body before being digested, e.g., opium (*afima*).
Vikāśī (Slackening substances)	Causes laxity in the limbs and loosens the ligaments present in the joints, e.g., betel nut.
Pramāthī (Expelling substances)	Eliminate accumulated *doṣas* from the *srota* (body channels) due to their potency (*vīrya*), e.g., black pepper.
Abhiṣyandī (Obstructing substances)	Blocks the *srotas* and causes heaviness in the body due to their gravity and oiliness, e.g., yogurt.

7. Food-Lifestyle, Important Diseases and their Best Remedies

Food plays a major role in both fitness or health and disease. Along with food, our behavioral conduct or lifestyle also affects the body differently. Keeping the focus on both these aspects of diet and lifestyle, *Āyurvedic* experts have prescribed and prohibited specific types of diets, medicines and conduct in special situations. *Āyurveda* texts prescribe some of the best remedies for specific diseases along with their particular herbal medications. Among them, the best ones are as follows:

- Milk is best to promote energy and strengthen the body. A glass of warm milk with dry ginger taken at bedtime nourishes the body and calms the mind.
- Clarified butter (*ghee*) is best to pacify *Vāta* and *Pitta doṣa*.
- A teaspoon of *ghee* with cooked rice promotes digestion.
- Milk and *ghee* are the best rejuvenators.
- Salt is best to provide taste to food.
- Based on need, addition of sour substances enhances the taste of food.
- Honey is best to pacify *Kapha* and *Pitta doṣa*.
- Regular intake of buttermilk is best for the treatment of sprue, edema, hemorrhoids and diseases which occur due to inappropriate use of oleation therapy. Buttermilk in different forms is best for dysentery and chronic sprue.
- Buttermilk with a pinch of ginger and cumin powder promotes digestion.
- Sesame oil is best to pacify *Vāta* and *Kapha*. Regular gargling with sesame oil is best to create an interest in food and also to strengthen the teeth.
- *Aṣṭavarga* group of herbs are best among vitality-promoting and life-enhancing rejuvenators.
- Fasting or lightning therapy is best among all treatment procedures.
- Lac is the best medicine for healing the fractured bones.
- Distilled cow's urine is best for obesity, constipation, cholesterol, dermatological diseases and cancer.
- External application of sandalwood paste is best to alleviate body odor and burning sensation.
- Coconut oil processed with wasp hive is best for baldness.
- Sugar cane and its juice are best to increase urination.

- Germinated barley is best to increase the fecal volume and promote defecation.
- Ginger is the best digestive that alleviates indigestion. One teaspoon of grated fresh ginger with a pinch of salt is a good appetizer.
- Garlic is the best herb for the treatment of the nervous system.
- Turmeric is best to reduce cysts.
- Cumin seeds and asparagus are best for increasing milk in lactating mothers.
- Roasted and flattened parched rice flakes (*lāvā* or *khīla*) are best for the treatment of emesis (vomiting).
- Pomegranate is best for dysentery, colitis, chronic cough and cardiac diseases.
- Juice of ginger and white onion mixed with margosa ash, 1 part each with 3 parts of honey is best for eye problems.
- Bottle gourd juice is best for cholesterol, cardiac diseases and obesity.
- Cucumber, bitter gourd and tomato juice is best in diabetes.
- Wheat grass, aloevera, *guḍūcī*, holy basil and margosa leaves juice is best in cancer treatment.
- Juice of *guḍūcī* (*Tinospora*), wheat grass, aloe vera and papaya is useful in dengue and deficiency of platelets.
- *Guḍūcī* is the best rejuvenator and herb to alleviate fever, gout and *Kapha* disorders.
- Liquorice root (*Mulethī*) is best for good vision, hair and voice, to enhance complexion and the healing of wounds.
- Juice of Indian rosewood (*Śīśama*) leaves is best to stop bleeding.
- Indian gooseberry (*Āṁvalā*) is the best rejuvenating herb, taken in any form.
- Indian gooseberry and turmeric are best for diabetes, prameha and tough to cure urinary diseases.
- Asafoetida (*Hīṅga*) is best for the downward movement of *Vāta* in the abdomen, good for digestion, and alleviates *Vāta* and *Kapha doṣa*.
- Myrobalan (*Harara*) is best for treating *Vāta* and *Kapha* disorders, chronic abdominal disorders and constipation.
- Long pepper (*Pippalī*) is best for hepato-splenic disorders.
- Use of root of long pepper is best to enhance digestive power, for the carmination of *Vāta* and to alleviate constipation.
- False pepper (*Viḍaṅga*) is the best herb to alleviate worm infestation

(including bacterial, viral and intestinal worms) and diseases associated with it.

- Bengal quince (*Bel*) is considered as the best binding agent or anti-diarrheal. It improves digestive power, pacifies *Vāta* and *Kapha* and is very effective in chronic abdominal disorders.
- Indian laburnum (*Amalatāsa*) is best used as a mild laxative.
- Telicherry bark (*Kuṭaja*) is the best medicine for diarrhea and dysentry.
- Indian *jalap* (*Trivṛt*) and gentian (*Kuṭakī*) are best to facilitate purgation.
- Latex of Indian spurge tree (*Snuhī*) is best used as a drastic purgative.
- Garcinia (*Amlavetasa*) is a best herb for purgation, to enhance digestive power, carmination of *Vāta* and to pacify *Kapha* disorder.
- Water hyssop (*Brahmī*) is the best herb to enhance memory power and intellect.
- Prickly chaff flower (*Apāmārga*) is a best drug used in errhine therapy, to treat head ailments.
- Medicines prepared from the catechu tree (*Khadira*) are best for treating dermatitis and leprosy.
- External and internal application of Indian fleabane (*Rāsnā*) is a best remedy for *Vāta* and diseases associated with its vitiation.
- Medicine prepared from castor root (*Eraṇḍa*) is best for alleviation of vitiated *Vāta doṣa.*
- To enhance the digestive power, for carmination of *Vāta*, for the treatment of hemorrhoids (bleeding piles) and shooting pain, medicine prepared from the root of white leadwort (*Citraka*) is the best.
- Fragrant swamp mallow (*Udīcya*) is the best refrigerant herb, brings coolness to the body.
- Aconite (*Atīsa*) is the best medicine for carmination of *Vāta* and also to alleviate *Tridoṣa*.
- Caltrope (*Gokharū*) is the best herb to treat dysuria and also to alleviate *Vāta doṣa*. Use of black bitumen (*śilājīta*) is also the best cure for urinary disorders.
- In all types of fever nutgrass (*Nāgaramothā*) and fine leaved fumitory (*Pittapāpaṟā*) are best.
- Gum guggula is the best medicine for obesity and diseases due to increased *Vāta*. It is also a very good healing medicine for wounds and ulcers.
- Marking nut (*Bhilāvā*) is the best medicine for treatment of hemorrhoids,

leprosy, painful skin diseases, tumors and cancer.

- Yellow-berried nightshade (*Kaṭerī*) is best for the treatment of bronchial asthma and bronchitis.
- Wintercherry (*Asvagandhā*) powder, velvet bean or cowhage (*Krauñca*) seed powder, asparagus (*Śatāvarī*) and muscle (*Mūsalī*) are the best aphrodisiacs.
- Juice of stone breaker (*Bhuī ām̐valā*), roots of hogweed (*Punarnavā*) and bark of Indian trumpet plant (*Śyonāka*) are best for hepatitis and liver cirrhosis.
- Hogweed (*Punarnavā*) is a drug of choice for edema.
- Hedge mustard (*Khūbakalā*), currants and figs are drugs of choice for typhoid.
- Horse gram (*Kulathī*) and Siberian tea (*Pattharacaṭā*) are best for calculi (gall stone).
- Elephant creeper (*Vidhārā*) is best for wound healing.
- Juice of marjoram (*Maruā*) or peach leaf juice is best for worm infestation.
- Lollipop plant (*Śivaliṅgī*) and *Putrajivaka* are drugs of choice for enhancing female fertility.

Lifestyle and routine for healthy and exhilarated life

Besides the above prescribed foods and medicines, if one focus on their daily habits and mental equilibrium, the following also result in promoting good health and longevity:

• Compatible and balanced diet	-	The key factor of good health
• Natural, easily available, simple,	-	Assure stability in life
		sāttvika food and balanced diet
• Diet as per digestive power	-	Further strengthen the digestion
• Overeating	-	Causes severe indigestion
• Eating on time	-	Maintains health
• Irregular eating	-	Results in abnormal digestion
• Fasting (once in a week)	-	Reduces toxins in the body
• Prolonged fasting	-	Unhealthy
• Intake of water	-	Best for maintaining equilibrium in the body
• Drinking water immediately before	-	Adversely affects digestion
		and after meals

- Excess of cold drinks - Weaken immunity and causes excess phlegm formation
- Water stored in a copper vessel - Good for liver and spleen
- *Prāṇa* or life-force - Most authentic, scientific, undisputable, effective and best health remedies
- *Prāṇāyāma* (regulated breathing) - Creates freshness in the mind and body
- Exercise - Best for energy and sturdiness in the body
- Fresh air environment - Best to refresh and remove fatigue
- Lying in *śavāsana* for 15 minutes - Calms the mind and relaxes the body
- Mental peace and happiness - Best to lead a disease-free life

Bad habits and their negative effects on the health

- A nap after lunch - Increases *Kapha* and body weight
- Reading in bed - Injures the eyesight
- Delayed urination and excretion - Extremely harmful
- Excessive talking - Dissipates energy and aggravates *Vāta*
- Working beyond capacity - Reduces life-span
- Celibacy - Increases longevity
- Promiscuity - Affects longevity
- Repeated masturbation and sex immediately after meals - Injurious to the body, causes *Vāta* derangement
- Oral and unnatural sex and homosexual activity - Unhygienic, injurious to the body, causes derangement of *Tridoṣa*
- Bad breath - Indicates constipation, indigestion and toxins in colon
- Bad odor - Indicates toxins in the system
- Unhappiness - Destroys vitality
- Depression and worry - Invites diseases and weakens the heart
- Fear and nervousness - Dissipates energy and aggravates *Vāta*
- Hate and anger - Creates toxins in the body and aggravates Pitta
- Possessiveness, greed and attachment - Enhances *Kapha*

8. Home Remedies from the Kitchen Pharmacy

Asafoetida

- When applied externally over the region around the navel, relieves spasm and flatulence.

Black pepper

- Chewing 1-2 black peppercorns relieves cough and also helps in sleep, especially if coughing.
- Intake of 4-5 pounded black peppercorns mixed with one teaspoon of warm *ghee* and sugar is beneficial in urticaria.
- Store the powder of 20 gm black pepper, 100 gm almond and 150 gm crystal sugar in a bottle. Use it regularly along with warm milk or water in cough and associated debility.
- For hiccoughs or headaches, inhale smoke of 3-4 burnt black peppercorns.

Cardamom

- Application of cardamom powder mixed with honey inside the oral cavity cures stomatitis (mouth ulcers).
- 2-3 gm cardamom powder mixed with crystal sugar provides immediate relief in burning micturition and oligouria (reduced urination).
- In continuous hiccoughs, boil 2 cardamoms and 3 cloves and sip it as a tea. If not relieved, one can take this drink 3-4 times a day. It freshens the breath and also relieves flatulence.

Cinnamon

- It promotes digestion and relieves cold, cough and congestion when used as a decotion along with cardamom, ginger and clove. It also relieves *Vāta* and *Kapha* disorders. It strengthens and energizes the tissues. It is an antiseptic and a good detoxifying herb.

Cloves

- Application of 4-5 gm clove powder mixed with water over the forehead or temples relieves headache including migraine.
- Chewing a slightly roasted clove gives relief from cough.
- Application of 5-7 pounded cloves and turmeric over the sinus or furuncles on any part of the body is useful.
- Application of powdered clove or clove oil relieves toothache.

Coriander

- Store dry coriander powder mixed with 4 parts of crystal sugar in a bottle. Take one teaspoon twice daily along with water in acidity. It also acts as a diuretic.
- In metrorrhagia and excessive heat in the body, boil 3-4 gm coriander seeds in 400 ml of water until it is reduced to 100 ml. Strain it, mix with honey and drink.
- Soak 2-3 gm of crushed coriander in 400 ml of water. Strain it and mix with a small quantity of honey. Taken frequently at certain intervals, this is useful for hyper-emesis during pregnancy and also in emesis in children. It also reduces restlessness and stops vomiting.
- Above remedy is also useful for diarrhea and blood dysentery.
- External application of 4-5 gm fine powder of dry coriander and some coriander leaves is useful for clearing up acne and blemishes. It also increases facial glow and complexion.
- Regular intake of 2-3 gm of coriander powder along with cold water is useful for reducing excessive libido.

Cumin seeds

- Intake of 4-6 gm powdered roasted cumin seeds along with yogurt or diluted yogurt (*lassī*) gives immediate relief in diarrhea.
- An equal quantity of roasted cumin and fennel seed powder (in a dose of one teaspoon, 3-4 times a day) is useful in diarrhea which is followed by colic pain.
- Boil 5-7 gm of cumin seeds in 400 ml of water until it is reduced to one-fourth the volume. It is useful in intestinal worm infestation when taken twice daily.
- In urinary diseases and leucorrhea, boil 3-4 gm of cumin seeds in water, strain the solution and take it with crystal sugar.

Fenugreek seeds

- Soak one teaspoon of fenugreek seeds in a cup of water overnight, next morning drink the water and chew the seeds. This is useful in diabetes and debility due to diabetes, *Vāta* diseases and cardiac diseases.
- Store the powder prepared from an equal quantity of fenugreek, turmeric and dry ginger in a bottle. Use one teaspoon of this powder along with warm water or milk in arthritis, inflammation and *Vāta* disorders. This preparation is very useful for chronic arthritis, if taken regularly for a long time.

- Regular intake of sprouted fenugreek seeds is also benefical in arthritis and diabetes.
- Decoction prepared from roasted and ground fenugreek mixed with small quantity of ginger during autumn is useful in common cold and cough.

Mustard

- Application of finely ground mustard paste over any inflammation, reduces the inflammation.
- In headache apply ground mustard over the forehead.
- Application of ground mustard mixed with vinegar is useful in many dermatological diseases such as ringworm, pruritus, itching and so on.

Thymol or carom seeds (*Ajawāyana*)

- In addiction to alcohol, boil 1/2 kg of thymol seeds in 4 liters of water until reduced to 2 liters. Strain it and store. Use one cup of this drink before meals regularly. It also protects the liver and reduces the desire for alcohol.
- For common cold and other stomach diseases, take 2-3 gm of lightly roasted *ajavāyana* twice daily along with hot water or milk.
- To prevent post partum (after delivery) diseases, boil 10 gm of *ajavāyana* in 1 liter of water until reduced to one-fourth. Strain and drink it twice daily.
- Application of 10 gm of fine *ajavāyana* powder mixed with half lemon juice, 5 gm of alum powder and buttermilk over the scalp helps to get rid of lice.

Turmeric

- In pyorrhea, halitosis (foul breath) and tooth diseases, massage the gums regularly with a mixture of turmeric, salt and a small quantity of mustard oil.
- Intake of one teaspoon of turmeric powder with a glass of milk enhances immunity, helps in the prevention of common cold and cough. It also relieves body ache and pain due to injuries.
- Half a teaspoon of parched turmeric powder along with honey is useful in hoarseness of the voice and cough.
- Sprinkling of turmeric powder over cuts or burns checks bleeding and also prevents blister formation.
- Wrap hot thick wheat flour bread (*capātī*) smeared with mustard oil and turmeric powder in cases of sprain. It relieves swelling and pain.
- In blemishes and boils, apply face pack made of turmeric powder, sandalwood powder and margosa leaves. This also enhances the healthy glow of the skin.

Garlic

- Soak overnight 1 bud of chopped garlic in water. Take it on an empty stomach in the morning to reduce cholesterol, for cardiac diseases and for osteoarthritis.
- Cook 50 gm of crushed garlic with mustard oil, sesame oil or olive oil and strain the oil. Its external application is good in reducing inflammation and pain. It is a very good remedy.
- External application of garlic oil (3 drops) is also very useful in earache.
- In an oxygen deficient environment, wear a piece of garlic around the neck as a charm. It provides relief.

Ginger

- Take a small quantity of ginger alongwith 3-4 morsels of food to enhance appetite. Ginger taken just after meals helps in easy digestion of food.
- Two teaspoons of ginger juice mixed with a small quantity of honey is useful in common cold and cough.
- Keeping a piece of ginger between the teeth is useful in toothache caused due to cold or sinusitis.
- Chewing a piece of roasted ginger is useful for suppressing cough.
- Dry ginger powder (2-3 gm) mixed with 1/2 or 1 gm of cinnamon powder taken along with milk or water helps to reduce pain due to angina. It also strengthens the heart and balances the digestive system.
- Drinking ginger juice mixed with lemon juice cures indigestion, as well as increases the appetite.
- Boil 5 gm of crushed ginger in two glasses of water and add lemon and honey to it. Taking it on an empty stomach in the morning reduces obesity.

Lemon

- For pimples apply lemon juice mixed with honey on the face.
- In metrorrhagia (excessive bleeding) and hemorrhoids (piles), take one cup of luke warm milk, add in it the juice of half lemon, drink it, before the milk curdles, early in the morning on an empty stomach. It acts as a haemostyptic and is a quick remedy. Continue its use for 3-4 days, but if the patient does not get relief, consult a physician.
- 10 ml lemon juice mixed with 20 ml onion juice and a small quantity of honey is useful in liver diseases, dyspepsia and indigestion.
- Lemon juice mixed with a small quantity of ginger and salt acts as an appetizer. It improves the digestion.

- Those having a tendency to vomit and who feel nauseated while travelling are advised to lick or suck a lemon with salt sprinkled over it.

Onion

- External application of lukewarm onion juice as an ear and nasal drop (4 drops) quickly relieves earache and common cold, respectively.
- Keeping an onion in the pocket or wearing it around the neck prevents heat stroke.
- To prevent airborne bacterial and viral infections in children, tie 8-10 onions in a cloth bag and hang it outside the house.
- In chicken pox, one teaspoon of onion juice mixed with 2-3 pounded black peppercorns, taken 2-3 times a day for a few days is beneficial. This also wards off marks on the skin after the pox.
- Tying a cloth soaked in the warm juice of an unripe onion quickly relieves painful furuncles, enhances suppuration and easily expels pus.
- Drinking onion juice mixed with lemon juice and salt quickly relieves abdominal pain.

Aloe vera

- Eating a vegetable stew prepared from inner pulp of aloe vera plant alleviates arthritis, diseases caused due to vitiated *Vāta*, abdominal and hepatic diseases.
- Aloe vera gel or juice externally applied on cuts or burns prevents blister formation, stops bleeding and causes quick healing of ulcers and wounds.
- Daily intake of 4-6 teaspoons of aloe vera juice is useful for relief from all abdominal diseases and general weaknesses.
- External application of aloe vera gel enhances the facial glow. It is also useful in fading freckles and acne.
- External application of aloe vera gel is useful to alleviate dryness of hands and feet.

Honey

- Regular use of one-fourth teaspoon of cinnamon powder with 1 teaspoon of honey strengthens the immune system and relieves sinusitis and severe cold.
- Mix two teaspoons of honey with carrot juice and take it regularly. This improves eyesight.
- In cold, cough and congestion, mix two teaspoons of honey with an equal quantity of ginger juice and have it frequently.
- A mixture of black pepper powder, honey and ginger juice in equal quantities, when consumed thrice daily, helps to relieve the symptoms

of bronchial asthma.

- Regular use of one teaspoon of garlic juice with two teaspoons of honey helps to control blood pressure.
- One glass of warm water with two teaspoons of honey and one teaspoon of lemon juice taken early in the morning increases metabolism and 'burns fat' and also purifies the blood.
- Daily intake of one teaspoon of honey keeps a person healthy (except in case of diabetes).

Miscellaneous uses

- Intake of the brew prepared from 2-3 gm cinnamon and 2-3 gm cloves boiled in water is very useful for reducing angina pain and palpitations. It is also useful for viral infection.
- Powder prepared from cardamom, cinnamon and dry ginger taken with milk or water is useful to strengthen the heart. It also enhances immunity.
- Regular intake of one cup of fresh juice of bitter gourd, cucumber and tomato on an empty stomach is useful in treating diabetes. It is also good for digestion.
- Regular use of bottle gourd juice taken on an empty stomach is good for the heart and general health. It can also be taken in combination with apple juice. In case of common cold, use it after adding ginger juice or dry ginger. It also decreases cholesterol levels.
- In case of high body temperature, round slices of bottle gourd be placed on the soles of feet, provide relief and reduce fever. It should be followed along with the medicines that are needed.
- In cases of anemia, drink pomegranate juice mixed with apple and spinach juices.
- Eating papaya in large quantities relieves constipation and is good for liver.
- To boost memory and body strength, in the morning chew 5-7 almonds, 5-10 gm walnuts, 5-7 black peppercorns soaked overnight in water.
- In the morning take 10 gm raisins or currants, 4-5 figs and 8-10 almonds soaked overnight in water. This acts as a tonic and is also useful in abdominal disorders.
- Ingesting a mixture of raisins and figs cooked in milk improves digestion, enhances strength and wards off weakness.

Chapter 5

Health Horizons - An *Āyurvedic* Approach to a Healthy Life

The primary aim of *Āyurveda* is to promote health and prevent disease(1). Maintenance of health depends on the condition of *tridoṣa* in the body. It was stated earlier that the *doṣas* have a natural tendency to increase or decrease at different times of the day and in different seasons of the year. Therefore, to maintain the balance of *tridoṣa*, *Āyurveda* prescribes appropriate health and lifestyle rules known as '*svasthyavṛta*' (an approach to a healthy life), and the two categories of these rules are: *Dinacaryā* (behavioral patterns and food habits during the cycle of day and night) and *Ṛtucaryā* (behavioral patterns and food habits in different seasons of the year). A lifestyle modelled on these guidelines maintains health and protects against the disease.

1. *Dinacaryā*: Food Habits and Conduct during the Day Time

- **Early rising**

Āyurveda recommends that a healthy person wakes up about two hours before dawn. This ambrosial hour (*brahma muhūrta*)(2) is considered auspicious as there is peace, purity, freshness and happiness all around in the environment. One should first think of God and pray, chant a *mantra* or meditate. This brings mental peace and joy. At this hour (during the *Vāta* period), the body is free of fatigue, also one gets the advantage of *Vāta* qualities such as lightness, exhilaration and freshness. They get infused in the body, mind and brain and last throughout the day. Whatever is memorized is remembered and influences us the whole day. Rising early also gives adequate time for ablutions, *yoga*, exercise and other routine activities, which in turn ensures a disease-free and long life. Planning out the day's schedule before rising from the bed ensures that all work is completed successfully and timely.

1. *Iha khalvāyurvedaprayojanaṁvyādhyupasṛṣṭānāṁ vyādhiparimokṣaḥ, svasthasyasvāsthya rakṣaṇaṁ ca.* (*Su.sū.* 1/13)
2. *Brāhme muhūrte uttiṣṭhejjīrṇājīrṇa nirūpayan.* (*A.Saṅ.sū.*3.3)

- **Washing the face**

Washing the face in all seasons with fresh cool water immediately after leaving the bed cleanses the eyes, nose, mouth and face, also relieves early morning dullness and brings freshness. In winter lukewarm water can be used instead.

- **Water intake on an empty stomach**

At least one to four glasses of cool water should be taken after washing the face in the morning. Water should preferably have been stored in a copper container overnight. Obese people should drink warm water to 'speed up' the metabolism and in general it is also recommended during winter. Drinking cool water in the morning is beneficial and stimulates the digestive tract. It helps in smooth and regular elimination of feces in the morning, which is essential for the removal of body toxins and thus provides protection from ailments. This is known as '*uṣaḥpāna*.'

In the morning, water should be taken in a sitting position. Drinking water while standing may lead to knee and joint pain. It is best to drink water in an upright position, where the whole body weight is on the feet. Some people prefer drinking tea instead of fresh water for smooth bowel movement, but its action is very different from that of water. Tea, being a hot and stimulating liquid, mimics the effect of water. Tea pressurizes and stimulates the bowels, causing expulsion of wastes, but there is a subtle difference. The effect of tea on the bowels wanes after sometime and the person again suffers from constipation. Besides, the caffeine and tannin present in coffee and tea harms the stomach and intestines. Cold water, on the other hand, has no side-effects. Only people suffering from cold, cough and sore throat should take lukewarm water.

- **Relieving the Bowel**

Early morning, clearing of the bowels is essential after drinking water. Every person should make it a regular practice. Modern, busy and stressful living causes many people to suffer from lack of regular and proper bowel movements in the morning. The rush to reach the workplace on time also contributes to the problem. People do not give sufficient time to the activity and the bowels are not cleared properly. Besides, eating heavy and *Vāta* causing food (heavy pulses, fried foods) accumulates flatus and also obstructs the fecal movement in the intestine. As a consequence, only after a little elimination, one feels that the bowels have been cleared. Later, one needs to repeat the process. Some people need to clear the bowels three or four times every morning. Indigestion, lack of sleep, stress, anger, depression and imbalanced emotions can all lead to this problem.

Excessive intestinal gas formation causes pressure on the heart leading to an increased heart beat. Prolonged constipation and flatus leads to serious ailments like chronic cold, bronchial asthma, piles, joint pains and arthritis. It also leads to loss of appetite, flatus, indigestion, headache, depression, self-pity, discomfort, restlessness, fatigue, lethargy and insomnia. It is, hence, essential to properly clear the bowels every morning. Several precautions should be taken like avoiding or reducing a heavy diet and *Vāta*-causing foods (heavy pulses, kidney beans, Bengal gram, black gram and fried foods). Intake of green leafy vegetables (spinach, chenopodium and fenugreek leaves), bottle gourd, angled loofah and yams; fruits such as apples, guava, papaya, currants and figs; and other fiber-rich foods should be increased in the diet. If one needs to clear the bowels more than once, it should not be avoided. To alleviate constipation and other abdominal ailments permanently, perform *kapālabhāti prāṇāyāma* regularly in the morning on an empty stomach.

- **Cleaning of teeth**

After relieving, the next healthy habit includes the cleaning of teeth.

1. Teeth should be cleaned with twigs (*dātuna*) that have bitter, pungent or astringent qualities because they protect the mouth from oral diseases and related bacterial infections. Twigs with sweet, sour and saline tastes aggravate *Kapha* and should be avoided. The best teeth cleaners are margosa (*nīma*) and gum arabica (*babūla*) twigs. Other trees whose twigs can be used on the basis of taste essence and their action on oral hygiene are smooth-leaved ponga (*karañja*), peacock tail (*mālatī*), Indian kino tree (*asana*) and prickly chaff flower (*apāmārga*).
2. The twig (*dātuna*) should be carefully selected. It should be 6 inches long so that it can be held firmly and is easy to clean the tongue. It should be as thick as the little finger, erect or straight and fresh with the bark adhered to it. Very slender or very thick twigs are not feasible. A thicker twig will injure the gums. The front end of the twig should be soft (not dry and hard) so that it can easily be fashioned into a brush with a little chewing. It should be straight and not twisted.
3. The movement of the twig (*dātuna*) over each tooth should be from top to bottom and *vice-versa*. This cleans the teeth thoroughly and does not damage the gums. Tooth powder or pastes formulated from many *Āyurvedic* herbs can be used with the twig or separately. This morning activity cleanses the teeth, tongue and mouth. It keeps bad breath in check, makes the teeth clean and strong and also stimulates the taste buds(3).

3. *Nihanti gandhaṁ vairasyaṁ jihvādantāsyajaṁ malam. Niṣkṛsya rucimādhatte sadyo dantaviśodhanam. Tathāsyamalavairasyajihāgandhā,, syadantajāḥ.*(*Ca.sū.* 5/72)

Nowadays, various kinds of tooth brushes and toothpastes are available for sale and are used more than naturally available twigs. There are many good tooth powders for this purpose as well. One should not use the same brush for a long time and for protection from oral disease, brushes should be kept in hot water for some time so as to kill the bacteria.

A white coating on the tongue, if has appeared overnight should also be cleaned after the teeth. This is the residue of *āma*, either from last night's meal as food gets deposited on its surface or due to a deeper imbalance. If not cleaned regularly, there may be an unpleasant odor and the sense of taste is reduced. The twig used to brush teeth can also be used to clean the tongue from the back side. Tongue scrapers made of wood, gold, silver, brass, copper and steel can also be used. The scrapers should be soft, smooth, curved in the center and flexible. The edges should not be sharp or pointed as they might cause injury to the tongue[4].

It has been suggested that cleansing of teeth with a twig (*dātuna*) should be avoided if one is suffering from indigestion, nausea, bronchial asthma, fever, stroke or paralysis, excessive thirst, stomatitis (mouth ulcers) and ailments of the heart, eyes, head and ear, as there is a possibility of aggravation of disease if twigs are used under such conditions.

- **Gargling**

If for some reason such as travelling one is unable to clean the teeth in the morning, gargling with water will help. This also cleans the teeth and the tongue and refreshes the mouth to some extent. It removes unpleasant odor and stickiness in the mouth and any *Kapha* accumulated in the throat and mouth. Ideally, after brushing the teeth, the mouth should be rinsed with sesame or mustard oil. This process is called *kavalagraha*. It strengthens the teeth and gums, prevents toothache, reduces sensitivity to hot, cold and sour substances (that sometimes cause toothache), helps chew tough and hard substances easily, improves the quality of voice, and boosts taste perception and appetite. Regular rinsing of the mouth, gargling and *kavalagraha* prevents drying of the throat and chapping of the lips.

Substances with pungent essences boiled in water are excellent for gargling, after straining them and when lukewarm. They clean the mouth and reduce any unpleasant odor. Witholding of decoction in the mouth is referred to as '*gaṇḍūṣa.*' When the liquid in the mouth can be moved around,

4. *Jihvānirlekhanaṁ raupyaṁ sauvarṇaṁ vārkṣameva ca.*
Tanmalāpaharaṁ śastaṁ mṛduślakṣaṇaṁdaśāṅgulam. (*Su.ci.* 24/13)
Suvarṇarūpyatāmrāṇi trapurītimayāni ca. Jihvānirlekhanāni syuratīkṣṇānyanṛjūni ca.
Jihvāmūlagataṁ yacca malamucchavāsarodhi ca.
Daurgandhyaṁ bhajate tena tasmājjihvāṁ vinirlikhet. (*Ca.sū.*5/74-75)

the process is called '*gaṇḍūṣa.*' *Kavala* helps to treat ailments of head and ear, dullness, sleepiness, anorexia, spasmodic torticollis, sinusitis, chronic cold (rhinitis) and nausea.

- **Head care**

The head should be oiled daily with sesame, coconut, olive, almond or mustard oil. This prevents hair loss, graying, balding (alopecia, unless genetic), headache, drying of the scalp and other *Vāta* diseases. It strengthens the head, forehead, eyes, ears and other sensory organs. The quality of hair improves as the hair become stronger, smoother, longer and darker. Also, the glow of the face increases[5]. Application of sesame oil on the head brings good and sound sleep. Combing the hair after oiling cleanses and beautifies the hair[6].

- **Body massage: *Abhyaṅga* (oleation)**

Just as applying oil to pots, dry leather and axles of wheels lubricates and strengthens them, oiling the body makes it stronger and softens the skin. Oil protects the body against diseases caused by *Vāta*. Skin is an important organ where *Vāta* accumulates. The pores in the skin are filled with the heat of *Pitta* which absorb the oil applied and calms the *Vāta*. Applying oil also prevents premature aging, fatigue, wrinkles, roughness and dryness. It clears the vision, strengthens the body and smoothens the skin, making it soft and attractive. It also provides relief from body odor, dirt, itching, heaviness, dullness and fatigue.

Strokes during body massage should be in the direction of hair growth on the skin. Too much force should not be used while massaging. Soft, smooth strokes are adequate. Applying oil in the sunlight speeds absorption. Massage not only gives disease-free skin, but also strengthens the muscles. Massage or *abhyaṅga* (oleation) is extremely beneficial in neuro-muscular weakness, arthritis and muscular tension.

- ***Karṇapūraṇa*: Oil as an ear drop**

According to *Āyurveda*, apply oil in the ears daily. This prevents ailments like deafness, defective hearing, spasmodic torticollis, lockjaw (tetanus) and

5. *Nityaṁ snehārdraśirasaḥ śiraḥśūlaṁ na jāyate. Na khālityaṁ na pālityaṁ na keśāḥ prapatantica.*
Balaṁ śiraḥkapālānāṁ viśeṣeṇābhivardhate. Dṛḍhamūlāśca dīrghāśca kṛṣṇāḥ keśā bhavanti ca.
Indriyāṇi prasīdanti sutvagbhavati cānanam.
Nidrālābhaḥ sukhaṁ ca syānmūrdhni tailaniṣevaṇāt. (Ca.sū.5/81-83)
6. *Keśaprasādhinīeśyā rajojantumalāpahā.* (*Svasthavṛtta samuccaya*)
Śirogatāṁstathā rogāñchirobhyaṅgo, pakarṣati.
Keśānāṁ mārdavaṁ dairghyaṁ bahutvaṁ snigdhakṛṣṇatām.
Karoti śirasastṛptiṁ sutvakkamapi cānanam.
Santarpaṇaṁ cendriyāṇāṁ śirasaḥ pratipūraṇam. (Su.ci.24/25-26)
Rucivaisadyalaghutā na bhavanti bhavanti ca. (A.saṅ.sū. 3/18)

other *Vāta* related ear problems. In a healthy ear, oil should be retained for two minutes. When suffering from earache, oil should be retained in the ear till the pain is relieved. This can be done by rubbing the painful area and pressing at the base of the ear.

- **Feet massage**

Applying oil on the feet every day is also very beneficial. It reduces and prevents roughness, dryness, fatigue, numbness, laxity, 'cracked heels,' reduced blood flow, tense muscles, sciatica and other *Vāta* ailments. It also improves the eyesight. In ancient times, its beneficial effects led the experts to make it a religious ritual to be performed daily after morning relieve, every time after urination, before meals and before bathing. Besides oil, ice, bottle gourd, cucumber and other medicinal substances are used for foot massage to alleviate many kinds of diseases or deformities.

- ***Nasya kriyā*: Oil as a nasal drop**

The nose is considered a pathway to the sinuses. Hence, medicinal preparations poured into the nostrils can reach every part of the head. Normally, oil drops should be added to the nostrils during monsoon, winter and spring seasons when there is no cloud cover.

This should be done daily after clearing of the bowels, cleaning of teeth and oiling the hair. The head should hang backward on the back of a chair, and a few drops of warm oil (indirectly heated by steam or by keeping it in hot water) should be placed in each nostril using a dropper and then inhaled. Oil should be applied in the nostrils drop by drop, in one nostril and then the other. While putting drops into one nostril, the other nostril should be closed. Any nasal secretions during *nasya* should be discharged from the mouth.

> Lukewarm clarified butter made from cow's milk is best for nasya. It provides relief in common cold, headache and other cephalagic disorders. It also enhances memory power. Olive oil and Almond oil are also good for nasya.

After *nasya*, lie down on your back for a minute or so, but do not fall asleep. *Nasya* cures all ailments that are caused above the neck. It is effective in ailments like spasmodic torticollis, paralysis (strokes), headache, migraine, swelling in the nose, shivering of the head and lockjaw (tetanus). It also prevents early signs of aging on the head and other organs and reduces graying of the hair. If a healthy person, free of diseases takes in the oil or distilled cow's urine, when poured in the nose during *nasya*, it is best for good health. It should not be spat out.

According to *Āyurveda*, in a healthy state, the best time for *nasya* therapy is generally autumn and spring (when it is neither too hot, nor too cold). Different times suggested for *nasya* treatment according to *doṣas* and seasons is as follows:

- *Kapha* aggravation - in the morning
- *Pitta* aggravation - in the afternoon
- *Vāta* aggravation - in the evening
- During autumn and spring - in the morning
- During winter - in the afternoon
- During summer - in the morning and evening
- During monsoon - in the afternoon

In case of headache due to *Vāta* disorders, hiccoughs, hysteria, spasmodic torticollis and hoarseness of voice, *nasya* should be given twice a day (every morning and evening).

- **Exercise**

Exercise is a physical activity for the purpose of conditioning the body. Physical activity that causes exertion and fatigue is exercise(7). Exercise lends strength and stability to the body. It should be performed daily, in all seasons and according to one's capacity. During winter and spring, it should be performed upto fifty percent of the body strength or maximum capacity until light sweat appears on the forehead and underarms, and the person starts to mouth breathes. These are the natural signals of the right limit of exercise. Do not exert to the point where one sweats heavily and pants for breath. During summer, rain and autumn, the force applied should be further reduced because these are the seasons of *Vāta* aggravation and accumulation. To relieve tiredness, the body should be massaged lightly afterwards. Exercise is highly appreciated in *Āyurvedic* texts. According to *Caraka* "from physical exercise one gets lightness, capacity to work, firmness, tolerance to difficulties, elimination of impurities and stimulation of digestion". Scientifically, beneficial exercise should be performed to strengthen the musculature of the body. Except in certain conditions or diseases, if 30 minutes of rigorous physical exercise is carried out regularly, not only the lungs, heart and brain become healthy and energetic, but it is extremely beneficial in obesity, type 2 diabetes, hyper-cholesterol, bronchial asthma, bronchitis, allergies and other diseases too. It balances the whole system, mind and body, the three *doṣas*, seven *dhātus* and *agnī* to provide complete health.

If done properly and within appropriate limits, exercising is very beneficial. It is important to note that exercise gives more energy than it takes. It tones and strengthens every muscle, reduces fat accumulation and

7. *Śarīrāyāsajananaṁ karma vyāyāma ucyate.* (*A.saṅ.sū.* 3/62)
Śarīraceṣṭā yā ceṣṭā sthairyārthā balavardhanī.
Deha vyāyāmasaṅkhyātā mātrayā tāṁ samācaret. (*Ca.sū.* 7/31)

brings the body into shape. Exercise followed with oil massage aids in the absorption of oil. Exercise results in sweating, which brings lightness and provides energy to the body. The capacity to work and to bear pain increases, digestion is strengthened and the body becomes more stable. Aggravated and corrupt *doṣas*, especially *Kapha*, get pacified.

- **Avoid over-exertion while exercising**: Exercising more than the body's strength causes breathlessness, cough, fever, intrinsic hemorrhage (bleeding), debility of both sensory and sexual organs and their physiological activities, fatigue and vomiting(8). Excessive exercise harms the body. In contrast, lower limits are not detrimental to fitness. In fact, they make exercise more efficient as it does not give the body much repair work to do afterwards and the cardio-vascular system does not have to put extra-efforts to return back to normal after the workout.
- **Exception to exercise**: *Vāta-Pitta* patients, those who suffer from severe ailments, small children, aged persons, people suffering from indigestion and malnutrition should avoid strenuous exercise(9). It should also be avoided by people who have turned feeble and lost weight due to too much of walking, weight-lifting or excessive sexual activity.Also, people under the strain of anger, sorrow, fear and fatigue should be careful with physical exertion. This is because *Vāta* and *Pitta* increases during exercise and in the above-mentioned conditions,*Vāta* and *Pitta* are already aggravated. Therefore, such conditions are unsuitable for exercising. Children are naturally very energetic, they are active throughout the day, hence doing strenous exercise such as wrestling and other such activities are contra-indicated for them.

- ***Ubaṭana (udvartana)***

In *Āyurveda,* massaging tthe body with medicated powders and herbal pastes or lotions is called *ubaṭana*. It supports detoxification and smooths the skin. It is applied externally to the body and is also helpful if done before bathing. It reduces mental fatigue, enhances the activity of sensory organs, lends stability to organs, helps to open and clean body pores and softens the skin. *Ubaṭana* can be prepared with a mixture of mustard powder, gram flour, milk and sesame oil or yogurt cream with mustard oil.

- **Face packs**

Herbal face packs applied before bathing helps to prevent wrinkles, freckles, spots and blackheads. Face packs increases the softness, smoothness and glow of the skin, and also enhance the complexion. They also improve eyesight. Ideally, only a cold face pack should be used. Only during *Vāta*

8. *Śramaḥ klamaḥ kṣayastṛṣṇā raktapittaṁ pratāmakaḥ.*
Ativyāyāmataḥ kāsovaraśchardiśa jāyate. (*Ca.sū.* 7/33)
9. *Vātapittāmayī bālo vṛddho, jīrṇī ca taṁ tyajet.* (*A.saṅ. sū.* 3/63)

and *Kapha* aggravation a warm pack should be applied. The pack should be removed when still wet. If it dries, it should be moistened before removal. Removing a dry pack destroys the glow (luster). Avoid activities such as sleeping, talking, sitting in the sun or near the fire, anger and worry during face pack application because these lead to wrinkle formation. Also avoid applying a face pack during indigestion, sinusitis, anorexia, during *nasya* therapy and at night. Different types of face packs are recommended in *Āyurveda*, during the six different seasons, which are as follows:

Seasons	Face Packs
Early Winter	Indian jujuba seed, root of malabar nut and yellow mustard
Late Winter	Roots of yellow berried night shade, black sesame and Indian berberry with its peel
Spring	Roots of woolly grass, sandalwood, vetiver, lebbeck and fennel seeds
Summer	Waterlily, blue waterlily, rose flower, couch grass, sandalwood and liquorice root
Monsoon	Yellow sandalwood, sesame, vetiver and Indian spikenard
Autumn	Indian valerian, Himalayan silver fir, lotus, eagle wood and liquorice root

- **Bathing**

Bathing daily is essential for cleaning and refreshing the body. It rejuvenates the body. The nose, ears and feet should be specifically cleaned during bathing. While taking a fresh water bath, coolness of the water helps to absorb the heat of the body through the body pores, which then enters the abdomen, thus boosting the digestive power. Bathing thus, exhilarates the mind and helps prolong life. It makes the body and mind enthusiastic and increases strength. It relieves fatigue, itching, body odor, sweating, lethargy, burning, thirst and irritation.

Bathing should be avoided immediately after meals; when suffering from ailments of eyes, mouth and ears; and in diarrhea, flatulence, chronic cold and indigestion. Bathing aggravates these conditions(10).

- **Clothing**

Clean clothes must be worn after bathing. Good, clean and appropriate clothes not only adorn the body, but also bring joy, make one beautiful and attractive and enhance the personality. They also protect the body from the harshness of the season. Hence, it is wise to wear clothes according to the

10. *Pavitraṁ vṛṣyamāyuṣyaṁ śramasvedamalāpaham.*
Śarīrabalasandhānaṁ snānamojaskaraṁ param. (*Ca.sū.* 5/94)
Nidrā dāhaśramaharaṁ svedakaṇḍūtṛṣāpaham. Hṛdyaṁ malaharaṁ śreṣṭhaṁ sarvendriyavibodhanam.
Tandrāpāpmodaśamanaṁ tuṣṭidaṁ puṁstvavardhanam.
Raktaprasādanaṁ cāpi snānamagneśca dīpanam. (*Su.ci.*24/57-58)

season, such as white or light-colored, thin clothes in summer and dark, heavy and thick clothes (woollens) during winter.

- **Perfumes, aromas and natural scents**

The body should be adorned with seasonal flowers and perfumes. Apart from adding fragrance and attractiveness to the body, aromatic oils also raise the spirit and increase strength and the desire to work. They help in combating insomnia. All of this ultimately improves the quality of life, longevity and develops interest in the work.

In *Āyurveda* each *doṣa* can be balanced with aromas that are matched to it. The odors detected by the nose first dissolve in the moisture of the nasal tissue and are then passed on by specialized olfactory cells straight to the hypothalamus in the brain. Thus to smell anything is to send an immediate message to the brain and from it to the whole body. This way it regulates dozens of bodily functions including temperature, thirst, hunger, blood-sugar levels, growth, sleeping, waking, sexual arousal, memory and emotions such as anger and happiness. Hence, aromas are used to send specific signals that balance the three *doṣas*. In general:

Aromas that balance the dosas

Vata is balanced with a mixture of warm, sweet, sour aromas like basil, orange, rose, clove and other spices.

Pitta is balanced by a mixture of sweet, cool aromas like sandalwood, rose, mint, cinnamon and jaismine.

Kapha, similar to Vata is balanced by a mixture of warm aromas, but with spicier overtones like juniper, eucalyptus, camphor, clove and marjoram.

- **Adorning with ornaments and gemstones**

Wearing ornaments made of gold or silver not only adds to a person's beauty and attractiveness, but also enhances cheerfulness, the glow on the face, feel of success, auspiciousness and an increased life-span. It also increases the desire and strength for life[11]. Not only ornaments, but gems like diamonds, emeralds and hessonite (*gomeda*) are also excellent. Also wearing charms, medicinal herbs such as ash-colored fleabane (*sahadevī*) and others herbs is useful. They reduce fear and anxiety and counter the adverse effects of Stars and planetary positions. Pure metals emit an astral light that provides a powerful counteraction to the negative pull of the planets. Wearing different ornaments and gems is a part of touch healing (*sparśa cikitsā*). All metals contain tremendous healing energy. *Āyurveda* utilizes the healing properties of metals, gems and stones. Thus, metals, stones and gems are the outer

11. *Dhanyaṁ maṅgalyamāyuṣyaṁ śīmadvyasanasūdanam.*
Harṣaṇaṁ kāmyamojasyaṁ ratnābharaṇadhāraṇam. (*Ca.sū.* 5/97)

manifestations of certain forms of energy and these metals contain *prāṇika* energy reservoirs. Adverse influences upon the normal functions of the body, mind and consciousness may be counteracted through the use of gems and metals. When they are applied to the skin, they induce an electromagnetic influence which acts on the physical cells and deeper tissues.

- **Chewing fragrant substances**

To keep the mouth fresh and fragrant, and for good taste, spices like nutmeg, betel nut, cardamom, cloves, betel leaves and essence of camphor can be chewed. They increase taste and provide protection against diseases of the oral cavity and throat. But one should not use cancer causing narcotic substances, tobacco, *pāna masālas* and so on.

- **Footwear**[12]

Footwear protects the body against heat, cold, thorns, insects and germs and provides comfort to the feet. It also protects the skin and keeps it healthy. Footwear should always be comfortable and of an appropriate size. High heeled shoes are uncomfortable and they also cause postural problems. Footwear should be selected according to the season. Appropriate footwear provides strength to the feet and makes movement quick and easy.

- **Nail and hair care**[13], [14], [15]

Trimming of hair, moustache, beard and nails should be a regular habit. Long nails accumulate dirt, germs and toxins. Hence they should be kept as short as possible. This not only ensures hygiene, health, beauty and freshness, but it keeps the body strong and promotes longevity.

- **Kohl application**

The eyes should be 'nourished' regularly with kohl or eye drops to keep them healthy and to improve the vision. The eye is a sense organ dominated by the element of fire. *Kapha doṣa* being the opposing force against *agni*, it constantly attacks the eyes. To maintain proper vision and health of the eyes and to prevent diseases, regular application of *Kapha* opposing collyrium[16] is very beneficial. Therefore, once every 5-8 days such extracts and *rasāñjana*

12. *Pādarogaharaṁ vṛṣyaṁ rakṣoghnaṁ prītivardhanam. Sukhapracāra maująsyaṁ sadā pādatradhāraṇam.*
Anārogyamanāyuṣyaṁ cakṣuṣorupaghātakṛt.
Pādābhyāmanupānādbhyāṁ sadā caṅkramaṇam nṛṇām. (Su.ci. 24/71-72)
Cakṣuṣyaṁ sparśanahitaṁ pādayorvyasanāpaham.
Balyaṁ parākramasukhaṁ vṛṣyaṁ pādatradhāraṇam. (Ca.sū. 5/100)
13. *Tripakṣasya keśaśmaśru nakharomaṇi vardhayet.*
Na svahastairna dantairvā snānaṁ cānusamācaret. (A.saṅ.sū. 3/55)
14. *Pāpmopaśamanaṁ keśanakharomāpamārjanam.*
Harṣalāghavasaubhāgyakaramutsāhavardhamam. (Su.ci. 24/73)
15. *Pauṣṭikaṁ vṛṣyamāyuṣyaṁ śucirūpavirājanam.*
Keśaśmaśrunakhādīnāṁ kalpanaṁ samprasādhanam. (Ca.sū. 5/99)
16. *Cakṣustejomayaṁ tasya viśeṣācchaleṣmato bhayam.*
Yojayet saptarātre, smātsrāvaṇārthaṁ rasāñjanam. (A.saṅ.sū. 3/26)

*(rasota)** should be applied. This promotes watery discharge from the eyes, cleaning them in the process. This paste is very beneficial for the eyes and also relieves eye pain. It should be mixed with honey or diluted with water and a few drops should be applied in the eyes at a time. It stimulates the eyes and causes tearing.

*Procedure for *Rasanjana* Preparation

Boil and thicken goat milk and decoction of Indian berberry in the ratio 4:1, cook until it becomes a paste.

A few precautions should be taken while using kohl or a collyrium. Strong kohls should be used only at night before sleeping as *Kapha* formation is low at this time. During the daytime, it causes excessive watering and exposes the eyes to the harmful rays of the sun and weakens them. Normally the best time to apply regular kohl or collyrium is in the morning as it keeps the eyes smooth and soft during the entire day. Kohl made from the soot of mustard oil, burnt in an earthen lamp lends luster to the eyes, makes the eyes attractive, darkens and thickens the eyelashes and protects the eyes from external infections.

- **Diet***

Diet is crucial to maintain health. Food should be taken in adequate amounts, at appropriate time, and should be favorable to your body constitution. The quantity of food taken should depend on your digestive strength and ability, and also on your metabolic activity.

Some foods such as green gram, rice, porridge and soups are light and easily digestible. The elements of air and fire are predominant in these ghlight° foods. These not only improve the appetite, but are also easily assimilated. Hence, if taken in slightly large quantities they do not cause much harm, but if taken in excess they produce ill-effects on digestion and metabolism. In contrast, several food substances such as black gram, ground pulse stuffing and so on are heavy and require time for complete digestion. They are dominated by water and earth elements. They also reduce appetite. Even a slight overeating of heavy food throws the digestive system out of balance and also affects the metabolism. Though a person with a very strong digestive fire can easily absorb and assimilate heavy foods, it is advisable that these heavy foods should be consumed only as much as is sufficient to fill half or three-quarter of the stomach, and the remaining half or one-fourth of the stomach should remain empty. In this way, these foods also do not cause harm.

Food should be nutritious, simple (*sāttvika*), complete and balanced, suitable for the body type (*prakṛti*). One must eat only after the digestion

*For detailed analysis on diet consult Chapter 6 - Dietary Facts and Rules

of the previous meal. If one pays attention to these points, food builds and supports the body, improves the complexion and general appearance, and increases the life-span. It also keeps all the *doṣas* and *dhātus* in balance, leading to a body that is stable and in harmony. In *Āyurveda* food intake is prohibited while doing any distracting activity because at the time of eating the mind should be calm, peaceful and stable for the proper digestion of food. Only then, one can derive maximum benefit from food.

- **Medicated smoking**

Āyurveda recommends medicated smoking in case of heaviness in the head, headache, inflammation in the nose, migraine, pain in the eyes and ears, hiccoughs, bronchial asthma, sore throat, weak and painful teeth, watery discharge from the ears, nose and eyes, smell in the nose and mouth, loss of appetite, itching, infections, pale complexion, premature graying and shedding of hair, baldness, excessive sneezing, too much sleep, lethargy, dizziness, insomnia, heavy voice and several other disorders.

In *Āyurveda* various preparations using herbs and medicinal plants to prepare medicated cigars have been described. Narcotic drugs and tobacco are not used in these mixtures. Such medicated smoking provides nourishment to the hair, sinuses, voice and strengthens the sense organs. It also protects against throat, neck and head ailments caused by *Vāta* and *Kapha doṣa*.

Eight times in a day are considered suitable for smoking. Smoke can be inhaled after bathing, cleaning of the tongue, brushing of the teeth, after meals, after sneezing, after *nasya* therapy, after kohl or collyrium application and after sleeping. If smoking is carried out only after these eight phases, diseases will not be contracted. Inhaling three times consecutively is recommended at every smoking session.

When smoking is carried out properly, chest, throat and head feel lighter, and helps in loosening and eliminating catarrh. Too much smoking dries the tongue, throat, palate and head. The sense organs become heated up and thirst increases which might also result in syncope, loss of consciousness, dizziness, and intrinsic hemorrhage (bleeding) may also be experienced from any part of the body. Therefore, smoking should be done carefully and in the proper dose. Smoking for the sake of intoxication is prohibited in *Āyurveda*.

- **Behavior: Good conduct**

To remain healthy and happy, one must follow the path of spirituality and a proper code of conduct, that is decorum. *Dharma* (virtue), *artha* (wealth) and *kāma* (lust) should be viewed in a manner that does not cause mutual conflict. This way, one achieves happiness and bliss in any of the paradises in this world or the other. Contrarily, if a person earns wealth by wrong means, enjoys sexual indulgences and lust, adapts indecent manners and spends wealth insensibly, then *dharma, arth* and *kāma* mutually contradict each other. Such a person has to face difficulties in life and the downfall is sure. In this regard, one must memorize the warning given by saint *Vālmīki* that "A wise man is one who persues *dharma, artha* and *kāma* in a balanced and decent manner. In contrast, one who does not fullfill his duties of life properly and engrosses himself in lust and desire, comes back to his senses after his downfall in such a manner, just as one sleeping on a tree becomes conscious when he falls down(17)." One should always speak the truth. Even small creatures such as ants and insects must be treated equally. One must ever be ready to help the victimized, the sick and poor people who are saddened by bereavement. One must never disappoint those who need help or have contempt for them. God, cattle, noble people, aged persons, physicians and guests must be treated with respect and regard.

One must never try to grab other's properties and belongings or even desire to acquire them, nor should one have desire for other women. Keep away from wrong deeds and avoid ill-treating any individual with unrighteous conduct. Do not reveal the weaknesses and secrets of others. Company of people with unrighteous conduct, disruptive tendencies and tough-natured, violent individuals should be shunned. Be friendly with people working for universal welfare and approach them for their advice. On the other hand, one must always be careful of those who have disruptive tendencies.

- **Conduct to be avoided**

  The following conduct and habits need to be checked in the daily routine:

- Climbing trees, undergoing dangerous mountain rides, travelling in dangerous vehicles, bathing in a river with high currents.
- Sleeping on an uncovered, small, uneven and pillowless bed.
- Do not step over a relative, aristocratic people, teacher, guide and worthy person, sacred trees and the shadow of an unworthy person.
- Transgressing by keeping sacred things and worthy people on the left side while putting unholy things on the right side.
- Keep away from uncivilized public behavior such as laughing loudly in a gathering, loud belching, yawning, coughing or sneezing without covering the mouth, blowing the nose, teeth chattering, scratching private parts, cracking nails and joints, placing limbs in awkward positions and moving ungracefully. In fact any behavior which is wrong and troubles anyone else.
- Staring at the sun, and censured objects.

17. *Dharmarthaṁ ca kāmaṁ ca kāle yastu niṣevate.*
Vibhajya satataṁ vīra sa rājā harisattama.
Hitvā dharmaṁ tathārthaṁ ca kāmaṁ yastu niṣevate.
Sa vṛkṣāgre yathā suptaḥ patitaḥ pratibudhyate.(*Vālmīki Rāmāyaṇa, Kiṣkindhā kāṇḍa.* 38.20-21)

- Entering late in the night and staying in temples, sacred places, near holy and auspicious trees, gardens, crossroads, graveyards and lonely places.
- Venturing alone in a jungle or slaughter house.
- It is unwise to show effrontery, courage or work more than one°s potential.
- Bathing and sleeping more than required, staying awake at night, intake of excessive liquids.
- Bathing during fatigue. Bathing without removing all clothes and without cleaning the mouth, and wearing the same clothes after bathing.
- Maintain distance from snakes and animals with sharp horns and teeth.
- Keeping fire under the bed. Also, one must stay away from fire when upset or unstable and after meals, especially if hands and mouth are unwashed.
- Protect yourself against wind from the east, from sun, hail and wind storms.
- Other things that need to be avoided are improper conduct, criminal acts, befriending wicked people, alienating people of good character, sitting for a long period with the knees drawn up.

- **Precautions while studying**

Appropriate time and proper light should be arranged for studying. The main light source should be on the left or behind the person studying. Avoid studying at places where something is burning, in front of fire and during solar and lunar eclipses, important festivals, dusk and dawn. While studying, the body posture, distance and position of the book are very important factors. The reading material should neither be very close nor very far from the eyes and it should be at least one feet away from the body. Reading while lying down weakens the eyesight. Care should be taken to keep the pronunciation clear and complete when reading aloud. The voice should be neither too loud nor too soft or too harsh. Reading should not be done with too much or too little effort. Recitation should be neither too fast nor too slow and should have all the necessary intonations.

- **Norms of good conduct**

Follow the universally accepted code of conduct and obey general rules and regulations. Keep an abiding faith in the cause and effect theory and the law of *karma*, and this should become the guiding principle of all actions.

- Going to dangerous places late at night is not advisable.
- Do not eat, study, sleep and indulge in sex at dawn and dusk. This is the best time for self-realization, meditation, *yoga* and for spiritual and individual development.
- Avoid alcoholism, intoxication, gambling and going to prostitutes.

- Do not behave in an uncivilized manner and humiliate anyone. Being unfriendly and behaving rudely due to excessive pride is a wrong practice.
- Stay away from impolite and uncultured people, tale bearing and using abusive words for older people, teachers, leaders and against anyone in a gathering.
- Do not behave impatiently and too aggressively, and do not talk too much.
- Take care of dependants and subordinates and do not look down them.
- Complete trust, without a suspicious nature or without being unduly dependent on someone is good.
- Careful planning before undertaking a new project is highly recommended. Once a job is undertaken, avoid delaying, postponing and leaving it unfinished.
- Maintain dignity in both success and defeat.
- Avoid working with excessive happiness or anger. Being too sensitive about petty things is not wise and healthy.
- Free yourself from bondage to your senses and mind. However, do not practice overly forceful suppression of desires.
- Act according to your true nature and character.
- Stop constantly thinking about past insults.
- Your character, behavior and habits should not be a matter of ridicule. Dress appropriately.
- Share your happiness with others.

- **Who to befriend**

- Friendship should be with people having wisdom, intelligence, pure conduct, patience, strong memory and good concentration, as well as those who have attained knowledge and maturity and those who are in the company of such people, who add value to any conversation.
- Those who are calm, remain free from worries and stress, think with clarity and can differentiate between good and bad.
- Those whose behavior is impeccable and who always work for the common welfare.
- Those who support good conduct and whose name and philosophy is revered.

- **Persons not to befriend**

One should not befriend those who lack the qualities enumerated above and who are deceitful, of bad character, having unrighteous conduct, who use abusive language, have unethical thoughts and a destructive mind, indulge in criticism and slander, are quarrelsome, greedy, envious, have contempt for others, are fickle-minded, cruel, unkind and those who have disruptive tendencies.

2. *Rātricaryā*: Food Habits and Conduct at Night

A complete duration of 24 hours including day and night is referred to as one day. Hence, *rātricaryā* is also a part of *dinacaryā*. After a whole day, rest at night is a necessary requirement for the body. Sleep here is described first, since the primary activity at night is sleeping.

- **Sleep**

It is commonly known that in order to maintain good health, freshness and high spirits, sound and adequate sleep is crucial. After completing all tasks for the day, the mind and body become inactive due to fatigue and the sense and motor organs are drained. All this induce a desire to sleep. The state in which the mind loses connection and communication with sense and motor organs, when one becomes inert and inactive, is called sleep. During sleep, vital processes like breathing and blood circulation do not stop performing. Energy thus conserved, recharge the body. This accounts for the high energy level and the feeling of freshness and good health after a good sleep.

Night time is most conducive for sleep as the *Kapha doṣa* in the body and *Tamas doṣa* in the mind helps to induce sleep. The silence, darkness and low temperature during the night increases the level of these two *doṣas* in the body, leading to sound sleep. Before sleeping, it is advisable to switch off the television and keep the telephone or mobile phones out of the room or at a distance from the bed. As far as possible, one should sleep separately, which is very essential from the point of view of health. *Āyurveda* prescribes to sleep early at night and to wake up early in the morning, because at night the effect of *Vāta* helps to induce good sleep while early in the morning both *Vāta* and *Kapha* are prevalent which helps in the proper elimination of excretory wastes.Therefore, one should wake up early in the morning, as it keeps the mind exhilarated. The body remains energetic, fresh and enthusiastic. An early morning walk in fresh air and a peaceful environment is very important to keep the body healthy.

- **Types of sleep:** Sleep may be of two types

(a) ***Svapnāvasthā* (state of dreams):** This is the state in which a person dreams while sleeping and the unconscious mind remains active, engaged in thinking though randomly. This type of sleep is not a sound sleep and hence not relaxing. This stage of sleep is important for memories to form.

(b) ***Suṣuptāvasthā* (state of deep sleep):** In this state of sleep all sensory activities of the body and mind are suspended. Deep sleep for even a short duration is extremely refreshing and healthy. It reinvigorates both the mind and the body. On the other hand, even a long period of sleep in the dream state fails to provide rest and does not refresh the body.

Together with physical exertion and fatigue caused by hard work, mental peace (a mind free from anger, fear, grief, sorrow, worry, tension and so on) is absolutely essential to enjoy sound sleep. Those who lack sleep suffer from insomnia which causes several mental and physical disorders.

◆ **Insomnia: Reasons and Remedies**

Causes for insomnia

1. Behavioral causes: Mental disturbances like fear, worry, sorrow and anger; an uncomfortable bed or resting place; excessive *sattva guṇa* and low *tamo guṇa*; smoking; and a natural tendency towards sleeplessness.
2. Physiological causes: Bodyaches due to excessive physical exertion, old age and ailments caused by *Vāta* aggravation such as shooting pains and so on, and expulsion of *doṣas* from the head and body parts due to diarrhea and vomiting.
3. Therapeutical causes: Blood-letting therapy and too much fasting leads to insomnia.

Remedies to cure insomnia

1. Massage, application of *ubaṭaṇa* (medicated pastes), bathing and pressing of limbs.
2. Intake of slightly oily foods, yogurt and unpolished rice, milk and alcoholic drinks.
3. Mental peace and happiness.
4. Listening to music according to one's interest.
5. Applying soothing ointments and pastes over the eyes, head and face.
6. Sleeping in a quiet and comfortable place.
7. Inhaling aromas (perfumes or scents) and adorning the room with pleasing flowers.

"Brahmacaryaratergrāmyasukhaniḥspṛhacetasaḥ.
Nidrā santoṣatṛptasya svaṁ kālaṁ nātivarttate." (*A. Saṁ. sū.* 9.66)

"Inclination towards celibacy and withdrawal from sexual indulgence and gratification keeps one away from diseases related to insomnia."

◆ **Restrict day sleep**

Sleeping during the day is harmful for health as it increases *Kapha* and *Pitta doṣa*, which may result in disease. It might cause headache, heaviness, bodyache, weak digestion, congestion in the chest, anorexia, vomiting, nausea, inflammation in the nose, itching, drowsiness, lethargy, blunting of memory and loss of intellect, debility of sensory and motor organs and several other disorders such as severe jaundice, blockage in various body channels, fever, cough, throat ailments, migraine and increased vulnerability to toxins. Hence, sleep in the day is very harmful for health. People who are obese, who take oily foods in their diet, who suffer from *Kapha* related ailments on account of having *Kapha prakṛti* and those suffering from arthritis should not sleep during the day time.

- **Exceptions**

  In summer, due to shorter nights and loss of water from the body as perspiration, *Vāta* gets aggravated, thus sleeping during the day time in summer is not harmful. There are some other conditions when sleeping during the day is not restricted. Sleeping during the day is not contra-indicated after rigorous music practice, studying, walking or consumption of alcoholic substances, while travelling, after a lack of sleep at night, and after being drained due to anger, fear or sorrow. It is also recommended under certain physiological conditions such as suffering from weakness, fatigue, thirst, hiccoughs, a weak constitution during childhood and old age, and in diseases such as tuberculosis, diarrhea, shooting pains, bronchial asthma, and suffering from trauma or injury. Under such conditions, strength of the body is improved by sleeping during the day time and the *dhātus* come back in balance. Aggravated *Kapha doṣa* nourishes the organs and increases the life-span.

- **Dining habits and rules**

Digestion of food and sleep are inextricably linked. Keeping in mind the fact that indigestion hampers sleep, the last meal should be taken as early as possible in the evening. A two-hour gap between dinner and sleep is essential. Take only light and easily digestible food at night. Leisurely walking after dinner is recommended. It helps to promote digestion and therefore gives a more relaxing sleep.

- **Avoid yogurt at night**

Despite being beneficial normally, yogurt has a tendency to 'block the body's channels.' Hence, *Āyurveda* does not recommend eating yogurt at night as one has to sleep after dinner. The digestive process continues very slowly while sleeping. The chance of 'blockage in the body channels' increases. Consequently sleep, digestion and metabolism are disrupted. In healthy people as well, eating yogurt at night is not recommended. Patients of bronchial asthma, cough, cold and arthritis are not recommended to eat yogurt even during the day as these disorders are caused due to the 'blocking of channels.'

- **Night study**

Adequate light while studying is a must to ensure healthy eyesight. However, it must be remembered that sunlight is far better than artificial light, which weakens the eye power gradually overtime. As far as possible, studying at night should be kept to a minimum. Writing at night time is stressful for the eyes; hence it should be avoided as much as possible.

- **Sexual activity**

Āyurveda places certain limits on sexual activity dictated by health concerns and rules of social conduct. Avoid sexual activity under the following circumstances (These rules are the same for both sexes):

- During menstruation or when suffering from infection or disease.
- With a person who is ill-natured, of bad character, uncultured, undignified or those having unrighteous conduct and with those who are unattractive.
- In case of a lack of friendly feeling, lack of sexual desire, and attraction towards a person of the same sex or a person who is married.
- In sacred places, under holy trees, public areas, crossroads, gardens, graveyards, slaughter houses, water spots, hospitals, places of worship and residences of *Brahmins* (Priests and holy people), teachers and guides.
- At dawn, dusk, full moon nights, nights of the new moon and the eighth day of the lunar cycle (*aṣṭamī*).
- The male being in an impure or not in a pious state or suffering from low libido.
- If not consuming milk or some other aphrodisiac substances.
- Without eating or after overeating.
- While fasting, after physical exertion, when experiencing fatigue or a strong urge to urinate.
- At an inappropriate place or where there is a lack of privacy.

3. Improper Lifestyle: The Major Cause of Obesity and Emaciation

At present, due to unwholesome lifestyle and diet regimen, obesity and emaciation are spreading worldwide as major health problems.

(A) Obese or overweight individuals: Symptoms, etiology and treatment

Excess fat deposition on the hips, waist and chest, flabbiness and sagging fat is a clear sign of obesity. Another symptom is lack of enthusiasm, energy and body strength corresponding to an increase in body mass. 'The bodily channels' of an obese person are blocked due to accumulation of fat. This leads to breathlessness while walking, heaviness in the body, anxiety and discomfort. All this cause the circulation of *Vāta*, especially in the bowels,

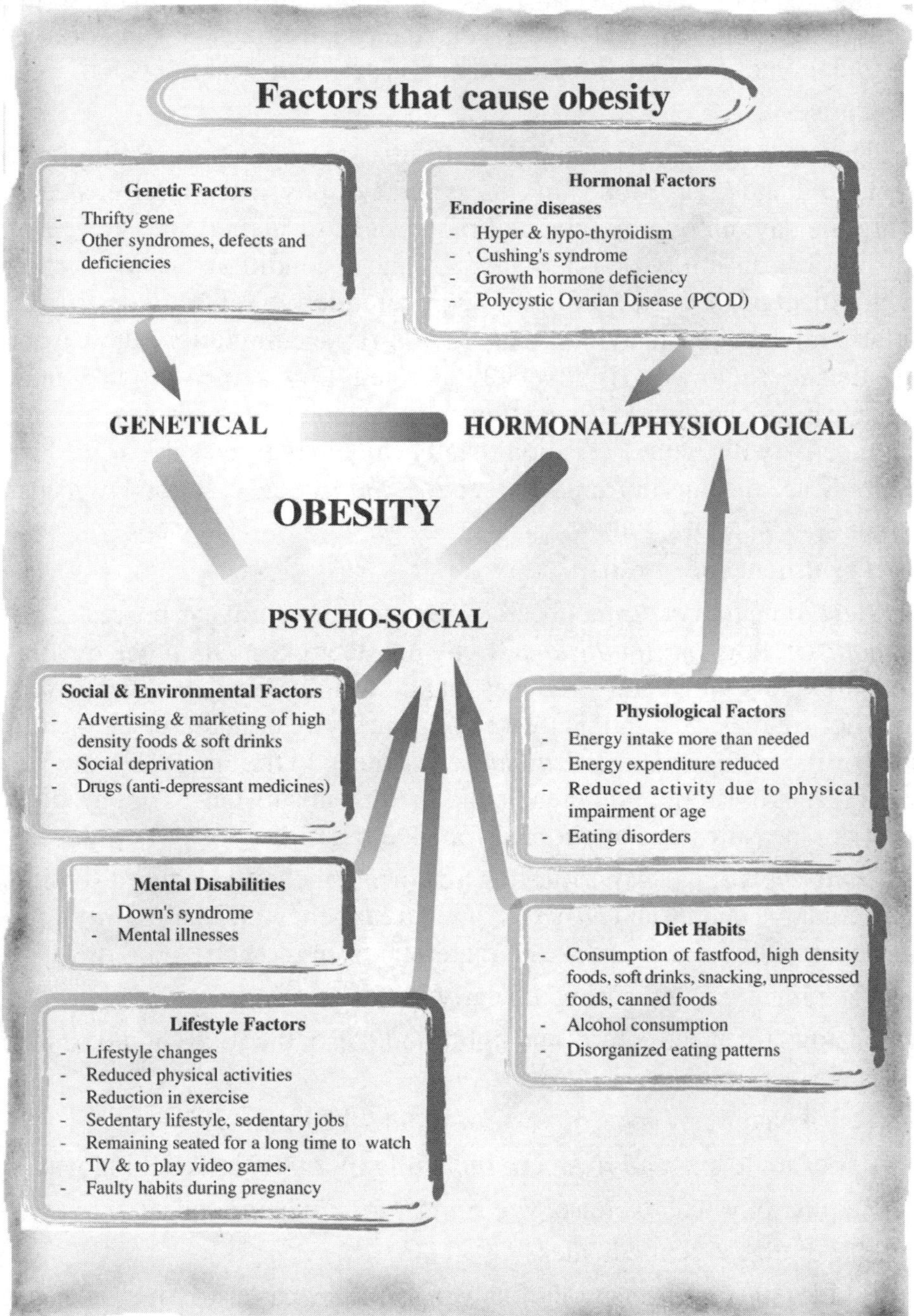
Factors that cause obesity
Genetic Factors
- Thrifty gene
- Other syndromes, defects and deficiencies
Hormonal Factors
Endocrine diseases
- Hyper & hypo-thyroidism
- Cushing's syndrome
- Growth hormone deficiency
- Polycystic Ovarian Disease (PCOD)
GENETICAL
HORMONAL/PHYSIOLOGICAL
OBESITY
PSYCHO-SOCIAL
Social & Environmental Factors
- Advertising & marketing of high density foods & soft drinks
- Social deprivation
- Drugs (anti-depressant medicines)
Physiological Factors
- Energy intake more than needed
- Energy expenditure reduced
- Reduced activity due to physical impairment or age
- Eating disorders
Mental Disabilities
- Down's syndrome
- Mental illnesses
Diet Habits
- Consumption of fastfood, high density foods, soft drinks, snacking, unprocessed foods, canned foods
- Alcohol consumption
- Disorganized eating patterns
Lifestyle Factors
- Lifestyle changes
- Reduced physical activities
- Reduction in exercise
- Sedentary lifestyle, sedentary jobs
- Remaining seated for a long time to watch TV & to play video games.
- Faulty habits during pregnancy

which aggravates the digestive fire. The digestive process speeds up, food gets digested soon and hunger increases in an unnatural way. In the form of digestive fire, both *Vāta* and *Pitta* get unbalanced, leading to disproportionate accumulation of fat. Due to *Vāta*, various types of diseases develop.

- **Causes**

The most common reasons for obesity are overeating; eating heavy, sweet, cold and greasy foods in excess; lack of physical exercise; sleeping during the day; an over-exhilarated mood, lack of mental strength, mental and physical disability and heredity. All these conditions cause increased development of fat (adipose) tissues compared to other bodily tissues. Due to flab and sagging, heaviness and excess fat accumulation, the capacity and intensity to do work is adversely affected. Low semen production and blockage in the channels of semen flow reduces their work capacity and makes sexual activity difficult. Fat is liquid and heavy in nature as it is mixed with *Kapha*. Since the equilibrium between the *dhātus* gets disturbed, it leads to weakness in spite of being obese.

- **Treatment for obesity**

According to *Āyurveda*, obesity or being overweight can be treated with *laṅghana* (fasting) or *asantarpaṇa* (lightning) therapies. *Laṅghana* treatment brings lightness to the body, reduces fat and weight. Medicinal herbs, foods and other sources used in this treatment principally contain the elements of *tejas* (fire), *vāyu* (air) and *ākāśa* (space or ether). In *laṅghana* therapy light, hot, dry, rough, subtle, liquid and solid medicinal substances are used. The following measures can be adopted for such treatment:

1. *Saṁśodhana cikitsā* (purification treatment), including induced vomiting, purgation, enema and *nasya* (errhine) treatment which helps to eliminate accumulated *doṣas* and waste materials from the body.
2. Sleeping early and getting up early in the morning.
3. Fasting, to take less food and light food. Also, the food should be taken at correct times.
4. To tolerate thirst and drink warm water when thirsty.
5. Exposure to sun and fresh air, including morning and evening walks.
6. Regular physical exercise, *yogāsanas*, *prāṇāyāmas* and so on.
7. Use of digestive medicines.

Besides *laṅghana* therapy, the following remedies can also be used to manage obesity:

1. Use of dry and hot substances.
2. Intake of buttermilk.
3. Along with buttermilk, eating bread made from barley with easily

digestible vegetables such as bottle gourd and so on.

4. Intake of one teaspoon of honey in luke warm water every morning and evening.
5. Intake of green vegetables and fruits along with a *Vāta* based diet.
6. Intake of 50-100 ml of herbal decoction of herbs like *guḍūcī* (*giloya*), nut grass (*nāgaramothā*), myrobalan (*harara*), belleric myrobalan (*baherā*) and Indian gooseberry (*āṁvalā*), every morning and evening.
7. Porridge prepared from wheat, rice, pearl millet and whole green gram with the skin (500 gm of each), after roasting them on a slow flame. Mix 50 gm sesame seeds and 20 gm thymol (carom) seeds to it. Add 50 gm of this porridge to 400 ml water and cook them together. Regularly eating this porridge instead of a meal is beneficial to reduce weight and obesity.
8. Regular use of one leaf of wintercherry (crushed by hand) daily in the morning and evening, on an empty stomach or an hour before a meal, with warm water. Use it for 7 days and then stop for 15 days and again start for 7 days.
9. Follow a regulated and balanced diet and lifestyle.
10. Soak one teaspoon of *triphalā* powder (powder of myrobalan, belleric myrobalan and Indian gooseberry) in 200 ml of water overnight. Boil it in the morning until it is reduced to half the amount, drink it warm after straining.

All the above methods are highly effective to overcome obesity. Related ailments such as cardiac disease, diabetes, cough and digestive disorders are also alleviated.

Improved material comforts and luxuries in life with consequent reduction in physical activity and changed lifestyles are chiefly responsible for widespread obesity in recent years, which has reached to epidemic level in the Western world, along with an increased rate of related diseases like diabetes, cardiac diseases and depression. Obesity breeds dangerous ailments and affects the vital systems of the body such as the circulatory, respiratory and digestive systems. The preventive and curative measures of obesity listed above can help to fight obesity.

(B) Emaciated or underweight individuals: Symptoms, etiology and treatment

Thin or underweight individuals have sunken stomachs, flat hips, thin necks and lack of muscles. Their veins and arteries are prominently visible and bones and joints are conspicuous. Their body look like a skeleton with a layer of skin covering.

Underweight people do not have sufficient strength for excessive physical exertion and do not have the capacity to tolerate excess hunger, thirst, pain, disease and strong medications. They cannot tolerate even severe summer or cold winter temperatures. Neither can they enjoy normal sexual activity. People like this most often suffer from cough, hemorrhoids, disorders of the spleen, abdominal swelling and disorders of the chest, stomach and intestines.

- **Causes**

The causes of being underweight or having a thin body are an unbalanced diet which is not nutritious, frequent fasting, insufficient diet and sleep, anxiety, worry, stress, anger, prolonged illness, suppression of natural urges, use of excess detoxifying therapies like emesis and purgation, use of body pastes (*ubaṭana*) made of dry substances, heredity and old age.

- **Treatment for emaciation**

To overcome the problem of emaciation or being underweight, *bṛṁhaṇa* (restorative) or *santarpaṇa* (stoutening) practices are brought into use. This type of treatment adds weight, nourishes, energizes and strengthens the body because of its calorie-rich food intake. Medicinal herbs, foods and other sources used in this treatment are rich in the elements of *prthvī* (earth) and *jala* (water). On this basis, food substances and beverages that are soothing, cooling, heavy, soft, slow, greasy, gross and dense in nature are used. Milk, *ghee*, cottage cheese, butter and other milk products, honey along with various natural sugars are important for the treatment of emaciation. Physical treatment involves the use of body pastes (*ubaṭana*) made of smooth and greasy substances, deep sleep for long hours, maintaining a good mood and happy frame of mind, avoiding anxiety, depression, worries, and enemas with oily medicines are all parts of *bṛṁhaṇa cikitsā* or restorative therapy. The use of such therapies and medication cures emaciation. The following measures are helpful in overcoming the problem of being underweight:

1. Sound sleep, cheerfulness, a comfortable bed, emotional satisfaction and peace of mind.
2. Avoiding anxiety, worry, excessive sex and too much physical work. These should be performed within limits.
3. Staying in a congenial environment with good friends and relatives.
4. Including yogurt, *ghee*, milk, sugarcane, rice, black gram, wheat and jaggery in the diet, and cooked food made from these ingredients.
5. Regular body massage with oil, application of medicated oily *ubaṭana* (pastes) and bathing with warm water.
6. Use of aromas and incense, and wearing gentle and soft clothes.
7. Use of rejuvenation therapy and aphrodisiac medicines (to increase the semen count and subsequently the strength).
8. Taking a balanced and nutritious diet at an appropriate time and keeping a tension-free attitude.
9. Regular practice of *āsanas*, *prāṇāyāmas* and a morning walk in fresh air.
10. Regular intake of milk with crystal sugar and one teaspoon of honey, everyday in the morning and evening. Eating easily digestible foods.

11. Use of a high protein and fat-rich diet and porridge prepared from protein-rich substances such as soyabeans, wheat, barley, Bengal gram and so on, and in general a balanced diet is a must.

The above remedies can help to overcome the problem of being underweight and the diseases related to it. In brief, avoiding anxiety and worry, living happily and cheerful, having adequate and deep sleep, eating nourishing and restorative food and herbs are helpful to overcome emaciation.

- **Obesity is more dangerous than emaciation**

As has been mentioned earlier, obesity and emaciation are both dangerous and harmful. In both conditions people suffer from one disease or another and the body remains unhealthy. Yet between the two, obesity is usually more dangerous. Obesity and emaciation can be corrected by appropriate dietary and lifestyle changes, but corrective measures for obesity are more difficult to adapt. There should be a treatment which alleviates accumulated fat, increases the digestive fire and reduces *Vāta. Bṛṁhana cikitsā* (restorative therapies) reduce *Vāta* and lower the digestive power in obese people, but increase accumulation of fat. In contrast, *laṅghana cikitsā* (fasting therapy) reduces fat but aggravate *Vāta* and increase the digestive fire, which is difficult to tolerate.

4. *Ṛtucaryā*: Food Habits and Conduct during Different Seasons

The season and environment also affects our health as much as our food habits. The condition of the *doṣas* in the body changes with the seasons. One *doṣa* gets aggravated in one season while the other gets pacified and *vice-versa*. Thus seasonal changes are intricately related with the health of a person. Due to the accumulation (deposition), aggravation and pacification of the *doṣas* as a result of seasonal changes, *Āyurveda* recommends different foods and behavior patterns for different times of the year. Following these rules are crucial to maintain health and to protect oneself from various diseases.

Table 15: The Natural Tendency of the *Doṣas* in Different Seasons

Doṣa	***Chāyā* (Accumulation)**	***Prakopa* (Aggravation)**	***Prasamana* (Normalcy)**
Vāta	*Grīṣma* (summer)	*Varṣā* (monsoon)	*Śarad* (autumn)
Pitta	*Varṣā* (monsoon)	*Śarad* (autumn)	*Hemanta* (early winter)
Kapha	*Śiśira* (late winter)	*Vasanta* (spring)	*Grīṣma* (summer)

India experiences three main seasons during a year - summer, winter and monsoon. These seasons bring many variations in the body. Each season is further divided into two, making six in all - *vasanta* (spring), *grīṣma* (summer), *varṣā* (monsoon), *śarad* (autumn), *hemanta* (early winter) and *śiśira* (late winter).

The Southern part of India receives a lot of rain; hence the monsoon is divided into two parts. The first is called '*prāvṛṭ*' and the second 'the rainy season.' The North of India has a shorter rainy season, but a longer winter which is divided into two phases: *hemanta* and *śiśira.**

Note: The Western world has a very different set of seasons with four pronounced seasons - winter, summer, spring and fall (autumn). In different countries, different seasonal routines need to be modified accordingly.

Two periods during a solar year depending on the direction of the sun are known as *ayana*. *Ayana* is of two types:

1. ***Uttarāyaṇa* (Northern solstice):** During *uttarāyaṇa*, the sun takes a northern course and gets progressively higher in the sky. Ascent of the sun in the sky is known as *uttarāyaṇa* or *ādāna* (absorbing) period as the sun's rays and the winds are hot, penetrating and dry, and absorb moisture rapidly. The effect of these conditions is felt by all vegetation and the human body as well. It depletes energy and causes debility. This period includes late winter, spring and summer.
2. ***Dakṣiṇāyaṇa* (Southern solstice):** During this period the sun takes a southern course and gets progressively lower in the sky. Descent of the sun in the sky is known as *dakṣiṇāyaṇa kāla*. Sun's rays and winds are neither hot and dry nor rough. The effect of the sun is mild and the moon is evident in the environment. The temperature decreases and the weather become pleasant and mild. Winds, clouds and rain have a cooling and soothing effect. This is called the *visarga* (releasing) period. Due to coolness in the environment, all sorts of vegetation (useful as food and medicinal substances) begin to grow and thrive. This results in an increase in physical strength in both animals and humans. This period includes the monsoon, autumn and early winter.

Visarga is *saumya* (calm) due to the predominance of *soma* (moon). On the other hand, *ādāna* is *āgneya* (fire) due to the predominance of *agni*. Thus the sun, moon and wind are responsible for the appearance of time, seasons, *rasas, doṣas* and strength in nature.

Due to the effects of *visarga* and *ādāna kāla*, the body becomes feeble, loses weight and experiences debility at the end of *ādāna* and beginning of *visarga kāla*. In the middle of *visarga* and *ādāna kāla*, the body strength is medium, neither too weak nor too strong. At the end of *visarga* and beginning of *ādāna kāla* the body tends to gain maximum strength. Taking into account all seasonal variations, *Āyurveda* recommends different foods and living habits for different seasons. [PLATE 18]

* This is described in *Suśruta Saṁhitā, Sūtrasthāna* 6.10

Table 16 : Natural Conditions According to Seasonal Variations

Ṛtu (Season)	Indian Months	English Months	Intensity of Sun	Intensity of Moon	Weather Conditions	Prominent *Rasa* (Taste)	Strength in a Person	Condition of *Doṣas*		
								Accumulation	Aggravation	Pacification
Śiśira (Late winter)	*Māgha, Phālguna*	January-February February-March	Hot ↑	Weak ↓	Dry	Bitter	Maximum	*Kapha*	—	—
Vasanta (Spring)	*Caitra, Vaiśākha*	March-April April- May	Very Hot ↑↑	Weaker ↓↓	Drier	Astringent	Moderate	—	*Kapha*	—
Grīṣma (Summer)	*Jyeṣṭha, Āṣāḍha*	May-June June-July	Hottest ↑↑↑	Weakest ↓↓↓	Driest	Pungent	Low	*Vāta*	—	*Kapha*
Varṣā (Monsoon)	*Śrāvṇa, Bhādrapada*	July-August August- September	Weak ↓	Cold ↑	Less Humid	Sour	Low	*Pitta*	*Vāta*	—
Śarad (Autumn)	*Āśvina, Kārtika*	September- October October- November	Weaker ↓↓	Very Cold ↑↑	Humid	Salty	Moderate	—	*Pitta*	*Vāta*
Hemanta (Early winter)	*Mārgaśīrṣa, Pauṣa*	November-December December-January	Weakest ↓↓↓	Coldest ↑↑↑	Very Humid	Sweet	Maximum	—	—	*Pitta*

Table 17: Different Seasonal Pattern in *Āyurveda* According to Indian Climate

Kāla (Semester)	*Ṛtu*	Season	*Sanskrit māsa*	Months
Ādāna Kāla (Northern solstice)	*Śiśira*	Late winter (cold and dewy season)	*Māgha-Phālguna*	Mid January-Mid March
	Vasanta	Spring season	*Caitra-Vaiśākha*	Mid March-Mid May
	Grīṣma	Summer season	*Jeṣṭha-Āṣāḍha*	Mid May-Mid July
Visarga Kāla (Southern solstice)	*Varṣā*	Rainy season (Monsoon)	*Śrāvṇa-Bhādrapada*	Mid July-Mid September
	Śarad	Autumn season	*Āśvina-Kārtika*	Mid September-Mid November
	Hemanta	Early winter	*Mārgaśīrṣa-Pauṣa*	Mid November-Mid January

Table 18: Different Seasonal Pattern According to Western Climate

Season	Months of the year	Climatic conditions
Spring	March-April-May	Days grow longer; the weather is warmer but it rains often and can get very windy.
Summer	June-July-August	Days are longer; the weather is usually warm and may even be hot.
Autumn	September-October-November	Days get shorter; the weather gets colder and leaves fall (hence Autumn = The Fall).
Winter	December-January-February	Days are shorter; cold, dewy and even snowy.

• Rejuvenating herbs in different seasons

In *Āyurveda*, for the upkeeping of health, different rejuvenating herbs are prescribed according to different seasons. Intake of these rejuvenating herbs with different substances helps to attain good health. The following herbs are prescribed in different combinations as follows:

Rejuvenating Herbs in Different Seasons

Early winter	:	Take half a teaspoon of myrobalan (*harara)* powder with an equal quantity of dry ginger powder.
Late winter	:	Take half a teaspoon of long pepper (*pippalī*) powder with fresh water.
Spring	:	Take myrobalan (*harara)* powder with honey.
Summer	:	Take myrobalan powder with an equal amount of jaggery.
Monsoon	:	Take myrobalan powder along with rock salt.
Autumn	:	Take myrobalan powder along with honey, crystal sugar or jaggery.

- ***Hemanta* and *Śiśira* (Winter season): Food regimen and living habits**

This is the best season as far as health is concerned. The body gains its maximum strength at this time. Shorter days and longer nights ensure more rest and favor digestion. Due to better digestion, the body gains its maximum strength and the appetite also increases, which is a natural tendency in winter. Due to strengthened digestive power, even if heavy foods are eaten in larger amounts, they are easily absorbed and assimilated.

Therefore, staying hungry or eating dry, rough and inadequate food during this season is harmful. The digestive fire in the absence of adequate food, attacks and destroys the essential digestive juices. It results in the aggravation of *Vāta doṣa*, which is characteristically cold and dry in attributes.

- **A compatible diet**

During winter, the diet should include food that is oily; sweet, salty and sour in taste; and nutritious. The following food items should be a part of the winter diet:

Milk and milk products such as clarified butter (*ghee*), cream, butter, rice pudding, black gram porridge, sweetened condensed milk (*rābaṟī*), honey with cold milk and oil. Sugar and sweets such as crystal sugar, sugarcane juice, sweets made of flour (*halavā*), apple and gooseberry succade (*murabba*), sweets and other delicacies made with ground pulses and dried fruits. Pulses like sprouted Bengal gram, black gram and green gram. Grains such as bread made from wheat or gram flour, cornflakes, new rice and porridge. All seasonal fruits like apple, gooseberry, oranges and so on. Vegetables such as pointed gourd (*paravala*), brinjal, cauliflower, cabbage, yams, ripe red tomatoes, carrots, beans, peas, spinach, fenugreek leaves, chenopodium, all other green leafy vegetables and dried ginger. Warm water, hot foods and all dried fruits can be incorporated in the diet as they are nutritious and good for promoting health.

- **A compatible living**

Along with the diet, it is necessary to follow a healthy lifestyle. The very first thing for a healthy lifestyle is to remain exhilarated, mentally fresh and stress free. It is best to wake up before sunrise and complete all routine morning activities like the intake of water (*uṣaḥpāna*), cleaning of the bowels, bathing and a brisk walk in fresh air. The speed of walking should be maintained based on your physical strength. Walking is ideal for good health, because it is a natural activity that satisfies all three *doṣas*. After a walk, rest for a while and go ahead with exercise and *yoga*. In this season exercising is essential. It tones the body, keeps it strong and makes digestion more efficient. During winter the skin becomes dry. Therefore, a body massage with oil and medicated paste (turmeric *ubaṭana*) and application of oil to the hair should be a part of the daily routine. It is very beneficial in winter. Massaging with mustard oil keeps the skin beautiful and healthy, and cures boils and pimples. A massage with oil medicated with camphor relieves arthritis and joint pain. Oil massages should be followed by *ubaṭana*. Exercise can also precede the body massage.

Exposure to cold winds may cause cold, cough, bronchial asthma, arthritis, pain in the joints, itching, fever and pneumonia. Hence, cold winds must be avoided to prevent diseases. Try to stay in warm places. Heavy, warm, silken and woolen clothes, blankets and quilts should be used. The home and vehicle should also be kept warm. Sit in the sun and near the fire to keep the body warm. Warmth from the sun should be taken on the dorsal (back) side of the body, while that from fire should be received on the ventral (front) side. Room heaters can be used for this purpose as well. Sexual activity within limits is advisable during this season. Consuming milk and aphrodisiac substances at night is advantageous.

- **Incompatible food and living habits**

In this season avoid light, dry and *Vāta* provoking foods, food and drinks with bitter, pungent and astringent tastes, and stale and cold substances such as cold drinks, ice cream and 'cool potency' substances. Also avoid sour items such as tamarind, dry mango powder, sour yogurt and mango pickle as much as possible.

An unfavorable lifestyle includes staying awake till late at night, rising late in the morning, laziness, avoiding workouts and exercise, bathing too much, exposure to cold, late dinners and sleeping immediately after a meal, as well as starving oneself or eating inadequately.

- **Difference between *hemanta* (early winter) and *śiśira* (late winter)**

Generally, the weather conditions during both these seasons are similar. During *hemanta* (early winter), the sun takes a Southward course. Hence, food and medicinal substances gather smoothness, a sweet taste and are nourishing. *Doṣa* accumulation reduces during this period. During *śiśira* (late winter), the sun takes a Northward course. Due to the beginning of *ādāna kāla*, the environment all around has coolness and dryness. The coolness, heaviness and sweetness gathered by the vegetation during this period accumulate *Kapha doṣa* in the body. Therefore, take only appropriate food, protect yourself from the cold and stay in a warm place during late winter. Refrain from the use of cold, light and dry foods and from fasting.

An appropriate diet and habits adopted during winter helps the body gain enough strength to keep fit and healthy throughout the year, with increased immunity to fight disease.

***Hemanta* and *Śiśira* (Winter)**

	***Hemanta* (Early Winter)**	***Śiśira* (Late Winter)**
Predominant *Rasa* (Taste)	- *Madhura* (Sweet)	*Tikta* (Bitter)
Predominant *Mahābhūta* (Element)	- *Pṛthavī* (Earth) + *Jala*(Water)	*Ākāśa* (Space/Ether)
Condition of *Doṣa*	- Vitiated *Pitta* gets pacified	Deposition of *Kapha doṣa*
Activity of *Agni* (Digestive fire)	- Increased	Remain in a higher state
Strength	- Maximum	Maximum

• *Vasanta* (Spring season): Food regimen and living habits

Spring is the most pleasant of all seasons. A profusion of multi-colored flowers and natural fragrances characterize this season, and pleasure, joy and the beauty of nature blossoms everywhere. It appears as if nature is in an exhilarated mood. This season beautifully expresses the transition from winter to summer. During spring, the weather is mild and pleasant, neither very cold nor too hot, the days are warm and nights are cool, with a steadily rising temperature.

***Vasanta* (Spring)**		
Predominant *Rasa* (Taste)	-	*Kaṣāya* (Astringent)
Predominant *Mahābhūta* (Element)	-	*Pṛthavī* (Earth) + *Vāyu* (Air)
Condition of *Doṣa*	-	Vitiation of *Kapha doṣa*
Activity of *Agni* (Digestive fire)	-	Slow or mild state
Strength	-	Moderate
Purification Therapy	-	*Vamana* (Emesis) and *Nasya* (Errhine) to pacify *Kapha doṣa*

• Effects on the body

The intensity of the sun's rays increase gradually, but steadily during this season. The warmth from the sun liquefies the *Kapha* accumulated in the body during winter. This vitiates *Kapha doṣa* and is the cause of cough, cold, a sore throat, low digestive power, nausea and the cause of diseases such as bronchial asthma, tonsilitis and sinusitis. Due to the changing environment, with an increased intensity of the sun and decrease in coolness of the moon, the moisture content and smoothness of the body reduces. This affects the body, which in turn causes a decline in body strength. Hence, one must be particular about diet. Eating sour, sweet and salty foods aggravates *Kapha* further.

• A compatible diet and living habits

The diet should be fresh, light and easily digestible. A diet including pungent, bitter and astringent tastes is recommended. The following food items are beneficial during spring:

Grains including *chapatis* (Indian bread) made of green gram, Bengal gram and barley flour, old wheat and rice, barley, Bengal gram, sprouted whole lentils, *chapatis* and bread spread with butter, roasted and flattened parched rice flakes. Vegetables such as green vegetables and their soup, bitter gourd, spinach, banana flowers, yams, radish, lemon and garlic are good. Spices and oils including dried ginger, long pepper, black pepper, mustard seed and mustard oil. All seasonal fruits and gooseberry. Medicinal herbs like myrobalan, belleric myrobalan, new leaves of margosa (*nīma*) and honey. Flavored water, vetiver (*khasa-khasa*) flavored water, water with ginger juice or honey is nourishing. Plenty of water should be drunk during spring. Rainwater can also be drunk.

Do light exercise and *yoga* regularly. A morning walk before sunrise improves health, massage with oil and medicated pastes followed by a warm water bath (or with fresh cold water, if one has the habit). Using fragrances like camphor, sandalwood, eagle wood (*agaru*), vermillion powder (*kuṁkuma*) and other aromatic substances after bathing keeps one fresh. Medicated smoking to reduce Kapha, and collyrium application in the eyes are beneficial. Induced vomiting (*vamana*) also reduces Kapha. Maintain proper hygiene in the excretory orifices. Use caps and umbrellas as a shield against the sun's rays whose intensity increases during this season.

- **Incompatible diet and living habits**

Do nnot consume heavy, oily, sour (such as tamarind, dry mango powder), sweet (sugar, jaggery) and cold foods. Avoid heavy foods such as new grains, black gram pulse, sweetened condensed milk (*rābaṟī*), cream and so on. The use of dates is also not recommended. Sleeping under the open sky (in the mist) and sleep in the day time are contra-indicated. Exposure to cold and sun is harmful.

- ***Grīṣma* (Summer season): Food regimen and living habits**

During this season the intense heat and powerful rays of the sun absorb all moisture content and oil from the body. The temperature suddenly shoots up increasing dryness and dullness. This is the peak of the *ādāna* period. Every living thing, from humans, animals, vegetation to water bodies which are inanimate get affected by the heat, dry and hot winds. Everything, everywhere experience only heat and high temperature.

***Grīṣma* (Summer)**		
Predominant *Rasa* (Taste)	-	*Kaṭu* (Pungent)
Predominant *Mahābhūta* (Element)	-	*Agni* (Fire) + *Vāyu* (Air)
Condition of *Doṣa*	-	Deposition of *Vāta doṣa*
		Pacification of *Kapha doṣa*
Activity of *Agni* (Digestive fire)	-	Mild state
Strength	-	Low

- **Effects on the body**

Summer is the season of dehydration, exhaustion, lack of energy and lethargy. In order to maintain health, strength and fitness, softness, smoothness and coolness are the prime requirements of the body. Just as vegetation becomes lifeless and dries up, so does the body in the absence of the above-mentioned qualities. Consequently, it corresponds to the weakening of all seven *dhātus* in the body, leading to depletion of strength. Sweat increases and so does thirst. Excessive water intake dilutes the acid content in the intestines, increasing the chances of bacterial colonization which might cause diarrhea, dysentry, vomiting, cholera and so on. Aggravated *Pitta* increases susceptibility to excessive thirst, fever, burning sensation, bleeding from the nose and other organs, dizziness and headache. For relief from these ailments and to maintain sufficient body strength during summer, *Āyurveda* recommends the following diet and living habits as a preventive measure from these effects on the body.

- **A compatible diet and living habits**

The diet in summer should include light, oily, sweet, easily digestible, cold and liquid foods in a higher ratio. Use boiled water after cooling in earthen pots.The following food items are recommended. The dairy products such as *ghee* (clarified butter), milk, buttermilk either with sugar or with salt and roasted cumin in the morning and afternoon (contra-indicated at night), milk with added *ghee* and crystal sugar, buffalo milk, *rāyatā* (a yogurt preparation including chopped fruits or vegetables and seasoning) and ice-creams are good. Grains include old barley, diluted coarse grain flour of barley and gram (*sattū*). Vegetables such as red leaved spinach, bitter gourd, chenopodium, pointed gourd, ripe tomatoes, unpeeled potatoes, unripe banana fruit curry, drum-stick, onion, ash gourd (*peṭhā*), mint, lemon and so on. Pulses like polished green gram, pigeon pea and lentils. Fruits such as watermelon, muskmelon, sweet mangoes, oranges, grapes, snake cucumber, mulberry, *phālasā* (berry of *grewia asiatica)* and pomegranates are healthy. Sweets such as gooseberry succade (*murabbā*) and sugar, and dryfruits such as raisins, currants, calumpang (charoli kernel), figs and soaked almonds are beneficial. Drinks including sweet fresh lime juice, juice of green unripe mango, sherbets, sweet diluted yogurt (*lassi*), Bengal quince sherbet (syrup), *ṭhaṇḍaī* (a cooling drink containing ground spices, musk melon seeds, almonds), sandalwood, *khasa-khasa* (vetiver) and rose sherbet, sugarcane, apple and sweet orange juice, water cooled with camphor and flavored with yellowsnake tree (*pātalā*) flowers, coconut water, and water cooled in the moonlight quenches thirst and heat. Pigeon pea pulse is dry, so garnish it with little *ghee* (clarified butter) and cumin seeds.

During summer, the diet should be reduced and food must be properly chewed. Only freshly cooked and warm food should be eaten. Eating refrigerated food after heating and reheating is harmful. Intake of food stored and refrigerated for a long period is unhealthy. Water cooled in an earthen pot is comparatively better than refrigerated water.

In order to avoid direct exposure to the sun's rays and prevention from heat, go for a walk in parks and gardens under the shade of tree as the sun's rays do not directly reach the ground. Rooms should be adequately cooled. The bedroom should have access to moonlight and fresh air. Sit on an 'Easy' chair, rest and enjoy the fresh air. Apply sandalwood paste to the body for coolness and adorn the body with pearl jewellery, as pearls have a cooling effect as well as calming and healing vibrations. They have anti-*Pitta* properties and also purify the blood. They are hemostatic; prevent hemorrhages from nose and gums. They have strengthening qualities and promote vigor and vitality. Cover the bed with banana and lotus leaves. Wear light-colored or white cotton clothes. Avoid moving out in the sunlight as far as possible.To prevent heatstroke, use comfortable and covered shoes, protective headgear and an umbrella. A glass of cool water before venturing out in the sunlight is helpful. It is believed (folk lore) that carrying an onion in the pocket also helps prevent heat stroke. If staying awake by late night, take a glass of cold water at frequent intervals to keep *Vāta* and *Kapha doṣas* in control and to prevent constipation. Dinner should be early, light and easily digestible. If possible, eat gruel in dinner, a couple of times in the week. Afternoon siesta in this season is not harmful.

- **Incompatible diet and living habits**

During summer, minimize the quantity of foods that are hot, dry, sour (tamarind, dry mango powder and so on), bitter, salty and astringent in tastes. Completely avoid heavy, fried, hot, spicy and stale foods, black gram pulse, garlic, mustard, brinjals, stale and sour yogurt, honey (honey can only be used as a medicine), ice and icy things. Savory snacks, *chutney*, other sour foods, sweets made of dried and condensed whole milk and ground black gram pulse preparations are harmful. Opposing foods must not be consumed. Drinking too much water at a time weakens the digestive fire. Instead, a glass of water at regular intervals is advisable. Sudden exposure to contrasting temperatures is dangerous. For example, walking out in the blazing sun from a cold room or drinking cold water immediately after being under the sun for a while. Drink water only when sweat evaporates and body temperature normalizes. It is ideal to mix refrigerated water with normal water kept at room temperature. Alcoholic drinks are completely prohibited. Those who are addicted to them must dilute the drinks as much as possible.

During summer, the following living habits must also be limited: awakening for long at night (as the nights are shorter in summer), prolonged exposure to the sun, being out in the sunlight without protective headgear, suppressing hunger and thirst for a longer duration, over exercising, suppressing the urge for urination and defecation, and sexual activity. *Āyurveda* prohibits sexual activity in summer; if the desire persists, as far as possible perform coitus in a regulated way.

- ***Varṣā* (Monsoon season): Food regimen and living habits**

The rainy season appears at the commencement of *visarga* period. It is characterized by greenery and humidity in the environment, and cloudy weather conditions. Humidity causes an increase in the number of insects such as mosquitoes and flies, and unhygienic conditions prevail around.

- **Effects on the body**

The increased humidity has its effect on the body. Increased moisture caused by the rain vitiates *Vāta doṣa* and reduces the digestive power that has already weakened during summer. The digestive power is also affected by environmental conditions, dust and smoke, increased sourness in food stuffs and gases released from the earth due to the rains. In between, if it does not rain for a few days, the intensity of heat increases causing accumulation of *Pitta doṣa*. The nutritive value of wheat, rice and other grains also reduces. Also more chances of infection increases susceptibility to malaria, filaria, coryza, diarrhea, dysentery, cholera, colitis, *alasaka* (retension of undigested food in the abdomen), arthritis, inflammation in the joints, high blood pressure, impurities of the blood causing pimples or boils, ringworm, itching and several other disorders.

***Varṣā* (Monsoon)**		
Predominant *Rasa* (Taste)	-	*Amla* (Sour)
Predominant *Mahābhūta* (Element)	-	*Pṛthavī* (Earth) + *Agni* (Fire)
Condition of *Doṣa*	-	Vitiation of *Vāta doṣa*, deposition of *Pitta doṣa*
Activity of *Agni* (Digestive fire)	-	Gets vitiated
Strength	-	Low
Purification Therapy	-	*Basti* (Enema) to pacify *Vāta doṣa*

- **A compatible diet and living habits**

The diet during the monsoon should include substances that are light, fresh, hot and easily digestible; and those that strengthen the digestive fire. They should be capable of pacifying *Vāta doṣa*. Hence, the diet recommended includes dairy products such as yogurt and buttermilk, sweet diluted yogurt or buttermilk flavored with cloves, *trikaṭu* (dry ginger, black pepper and long pepper), rock salt, thymol (carom) seeds and black salt which keeps digestion strong. Roasted corn is easily digested if followed by buttermilk. Also, old grains such as wheat, barley, unpolished rice and corn are reccommended; pulses such as green gram and pigeon pea; vegetables such as bottle gourd, lady finger, angled loofah (*turaī*), tomatoes, cucumber and mustard; and fruits such as apple, banana, pomegranate, pear, blackberry and ripe mangoes. Mangoes and milk are particularly beneficial. Mangoes must be ripe, sweet and fresh. They can cause harm if unripe and sour. Drinking milk after eating a ripe mango is nourishing. This combination helps the body gain strength and stability, so it can even replace a meal. Similarly, regular use of ripe blackberries heals boils and pimples, burning, and skin and urinary diseases. Garlic and mint *chutney*, salty dishes made in clarified butter (*ghee*) and oil, gruel, vegetable soups, linseed and honey in water or with other substances (that are not hot in potency) are also beneficial in this season.

To calm *Vāta* and *Kapha doṣa* in this season, substances with bitter, sour and salty taste should be included in the diet. Sour, salty and oily foods calm *Vāta*, especially when the weather cools down due to heavy rains and winds. Water purification should be ascertained before consumption. Properly harvested rainwater is the purest form of water and is beneficial. Underground water should preferably be boiled and cooled before drinking. Water can also be treated and purified by adding holy basil leaves and a pinch of alum powder. Nowadays, water filters, reverse osmosis and other modern techniques are very helpful for this purpose. Adding honey in purified and cold water is advantageous. Massage with oil, application of *ubaṭana* and fomentation is beneficial. Wear clean and light clothes and immediately change wet clothes. Sleep in a place which is not exposed to wind and rain. Take food on time and only when hungry. Dinner should be eaten early. To prevent mosquito bites use mosquito nets. Keep the surrounding area clean and use an insecticidal spray for stagnant water because it is a dwelling place for mosquitoes and other insects. Maintain proper environmental cleanliness.

- **Incompatible diet and living habits**

Cold and dry foods are incompatible. Harmful during this season are pulses such as black gram, Turkish gram, lentils and Bengal gram; grains such as Indian millet, barley, coarse grain flour of gram and barley (*sattū*); vegetables such as potatoes, jack fruit, bitter gourd, leafy vegetables and peas; and fruits such as water chestnuts. A lesser amount of rain in the monsoon aggravates *Pitta doṣa*. In such conditions, avoid sour, fried, hot and spicy, stale and other *Pitta* aggravating foods and eatables made from gram flour. According to a proverb, consumption of milk in *śrāvaṇa* (July-August), buttermilk in *bhādrapada* (August-September), bitter gourd in *kvāra* (September-October) and yogurt in *kārtika* (October-November) are not recommended. Incompatible habits include siesta, sleeping outside in sunlight, exposure to the sun, excessive sexual indulgence, excessive walking and exercising. Taking a heavy diet, eating frequently, and eating without hunger should also be avoided.

Completely avoid yogurt and buttermilk at night. Do not wear wet and damp clothes and avoid sleeping on a wet bed. Keep the joints of the body, especially the thigh joints and the genital organs dry. Wash vegetables and fruits thoroughly before use. Never use impure water from rivers and ponds, drink only purified water. Drive vehicles at normal speed to prevent skidding. Rubbing ice cubes or applying other effective medicines to the body gives relief from prickly heat. One can enjoy the rainy season to its fullest by following the above diet and lifestyle tips.

- ***Śarad* (Autumn season): Food regimen and living habits**

This season is characterized by the presence of clear clouds and a beautiful sky, the rays of the moon become effective, stronger, clean, smooth and pleasant which evoke contentment. Moonlight and the sun's rays lend purity to rivers, lakes and ponds. The sour taste becomes predominant in vegetation and medicinal herbss.

- **Effects on the body**

During the monsoon, the body gets accustomed to the seasonal effect and cool weather. After the monsoon, in the autumn, the sun shines with full intensity, resulting in the vitiation of *Pitta doṣa* which has accumulated in the body during monsoon. This also vitiates the blood. As a result, there is an increased susceptibility to *Pitta* and blood disorders such as fever, boils, pimples, rashes, scrofula, itching and so on. Being in the middle of the *visarga* period, physical strength is medium, neither abnormally high nor very low.

Śarad (Autumn)

Predominant *Rasa* (Taste)	-	*Lavana* (Salty)
Predominant *Mahābhūta* (Element)	-	*Jala* (*Water*) + *Agni* (Fire)
Condition of *Doṣa*	-	Vitiation of *Pitta doṣa*, pacification of *Vāta doṣa*
Activity of *Agni* (Digestive fire)	-	Increases
Strength	-	Moderate
Purification Therapy	-	*Virecana* (Purgation) and *Rakta mokṣaṅa* (Blood-letting) to pacify vitiated *Pitta*

- **A compatible diet and living habits**

Clarified butter *(ghee)* and foods with bitter taste are ideal to pacify vitiated *Pitta*. Other favorable foods include substances that are light and cool in their attributes, sweet and bitter in taste, and easily digestible. Good for this season are dairy products such as boiled milk, yogurt, butter, clarified butter (*ghee*), cream and *śrīkhaṇḍa* (sweet, flavored and condensed yogurt); grains such as unpolished rice, wheat and barley; vegetables such as red leaved spinach, chenopodium, bottle gourd, angled loofah, cauliflower, radish, spinach and beans; pulses and beans such as green gram and soyabeans; fruits and dried fruits such as pomegranates, water chestnuts, Indian gooseberries, currants and lotus seeds. Indian gooseberries should be eaten with sugar. Cook bitter things in clarified butter. Use water treated with the sun's rays during the day time and moonlight at night. In this season, due to the effects of the star canopus (*agastya*), water becomes free of impurities and is considered as good as nectar. Besides drinking, the use of such water in bathing and swimming is also good for health. Such water is called '*haṁsodaka*' by *Ācārya Caraka*.

Purgation (with laxative medicines) and blood-letting therapies pacify vitiated blood and *Pitta*. This guards against corresponding *doṣaja* ailments.

Use seasonal flowers as an ornament for adornment. Walking, sleeping or resting in the moonlight gives a good effect to the body.

- **Incompatible diet and living habits**

Reduce oily foods and mustard oil in this season. Avoid dairy products such as buttermilk and yogurt; spices and condiments such as fennel seed, asafoetida, black pepper, long pepper; vegetables such as garlic, brinjal and bitter gourd; heavy dishes made of black gram pulses; sour foods like *kaḍhī* (gram flour and yogurt curry), alkaline substances and strong alcoholic substances; and food with salty taste in the diet. Eating without hunger is harmful. Protect yourself from exposure to the sun, dew and the West winds. Excessive exercise and sexual indulgence is also harmful.

- **Suitable food types in different seasons**

Spring	Foods with pungent, bitter and astringent tastes; dry and hot foods and drinks.
Summer	Foods with sweet taste; oily and cool foods and drinks.
Monsoon	Foods with sweet, sour and salty tastes; oily and hot foods.
Autumn	Foods with sweet, pungent and astringent tastes; dry and cool foods and drinks.
Early winter	Foods with sweet, sour and salty tastes; oily and hot foods.
Late winter	Foods with sweet, sour and salty tastes; oily and hot foods.

Though food with all six tastes should be consumed during all seasons, the type of food based on the predominant taste in a particular season should be increased accordingly in the diet.

Ṛtusandhi is the transition phase between two seasons; it includes the last week of the preceding season and first week of the coming season. At this time, it is important to remember that diet and lifestyle should not be changed abruptly with the change in season. This will cause imbalance and disharmony in the body leading to ailments. Food and lifestyle habits should be modified gradually at the time of transition between two seasons (*ṛtusandhi*).

According to *Acāryas*, the transition phase between the two seasons, especially the last week of October and the first week of November is known as '*Yamadaṁṣṭrā*.' During this period strictly follow seasonal regimen because at this time due to seasonal changes aggravation of *Pitta* leads to the genesis of fever and other seasonal disorders. This is typically the time when seasonal cold and flu strike. These are the times where you want to especially adhere to your body-type regimen.

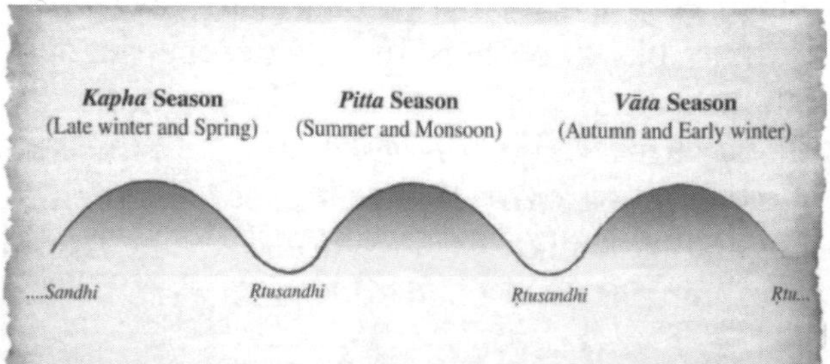

Ṛtusandhi

There is a continous transformation in the external and internal environment with the change in season. *Doṣas* accumulated in the previous season and our basic constitution governed by *tridoṣa* (internal environment) and the external environment constantly change with the change in season. Hence, at this time, special attention should be paid to food habits, lifestyle and *yoga* practice. These are the preventive measures, which keep oneself free from the effects of seasonal changes and the disorders provoked by these changes. The *Āyurvedic* seasonal routine is just another way to encourage your body's own natural instincts to emerge and match the rhythm of nature.

5. Suppression of Natural Urges: Unretainable Urges

It has been commonly experienced that to avoid eating when hungry leads to a sudden drop in energy level. Similarly, the body feels tired and lifeless if thirst is not quenched. Thirst might cause dizziness and syncope. To avoid urination or fecal elimination on experiencing an urge to do so, leads to pain in the bladder and one may develop flatus and other symptoms, respectively. Hunger and thirst, the urge to discharge body wastes and other such urges develop naturally in the body. These are the natural urges of the body. These urges are felt by all conscious people. Timely satisfaction of these urges is paramount to good health. Interfering with the natural action of the urges provokes *Vāta*, and thereby postponing or ignoring them can lead to various kinds of ailments. There are thirteen main urges listed in *Āyurveda,* which are as follows:

1. The urge for urination
2. The urge for defecation
3. The urge for seminal ejaculation
4. The urge for passing flatus
5. The urge for emesis or vomiting
6. The urge for sneezing
7. The urge for belching (eructation)
8. The urge for yawning
9. The urge for hunger
10. The urge for thirst
11. The urge for tears (weeping)
12. The urge for rapid breathing or hyper-breathing
13. The urge for sleep

There are some contradictory views regarding these 13 non-suppressible urges in some *Āyurvedic* texts. They count the non-suppressible urge to discharge urine and fecal matter (Nos.1and 2) as one and consider cough as a separate urge, thus maintaining the number of total urges to be 13. Hyper-breathing due to physical work is counted as number 12, and this is associated with the trachea. Therefore the urge to cough has been included in the urge for hyper-breathing and not as a separate identity.

Usually for the sake of good conduct, manners and etiquette, some urges are suppressed forcefully. Among these urges, sneezing and flatus in gathering or public places are commonly suppressed. Such tendency of suppression is more common in women. It is clearly specified in *Āyurvedic* treatises that when such natural urges develop, allow them to occur. Suppressing the urge to expel flatus, fecal elimination and urination develops a serious disease named *udāvarta* (circulation of flatus in the upward direction in the abdomen). Also, other diseases occur due to the inhibition of these non-suppressible urges.

- **Suppression of the urge to cough**

When a patient suppresses the urge to cough forcefully, it not only causes an increase in cough, but also results in hyper-breathing, anorexia and cardiac diseases. The chances of tuberculosis, emaciation and hiccoughs may also develop. For this, anti-cough treatment is required.

- **Incurable symptoms of urge suppression**

In *Āyurveda*, as a consequence of suppression of the above-mentioned urges, if a person is not benefitted even by medication and the following symptoms are also visible, then the patient is said to be incurable. These symptoms are:

1. Increased thirst and suffering from pain
2. Patient turning emaciated
3. Vomiting of toxic food

All these diseases are caused by the forced initiation or inhibition of urges. On the other hand, if one excretes forcefully, this also may result in disease. In such conditions, the majority of diseases develop due to aggravated *Vāta*. Therefore, to pacify them, carminative substances, certain foods, liquids and medicines should be used.

When natural urges are forcefully suppressed or not expelled in time, then they develop into suppressed urges. They are described below:

- **Suppression of the urge for urination:** Suppressing the urge to urinate leads to pain in the bladder, genital organs, lower abdomen, kidney, urethra and urinary canal. It causes dysuria, headache, flatulence, distension in the lower abdomen, drooping of the body and other complications such as bodyaches, calculi (stones), weakening of the urinary bladder, inflammation and infection in the urinary tract.

_**Treatment:** These can be treated with tub baths, abdominal massage, instilling drops of *ghee* in the nose and by three types of enema therapies (*āsthāpana basti*, *uttara basti* and *anuvāsana basti*). Besides, therapies to reduce inflammation in the urinary tract and medicines to strengthen the urinary bladder and to reduce the infection should be prescribed. According to *Āyurveda*, intake of '*avapīḍaka ghṛta*' is effective. The intake of *ghee* in a good amount before food and also after the digestion of food is termed as '*avapīḍaka ghṛta.*'

- **Suppression of the urge for defecation:** Avoiding or postponing defecation (at its natural call) can cause acute pain, headache, obstruction of flatus and feces, cold, constipation, cramps in calf muscles, distension in the lower abdomen, obstructed heart beat and toxic vomits.

  _**Treatment:** Treatment includes *sveda* (fomentation), *abhyaṅga* (massage), *avagāha* (tub-bath), *varti* (inserting suppositories in the anus) and *basti karma* (enemas). Purgative foods such as papaya, green vegetables, fruit juices and other laxative foods and drinks are helpful.

- **Suppression of the urge for seminal ejaculation:** Suppressing the urge for seminal ejaculation leads to pain in the genital organs and testicles, inflammation, fever, wheezing, pain in the cardiac region and retention of urine. It can also lead to bodyache, frequent stretching and yawning, hydrocele, calculi and impotency.

  _**Treatment:** Treatment for such complications includes massage, tub-bath, oil-free enema, eating unpolished rice and milk. Milk boiled with diuretic medicines such as caltrope (*gokharū*) is also effective. To prevent unnecessary seminal discharge, avoid sexual intercourse, and also avoid desire-provoking literature, videos, photographs and excited talks. Along with such regimen, refrain from heavy, spicy and *tāmasika* food, and consume *sāttvika* food.

- **Suppression of the urge for passing flatus:** Suppressing the urge to pass flatus (suppressing the urge to evacuate flatus, when it moves downward in the abdomen and gets accumulated there) aggravates the *Vāta doṣa*. It prevents elimination of urine, feces and flatus leading to constipation and pain with distension in the lower abdomen, exhaustion and other digestive disorders. It may also result in eye disorders, disturbed heartbeat and indigestion due to sluggish digestive fire.

_**Treatment:** Treatment includes intake of and massage with oily substances (*snehana*) like clarified butter (*ghee*) and oil, fomentation, suppositories and enemas. Consume digestive and carminative foods and drinks. Also avoid the suppression to pass flatus.

- **Suppression of the urge to vomit:** Suppressing the desire to vomit may cause itching, urticaria, dermatitis, anorexia, edema, freckles, fever, anemia, nausea, cough, bronchial asthma, eye disorders, erysipelas and other skin diseases.

  _**Treatment:** Treatment includes induced vomiting using medicines, gargles, medicated smoking, fasting, blood-letting, purgation, along with exercise and eating dry foods. In erysipelas, massage with oil containing a salt or an alkali is useful.

- **Suppression of the urge for sneezing:** Its obstruction may lead to headache, strokes or paralysis, migraine, weakness of the sense organs, and spasmodic torticollis (stiffness of the neck muscles).

  _**Treatment:** The treatment includes massage and fomentation between the head and neck, medicated smoking, use of nasal drops. Use of clarified butter (*ghee*) after food is especially beneficial. *Vāta* pacifying medication and food should be consumed.

- **Suppression of the urge for eructation or belching:** Its obstruction can cause hiccoughs, breathlessness, tremors, anorexia, malfunctioning of the heart and lungs, flatulence and cough.

  _**Treatment:** Treatment includes carminative herbs, purgation and other remedies to control hiccoughs.

- **Suppression of the urge for yawning:** Its restriction can cause convulsions, contractions, postural problems, numbness and tremors in the organs.

  _**Treatment:** Treatment consists of medicines and substances that pacify *Vāta*.

- **Suppression of the urge for hunger:** Avoiding food when hungry can create problems of emaciation, weakness, debility, anorexia, dizziness, wheezing and a change in complexion. Besides, it may also lead to spasmodic torticollis, facial paralysis, strokes, liver disorders and other related disorders.

  _**Treatment:** To get rid of such complications, take light and oily food at an appropriate time, when hungry.

- **Suppression of the urge for thirst:** Ignoring thirst may cause dryness of the throat and mouth, deafness, exhaustion, debility, cardiac pain and dizziness.

  _**Treatment:** Treatment consists of cool and refreshing drinks. Do not drink water in excess and at one time. Drink at intervals throughout the day.

- **Suppression of the urge for tears (weeping):** Tears are produced due to grief or when the heart is touched by other emotions. Avoiding crying can cause emotional disorders, rhinitis, eye disorders, cardiac diseases, anorexia, dizziness and other complications.

  _**Treatment:** Treatment consists of a good sleep, use of *āsava, ariṣṭa* and other medicines, staying exhilarated and cheerful, laughing and joking.

- **Suppression of the urge for hyper-breathing caused due to physical activities:** Excessive exercise, running or other physical activities increases the heart rate and also the breath rate. As a result, it causes breathlessness or increased heartbeat, which is known as hyper-breathing. When one tries to suppress this rapid breath forcefully, then *prāṇa* and *udāna vāyu* gets vitiated, resulting in the emergence of lung and heart disorders related to damage of the valves. At times, this practice obstructs the breath, resulting in syncope. It may also lead to other cardiac disorders and phantom tumors.

  _**Treatment:** It requires rest, along with food and a lifestyle that alleviates *Vāta*.

- **Suppression of the urge for sleep:** Suppression of the urge to sleep results in yawning, exhaustion, lethargy, malaise, drowsiness, headache, heaviness in the eyes, dark circles under the eyes and dizziness.

  _**Treatment:** Treatment requires sufficient and good sleep and complete rest. Also helpful is body massage, *Vāta* pacifying diet, drugs and lifestyle changes.

The interference in the natural action of these urges provokes *Vāta* and thereby causes ailments. Therefore, for healthy living, these natural urges should be eliminated at the correct time and in a proper manner. Do not suppress them. To keep healthy eliminate these urges at the time they 'give a natural call.' Otherwise, inhibition may lead to deterioration of health.

6. *Dhāraṇīya Vega*: Retainable Urges

Besides the above-mentioned irresistable urges, each one of us develops certain tendencies by nature that are harmful to ourselves and our society. They are the urges which can be retained. These negative tendencies spring from feelings of greed, fear, anger, grief, envy, pride, hostility, shamelessness and attachment. Actions are performed according to these tendencies, but to lead an exhilarated and contented life, it is very important to keep these urges under control and avoid acting under their influence.

- **Suppressible or retainable urges:** There are certain urges whose suppression is essential. These suppressible (retainable) urges are divided into three types:

1. **Mental urges:** Greed, malice, envy, infatuation, anger, grief, fear, ego, hatred, shamelessness, treason and so on.
2. **Vocal urges:** Undignified and uncivilized speech due to anger, unnecessary and excessive talking, backbiting, repeated talks, untimely and inappropriate or digressive talk. All these urges are related to speech. These are restrainable urges.
3. **Physical urges:** Violent attitude, indisciplined actions such as thrashing, robbing, rape, theft and such other urges are considered to be physical urges. Suppression of these urges will save you from illegal, undignified, unsocial and unethical conduct.

One can refrain from these urges if one contemplates the losses which will result from these impulsive urges. This will help maintain mental peace for oneself and one's family. People who control their behavior are dignified and respectable in society. By keeping a check on retainable urges and a good code of conduct, a person can fullfill all his duties related to *dharma* (religious and ethical principles), *artha* (material wealth) and *kāma* (desire or lust). So these suppressible urges, if retained and kept under control, can result in attainment of all these goals in life efficiently. Therefore, they are meant for the complete welfare of a human being.

Chapter 6
Dietary Facts and Rules

It is a well-known fact that food is vital for health, and it is important to know, that, what to eat, when to eat and how to eat? Only then, we can enjoy all the benefits that food offers us. Some important facts about food are given below. [PLATE 19]

1. Facts About Food

- **Oily food(1)**

Our diet should contain adequate amount of *ghee* (clarified butter), oil and other oily substances. In today's life, the fear of heart diseases, high blood pressure and obesity causes one to lean towards oil-free diet and to avoid oily foodstuffs. This is not a very rational approach. Clarified butter (*ghee*) and other oils stimulate the appetite, enrich taste, soften food, activate the digestive fire and hasten digestion, strengthen the body, stabilize the sensory and motor organs, enhance the complexion, help in the carmination of *Vāta* and aid in smooth elimination of waste materials. Hence, instead of abandoning *ghee* from the diet, ward off laziness and adopt the habit of exercise and physical workouts to enjoy the benefits of oily foods.

- **Fresh and warm food(2)**

Always take freshly prepared and warm food. Such food tastes pleasing, it is nourishing, easy to digest, increases digestive fire, boosts digestion and carminates *Vāta*. Cold and stale food is heavy, *tāmasika* and not nourishing. *Āyurveda* does not recommend the consumption of frozen food, neither does it recommend the use of canned foods, canned and bottled juices and other drinks, instant foods with added preservatives, and cakes and pastries which

1. *Snigdhamaśnīyāt, snigdhaṁ hi bhujyamānaṁ svadate, bhuktaṁ cānudīrṇamagnimudīrayati, kṣipraṁ jarāṁ gacchati, vātamanulomayati, śarīramupacinoti dṛḍhīkarotindriyāṇi, balābhivṛddhimupajanayati, varṇaprasādaṁcābhinivartayati.* (*Ca.vi.* 1/24 [2])
2. *Uṣṇamaśnīyāta uṣṇaṁ hi bhujyamānaṁ svadate, bhuktaṁ cāgnimaudāryamudīrayati, kṣipraṁ jarāṁ gacchāti, vātamanulomayati śleṣmāṇaṁ ca parihrāsyati, tasmāduṣṇamaśnīyāt.* (*Ca.vim.* 1/24 [1])

are commonly eaten nowadays. Packaged foods and other fast foods that are eaten with great enthusiasm and appetite are the cause for obesity. Nowadays, obesity is spreading like an epidemic in the entire world, because of these canned and preserved foods, packaged snacks and other high-density foods. The genesis of most diseases is a result of wrong food habits, inappropriate diet and a faulty lifestyle. Food habits which are not conducive to good health should be omitted. Drink natural and fresh juices and do not consume stale food.

- **Appearance and presentation of food**

The color, aroma, touch and taste of the food make it attractive, enhance our appetite and stimulate the secretion of digestive juices. Hence, to stimulate the appetite, attention must be paid to its presentation and garnishing. Besides, clean and attractive utensils and crockery with a pleasing dining area make eating a really enjoyable affair. This is particularly true for patients, as the regular intake of bland, restricted and simple diet reduces their appetite and may cause to develop anorexia.

- **A congenial environment**

Along with food, the place where food is eaten should be clean, pleasant and peaceful. When possible, food should not be taken alone. Eat along with others. Clean, spiritual and aesthetic places bring peace of mind, whereas unhygienic or disorganized surroundings disturb peace of mind, which adversely affects the appetite and the entire digestive process. Eating food should be considered a pious activity and be performed with earnestness and concentration. Avoid eating while watching the television, talking on the telephone or with any distracting activity. *Āyurveda* does not recommend eating food while wearing footwear. Footwear slows down the digestive fire due to the heat released from the feet, which can result in several disorders. Therefore, *Āyurveda* recommends washing the hands and feet, cleaning and wiping them and sitting on the floor while eating. Never eat food while standing. Pray before eating, be grateful to nature's unending gift in the form of food and respect it as you do yourself. Drink 2-3 sips of water before eating, which enhances the digestive fire and clears the passage from throat onwards, where *Kapha* is accumulated. Then peacefully eat with the fingers, which help one to feel the nature of the food; hot or cold, and the touch helps to develop interest and liking for the food. If it is not possible to sit on the floor to eat, then use a dining table, but restrain yourself from eating food while standing or moving.

- **Mental state**

Negative emotions have a harmful effect on digestion. Eat food in a pleasant and peaceful state of mind. One does not enjoy the taste of food when food is eaten in an emotionally disturbed state of mind. Also, the secretion of digestive juices is hampered, affecting digestion. Hence, eat food when at ease and avoid unpleasant discussions, watching television, reading or thinking about disturbing subjects while eating.

- **An appropriate time for food intake**

"***Kāla bhojanam-Ārogya karaṇam***" (*Caraka Saṁhitā,* source 25:40) means the best remedy for health or a disease-free life is to take food on time. For proper and complete digestion, it is of vital importance that food should be eaten only at appropriate and regular hours. A few things must be kept in mind while deciding the appropriate time to eat. Food should only be consumed under the following circumstances:

- When experiencing hunger.
- After complete digestion of the previous meal. If food is eaten before the complete digestion of preceding meal, its undigested *rasa* gets mixed with the rasa of the fresh meal, thus vitiating all the *doṣas* and making the body susceptible to a variety of ailments.
- If one does not experience eructation from the last meal.
- When there is no feeling of heaviness in the heart or stomach, after carmination of *Vāta*.
- After elimination of waste matter (urine and feces).

The body gains more strength if food is eaten during the period of *Pitta* aggravation (between 12 to 2 pm), as it gets digested very quickly. As a result, maximum nutrition is derived. Ignoring hunger at its natural time leads to migraine, weakness, fatigue, emaciation, body aches, lethargy, anorexia, changes in skin tone and weakening of the eyesight.

> It is a common practice that hunger naturally arises at definite hours of eating. Something must always be eaten at such a time as sufficient amounts of digestive juices are then being secreted. If nothing is eaten at that time, these secretions vitiate Pitta causing damage to the body. If food is eaten thereafter, it does not get properly digested, due to reduced activity of digestive enzymes owing to the effects of aggravated Vata after the regular mealtime.

- **Moderate quantity of food**

To obtain maximum nutrition, food should be taken in an appropriate quantity. A good practice in this context is to leave one-third to one-quarter of the stomach empty after eating, to aid digestion. This is essential for proper mixing of digestive juices and *Kapha* with food, so as to smoothen the food for proper assimilation. It also regularizes the movement of *Vāta* within the system. The following conditions indicate that the food has been consumed in a balanced manner and in an appropriate quantity:

- When hunger and thirst are satiated after a meal.
- The absence of heaviness and pressure in the stomach.
- The absence of heaviness and tightness in the chest.
- When one does not face any difficulty in various activities such as standing, sitting, sleeping, walking, laughing, breathing or talking.
- After complete digestion of the previous meal.
- Upon the carmination of *Vāta*.
- The absence of any kind of disturbance in the *doṣas*, *dhātus* and *malas*.

While deciding the appropriate quantity of food to be eaten, keep in mind your own body-type (*prakṛti*), age, digestive capacity, lightness of food, intensity of the digestive fire and digestibility of food. If a person with a strong digestive power overeats or consumes heavy food, he will not be affected much, but even a little overeating or heavy food consumed by someone with weak digestive power can be very uncomfortable. Larger quantities of light foods like unpolished rice and green gram are easily digestible, but if consumed in bulk, they also take a longer time to digest like the heavy foods. Similarly, heavier foods like black gram, if eaten in small portions, can be easily assimilated and also can be made more digestible by adding spices such as asafoetida, thymol seeds (*ajavāyana*) and ginger. In brief, an inadequate quantity of food results in dissatisfaction and does not satiate or provide complete energy. On the other hand, excessive eating causes lethargy, heaviness, obesity and indigestion. Hence, it is suggested to eat only when hungry, according to one's digestive capacity, niether inadequate nor in excess, but in a moderate amount.

- **Importance of chewing**

The first step in the digestive process is softening of food in the mouth by saliva. This is possible ofirst step in the digestive process is softening of food in the mouth by saliva. This is possible only when food is properly chewed. The more it is chewed, the more it gets liquefied and more easily it will get digested. On the contrary, if not chewed properly, the delicate digestive organs have to put in some extra- efforts in order to break down the solid food before absorption, which leads to the weakening of the digestive system. Besides, it hampers complete assimilation of food, resulting in acidity, constipation, indigestion, flatulence and other such disorders. Hence, one should swallow the food only after proper chewing and softening. It has been said that "drink solid foods and chew liquid foods," which means to chew the solid food so well that it gets churned and becomes smooth and liquefied, which can easily be sipped while eating; whereas do not drink liquids instantly, but take sip by sip, which gives an illusion of chewing food while drinking.

- **Suitability of diet**[(3)]

Suitability means usefulness or favorable or compatible diet. A diet that suits and benefits one person maymeans usefulness or favorable or compatible diet. A diet that suits and benefits one person may not necessarily be compatible for another. That is why it is important to match your *prakṛti*; your natural make-up, with the correct diet and carefully select your diet. The following table is about qualities of food that affect the *doṣas*.

Table 19: Selection of Food Types According to the *Prakṛti* (Constitution)

	Balances		Aggravates	
	Food taste	Food attribute	Food taste	Food attribute
Vāta	Sweet	Heavy	Pungent	Light
	Sour	Oily	Bitter	Dry
	Salty	Hot	Astringent	Cold
Pitta	Sweet	Cold	Pungent	Hot
	Bitter	Heavy	Sour	Light
	Astringent	Dry	Salty	Oily
Kapha	Pungent	Light	Sweet	Heavy
	Bitter	Dry	Sour	Oily
	Astringent	Hot	Salty	Cold

It is only through practice and experience that we learn what kind of diet suits us best. A compatible diet and favorable foods provide maximum nutritional benefits, whereas incompatible and unfavorable foods can harm the body. Suitability of food is dependent on the following factors:

- **Body:** There are suitable diets based on different body constitutions according to the predominant *doṣa*. For example, persons with a *Kapha* constitution should take hot and light food.
- **Region:** There are suitable diets with respect to geographical location. For example, rice is good for people living in Bengal, Kashmir and in the Southern part of India.

3. *Tatra sātmyaṁ nāma sahātmanā bhavatyabhyastaṁ tadaucityādupaśet ityeke. Sātmyaviparītamanupaśayādasātmyam.* (*A.saṅ.sū.* 10/27)

- **Season:** There are also diets which are favorable according to the season. For example, hot and oily foods are beneficial in winter while cold foods are suitable in summer.
- **Ailments:** A diet must be chosen keeping in mind the nature of the ailment one is suffering from. Food chosen according to the nature of the illness helps in quick recovery and regaining complete health. For example, ginger juice and honey for the common cold and gruel for diarrhea.

Food taken while keeping all these facts in mind preserves health and prevents ailments. Adopting the above-mentioned food habits and principles of eating helps to gain maximum nourishment from the food, maintains the health of all the *doṣas* and *dhātus* and aids in proper elimination of *malas* (waste products). All these rules together constitute the *'Āhāra Saṁhitā'* (dietary facts). Eating should be taken as a serious and personalized activity. Do not disrupt the diet routine in spite of being busy and this personal eating activity should be performed with sincerity and concentration.

An individual, who takes a compatible and appropriate diet, normally does not fall ill. However, if for some reason he is afflicted by a disease, merely controlling and regulating the diet ensures speedy recovery without any medication. Taking the right medication, but neglecting a compatible diet makes recovery very difficult. An incompatible diet and lifestyle aggravates the disease, negates the effect of medication, because without curing the cause, disease cannot be cured. Therefore, a combination of right medication and an appropriate diet is essential for overcoming ailments and regaining complete health. It is correctly said that "a person taking a compatible diet does not require any medication and with incompatible diet, even medication is of no use:"

"Pathye sati gadārtasya kimauṣadhaniṣevaṇaiḥ.
Apathye, sati gadārtasya kimauṣadhaniṣevaṇaiḥ".

or in other words:

"Vināpi bheṣaajairvyādhiḥ pathyādeva nivartate.
Na tu pathyavihīnasya bheṣajānāṁ stairapi."

"In the absence of medication, disease can be treated by taking the right kind of diet, but if the right diet is not maintained, all medicines turn ineffective."

2. A Compatible Diet[4]

While following all these rules for good food habits, one must also insure that the food taken is compatible and beneficial for health.

> A compatible and beneficial diet is one that nourishes all the dhatus of the body and keeps them in a state of equilibrium, and also helps to restore balance between them when disrupted, does not block the body channels and satiates the mind.

In a diet that blocks the body channels, is incapable of maintaining balance between the *dhātus*, causes harm and is non-satiating, is an incompatible and non-beneficial diet. A compatible and beneficial food and lifestyle are very important factors for a healthy life. Factors that determine whether a diet is compatible or incompatible vary from person to person. What is compatible for one person might be incompatible for another. The suitability of a diet varies according to a person°s age, body constitution, nature, season, region, quantity of a particular substance and its compatibility with other substances. For a person with a hot temperament, cool potency substances are compatible, but for a cool natured person they are considered incompatible. In diarrhea, milk is incompatible whereas yogurt is compatible, but in constipation it is *vice versa* - milk is compatible but not yogurt.

Some foods/substances are by nature compatible or incompatible. Unpolished rice, barley, green gram, rock salt, Indian gooseberry, currants, milk, *ghee*, honey and rainwater are compatible by nature. In contrast unripe fruits; bitter foods such as red chillies and sour foods such as tamarind, dry mango powder; fermented and preserved foods are harmful.

Also, if compatible foods are not eaten in proper quantity and according to their nature, in an appropriate way, they can also behave like incompatible. Hence, a compatible diet should be carefully selected with respect to the quantity, age, region, season and ailments. Food builds up the body, so it must be consumed sensibly by examining a compatible diet for oneself. Greed and ignorance must not be allowed to dictate our diet as it can only

4. *Pathyaṁ patho, napetaṁ yadyaccoktaṁ manasaḥ priyam.*
Yaccāpriyamapathyaṁ ca niyataṁ tanna lakṣayet. (*Ca.sū.* 25/45)
Mātrākālakriyābhūmidehadoṣaguṇāntaram.
Prāpya tattaddhi dṛśyante te te bhāvāratahā tathā. (*Ca.sū.* 25/46)
Tasmāt svabhāvo nirdiṣṭastathā mātrādirāśrayaḥ.
Tadapekṣyobhayaṁ karma prayojyaṁ siddhimicchatā. (*Ca.sū.* 25/47)
Āhitāgniḥ sadā pathyānyantargnau juhoti yaḥ.
Divase divase brahma jayatyatha dadāti ca.
Naraṁ niḥśreyase yuktaṁ sātmyajñaṁ pānabhojane.
Bhajante nāmayāḥ kecid bhāvino, pyantarādṛte. (*Ca.sū.* 27/346-347)

lead to disorders and imbalances, causing various ailments. Whatever food we take, ultimately becomes a part of the seven *dhātus* and it remains in our body throughout life. It is advantageous not to take the wrong food or substances even once. In a similar manner, whatever thought comes into our mind reaches the brain as a neuro-chemical, which then becomes a part of the body. The food we take (be it alcohol, tobacco, milk, vegetables, cereals, fruits and so on), and whatever thoughts, negative or positive (whether it increases pain, stress, misery, unhappiness, lust, anger, fear, happiness and contentment) deeply affects the body right from the DNA of an individual to the whole body structure and character. This makes us healthy or unhealthy. Therefore, to lead a happy and healthy life does not indulge in wrong food habits or thought processes ever, as far as possible.

3. Unfavorable Food Combinations

In the previous topic, it is discussed how compatible food safeguards human health and maintains the *doṣas* in their balanced state and in the same way an incompatible diet affects the health and aggravates the *doṣas*. Incompatible foods are of several kinds. Some foods are incompatible by nature and create a problem on consumption, because they are heavy, aggravate the *doṣas* and cause diseases. Some of these foods by nature are very beneficial and health-promoting when consumed alone, but become incompatible when taken along with other foods or when taken at a particular time, seasoned or cooked in a particular container, instead of benefitting the health, they may harm the body and become the cause of several diseases. This includes an opposing combination of substances which do not have an affinity for each other. Such foods are incompatible because they corrupt the *dhātus*, aggravate the *doṣas* and cause an imbalance in the constituents of useful body secretions. They do not allow wastes to be eliminated smoothly and lead to many serious health complications which sometimes create problems in right diagnosis. Prolonged use of unfavorable foods slowly and steadily affect the health of an individual by disturbing the *dhātus* and their normal functioning and may give rise to several diseases. Unfavorable foods are of several kinds:

1. **An unsuitable diet in a particular area**: Consuming watery and oily foods and those that are cool in attributes in humid areas.
2. **An unsuitable diet in a particular season**: Cold and light food in winter.
3. **An unsuitable diet according to one's digestive power**: Heavy, oily, cold and sweet food, if consumed by a person with weak digestive power.

4. **An unsuitable diet based on the quantity**: *Ghee* and honey in equal quantities act as poison, but consuming the same in small amounts and in different proportions, it becomes nectar.
5. **An unsuitable diet as per one's habit**: Wheat or barley being consumed by a person who used to eat rice every day.
6. **An unsuitable diet according to the *doṣas***: A person with a *Vāta* dominant constitution eating a *Vāta* aggravating diet and one with *Kapha*-type body consuming a *Kapha* provoking diet.
7. **An unsuitable diet according to cooking habits and tradition**: Cooking sour foods in a copper or brass vessel.
8. **An unsuitable diet according to the potency**: Eating hot and cold potency foods together. For example, taking orange, sweet lime or pineapple along with milk, yogurt or buttermilk.
9. **An unsuitable diet as per the bowel habits**: Fecal elimination naturally takes place with difficulty in persons with slow peristaltic movements in the gastro-intestinal tract (bowel movements). Due to aggravated *Vāta* such individuals suffer constipation and pass hard stools. Similarly, those having moderate bowel movements are *Kapha* dominated individuals. In such individuals the process of fecal elimination is moderate and still difficult. For such individuals, light, constipating, *Vāta* and *Kapha* provoking substances are incompatible. On the other hand, those having soft bowel movements are *Pitta*-dominated individuals. In them, fecal elimination takes place smoothly and easily therefore, pungent, purgative and laxative substances are incompatible.
10. **An unsuitable diet according to the condition of the body**: Obese people taking heavy and oily foods whereas dry and light foods being taken by emaciated person.
11. **An unsuitable diet as per the time and routine**: Eating before morning relieve, eating without hunger, not eating when hungry and so on.
12. **An unsuitable diet as per healthy diet principles**: Breaking rules regarding healthy food habits. To counter the bad effect of a particular substance, one must consume some other substance after the previous one, e.g., do not drink cold water after *ghee* (*ghee* must always be followed by warm drinks), do not exercise after a meal, and do not drink cold water after consuming food containing wheat or barley.
13. **An unsuitable diet based on cooking**: Taking uncooked or half cooked or overheated food, food cooked in a bad medium or with a polluted fuel source (heat).

14. **An unsuitable diet in a combination**: Combining wrong foods like sour things with milk, eating muskmelon, watermelon or salty foods with milk.
15. **An unsuitable diet based on the taste**: Forcing oneself to eat food that one dislikes, eating delicious food without interest.
16. **An unsuitable diet according to the properties**: Food without taste or bad in taste or food whose taste has been changed.
17. **An unsuitable diet as per classic texts**: Foods taken against '*Ācāra saṁhitā*' (dietetic facts).

- **Examples of some incompatible combinations**

- **Milk with**: Yogurt, salt, radish, radish leaves, green and raw salad, drum stick, tamarind, muskmelon, Bengal quince, coconut, Indian hog plum, lemon, monkey jack, cranberry, star fruit (carambola), blackberry, wood apple, pomegranate, Indian gooseberry, angled luffa, jaggery, sesame cake, horse gram, black gram, Turkish gram, Indian millet, coarse grain flour of barley and gram (*sattu*), oil, fish sour fruits and foods. Also, milk, wine and gruel eaten together.
- **Yogurt with**: Rice pudding, milk, cottage cheese, hot foods and other hot substances, cucumber, muskmelon, the fruit of the toddy palm.
- **Rice pudding with**: Jackfruit, sour foods (yogurt, lemon, tamarind and so on), coarse grain flour of barley and gram (*sattū*) and alcohol.
- **Rice with**: Vinegar.
- **Honey with**: Black nightshade, clarified butter (*ghee* along with an equal quantity of old honey), rainwater, oil, fat, grapes, lotus seeds, radish, very hot water, hot milk and other hot substances, safflower leaves, sugar (*sherbet* containing sugar syrup) and date wine. Warm honey is prohibited.
- **Cold water with**: Clarified butter (*ghee*), oil, warm milk and hot substances, watermelon, guava, cucumber, snake cucumber, groundnut, chilgoza (which is an edible pinenut).
- **Hot water or other hot drinks with**: Honey, ice cream and other cold items.
- **Ghee with**: Equal amounts of honey and cold water.
- **Ghee**: Kept in a brass container for more than 10 days.
- **Muskmelon with**: Garlic, yogurt, milk, radish leaves, water.
- **Watermelon with**: Cold water, mint.
- **Sesame paste with**: Cooked Malabar spinach.
- **Salt**: Its excessive and prolonged use.

- **Mustard oil with**: Mushrooms.
- **Sprouted pulses and grains with**: Lotus stems; also raw sprouts along with cooked food.
- **Black nightshade with**: Long pepper, black pepper, jaggery, honey, black nightshade kept overnight and cooked in a utensil in which fish has been previously cooked.
- **Black gram with**: Radish.
- **Banana with**: Buttermilk.
- **Radish with**: Milk, banana and raisins.
- **Mango with**: Cucumber, cheese and yogurt.

- **Incompatible non-vegetarian* combinations**

- **Fish with**: Milk.
- **Fried fish with**: Long pepper.
- **Cooked in fish oil**: Long pepper.
- **Pigeon meat cooked in mustard oil with**: Honey and milk.
- **Water animals with**: Honey, sesame, milk and raddish.
- **Parakeet bird flesh with**: Mustard oil and honey; roasted on turmeric wood.
- **Crane flesh with**: Alcohol and roasting in pork fat.
- **Mutton**: Roasted on coal.
- **Pork with**: Hot foods.
- **Egg with**: Milk, meat, melon, cheese, banana and fish.

4. Diseases Caused by an Incompatible Food & Lifestyle and their Treatment

All the *doṣas*, *dhātus* and *malas* get vitiated if one keeps on taking the above-mentioned incompatible foods and harmful combinations in the diet, resulting in innumerable problems like food poisoning, colitis and sprue syndrome, *Vāta* disorders, abdominal disorders, abdominal swellings, flatulence or distention in the abdomen, *alasaka* (retention of partially digested food in the abdomen), cholera, acidity, indigestion, anemia, debility, tuberculosis, declination of glow (*oja*) and energy, hemorrhoids (piles), *prameha* (urinary abnormality), sinus, common cold, fever, pharyngitis

*Non-vegetarian food is considered as *tāmasika* food in *Āyurveda*, which increases laziness, anger and makes one homicidal and violent in nature, but still some important facts are mentioned above for the non-vegetarians.

(a throat disorder), diminished vision, dizziness, syncope, insanity, loss of memory, unconsciousness, deterioration of brain power and intellect, intoxication, deterioration of sensory and motor organs, skin disorders, leucoderma, leprosy, erysipelas, ascites, boils or eruptions, fistulas, abscesses, intrinsic hemorrhage, calculi (stones), edema, impotency, infertility, reproductive deformities (miscarriage, abortion, foetal death immediately after birth or deformities in the offspring) and slow poisoning in the body, at times even leading to death.

- **Treatment**

Remedies for the above-mentioned disorders and other diseases that emerge as a result of incompatible food and harmful combinations can all be treated in the following manner:

1. Such disorders require detoxification or purification treatments like emesis and purgation. Emesis results only in alleviation of *doṣas* whereas purgation detoxifies the entire abdomen, making it possible to cure the disease completely.
2. Consuming food substances having opposing properties to those of the incompatible food, causing the disorder.
3. Be aware of compatibility and incompatibility of food based on physiology and constitution. Also be careful in selecting a compatible diet, clearing the root cause of the disease, so as to prevent a disease in the future.

- **People unaffected by incompatible diet**

1. One who exercises regularly; regular exercise improves immunity.
2. Those who regularly consume oily and smooth substances such as milk, clarified butter (*ghee*) and other such substances.
3. One with strong digestive fire.
4. A physically strong person with the habit of eating unfavorable foods and for whom such foods have transformed into a suitable diet.
5. Taking incompatible foods in small amounts does not affect a person much or if affected the result will be negligible.

Aṣṭāṅga Saṅgraha of *Vāgbhaṭa* (an *Āyurvedic* text) quotes that milk and yogurt having opposite qualities to those of *doṣa*, *dūṣya*, time and strength, if used together, are not harmful. They pacify the ailment. The text specifies that in combination, as a result of specific factors, compatible food sometimes transforms into incompatible food and *vice versa*. In a similar manner, in several different types of combinations, incompatible substances also surrender their opposing qualities. Therefore, through regular practice and experience, if one gets into the habit of eating and drinking incompatible combinations, then they may turn out to be suitable and favorable for them. Still, in the future there are chances that they may harm the body. Hence, it is recommended to use favorable and compatible foods, rather than incompatible and unfavorable ones.

Table 20: Effect of Excessive Intake of Food and its Antidotes

Edible Products	Effect of Overeating	Antidotes
Animal Products		
Egg	Provokes *Kapha* and *Pitta,* if taken raw	Black henbane *(Khurāsānī ajavāyana)*, coriander, turmeric and onion
Fish	Provokes *Pitta*	Coconut, limestone and lemon
Red meat	Heavy to digest	Red chilli and clove
Dairy Products		
Sour cream	Provokes *Kapha*	Coriander or cardamom
Yogurt	Provokes *Kapha*	Cumin or ginger
Cottage cheese	Provokes *Pitta* and *Kapha*	Black pepper, red pepper
**Kulfi*	Provokes *Kapha*	Clove or cardamom
Grains		
Oats	Provokes *Kapha*	Turmeric, mustard seed or cumin
Wheat	Provokes *Kapha*	Ginger
Rice	Provokes *Kapha*	Black pepper or clove
Popcorn	Causes dryness and provocate *Vāta*	Add *ghee*
Vegetables		
Legumes or pods	Provokes *Vāta* and causes flatulence	Garlic, clove, black pepper, red pepper, ginger, rock salt
Cabbage	Provokes *Kapha* and *Vāta*	Cabbage cooked in sunflower oil with turmeric and mustard seeds
Garlic	Provokes *Pitta*	Grated coconut and lemon
Green salad	Provokes *Vāta*	Olive oil mixed with lemon juice
Edible Products	**Effect of Overeating**	**Antidotes**
Onion	Provokes *Vāta*	Cook or add salt, lemon, yogurt and mustard seeds
Potato	Provokes *Vāta*	*Ghee* mixed with black pepper
Tomato	Provokes *Kapha*	Lemon and cumin

* *Kulfi*: An Indian dessert made by freezing milk that has been concentrated by boiling and flavored with nuts and cardamom seeds.

Fruits		
Avocado, Pear	Provokes *Kapha*	Turmeric, lemon, garlic or black pepper
Banana	Provokes *Kapha*	Cardamom
Mango	Causes diarrhea	*Ghee* with cardamom
Melon	Causes water retention	Grated coconut with coriander
Water melon	Causes water retention	Salt with red pepper
Dry Fruits and Nuts		
Dry fruits (in general)	Causes dryness or may provocate *Vāta*	Take after soaking in water
Groundnut	Provokes *Vāta* and *Pitta*	Soak overnight in water, cook it and use
Peanut butter	Heavy, provokes *Pitta* and causes headache	Ginger or roasted cumin powder
Stimulants and Depressants		
Various alcoholic drinks	Stimulant, depressant	Chew one-fourth teaspoon of cumin seeds or 1-2 cardamom seeds
Black tea	Stimulant, depressant	Ginger
Coffee	Stimulant, depressant	Nutmeg powder with cardamom
Chocolate	Stimulant	Cardamom or cumin
Tobacco	Provokes *Pitta* and *Vāta,* stimulant, depressant	Thymol seed or water hyssop (*brahmī)* and roots of sweet flag (*vaca*)

5. Favorable Food Combinations

Just as an unsuitable diet harms the body and may result in several ailments. In the same way, there are certain food substances which, if taken in combination, enhance each other°s qualities. They help in digesting food easily and are known for being a beneficial combination of food. If for the sake of taste, food has been overeaten, it results in indigestion or causes some other digestive problems. In such circumstance, the effect of overeating can be negated if it is followed by a combination that counters the effect of indigestion.

- **Examples of some favorable combinations**

Food Substances	Beneficial Combinations (that aids in digestion)
Black gram	Buttermilk and drained raw sugar
Bengal gram	Radish
Green gram	Indian gooseberry
Pigeon pea	Fermented digestive appetizer (*kāñjī*)
Wheat	Snake cucumber
Corn	Thymol (carom) seeds
Gruel	Rock salt
Milk	Green gram soup
Clarified butter (*ghee*)	Lemon juice
Coconut	Rice
Mango	Milk
Banana	Clarified butter (*ghee*)
Orange	Jaggery
Lemon	Salt
Grape fruit, currants, raisins, pista, walnuts and almonds	Cloves
Potato	Rice water
Yam	Jaggery
Salt	Rice broth
Crystal sugar	Dry ginger
Jaggery	Dry ginger and nut grass
Sugarcane	Ginger

Chapter 7

The Characteristics of Important Liquids and their Adjuvants (*Anupāna*)

Anupāna (anu+pāna), where *'anu'* means *'after'* and *'pāna'* means 'intake of a substance,' means liquids or substances that need to be taken after meals and medication[1]. *Anupānas* (adjuvants) are chiefly of two types, a drink taken immediately after food such as buttermilk, milk or juices, and others which are taken along with the medicines such as water or honey. It is a substance used as a medium for the administration of medicines or to increase the action of principal ingredients. It is a carrier of food and medicines. *Anupāna* is a supplementary item added to the main medicine as a suitable medium, to reduce its bad taste, to increase its natural power or to modify it. They are considered very important and occupy a specific place in *Āyurveda*. *Anupānas* boost taste. Appropriate adjuvants provide energy, strength and increase virility. They also provide freshness, joy and softness. They activate the digestive fire, brighten the complexion and reduce mental and physical fatigue. Appropriate adjuvants not only pacify all *doṣas*, but also prevent the accumulation of *doṣas* in all *dhātus*[2].

The most important substances used as adjuvants (vehicles)[3] are water (hot and cold), fermented medicated herbal decoctions (*āsava*), soup, sour fruit juices, fermented drinks made from grains and other sour substances, *kāñjī* vinegar, milk, fruit juices and extracts of medicinal herbs and decoctions. Selection of anupḍna is based on its qualities, according to the constitution, *doṣa* pattern, state of illness of a patient, time and age. *Anupānas* should be taken in an appropriate quantity to ensure quick and easy digestion of medicines and food. Taking more than the required amount leads to heaviness and *doṣa* aggravation, whereas a lesser quantity than required or its complete

1. *Anu paścāt saha vā pīyate ityanupānam. Alpadoṣamadoṣa vā, pyanupānena jīryate.* (A.hṛ.sū. 8/50)
2. *Anupānaṁ hitaṁ yuktaṁ tarpayatyāśu mānavam.*
   Sukhaṁ pacati cāhāramāyuṣe ca balāya ca. (Ca.sū. 27/326)
   Anupānaṁ karotyūrjāṁ tṛptim vyāptiṁ dṛḍhāṅgatām.
   Annasaṅghātaśaithilyaviklittijaraṇāni ca. (A.hṛ.sū. 8/52)
3. *Anupānaṁ himaṁ vāri yavagodhūmayorhitam.*
   Dadhni madye viṣe kṣaudre koṣṇaṁ piṣṭamayeṣu tu. (A.hṛ.sū. 8/47-48)
   Śākamudgādivikṛtau mastutakrāmlakāñjikam.
   Surā kṛśānāṁ puṣṭyarthaṁ sthūlānāṁ tu madhūdakam. (A.hṛ.sū. 8/48-49)

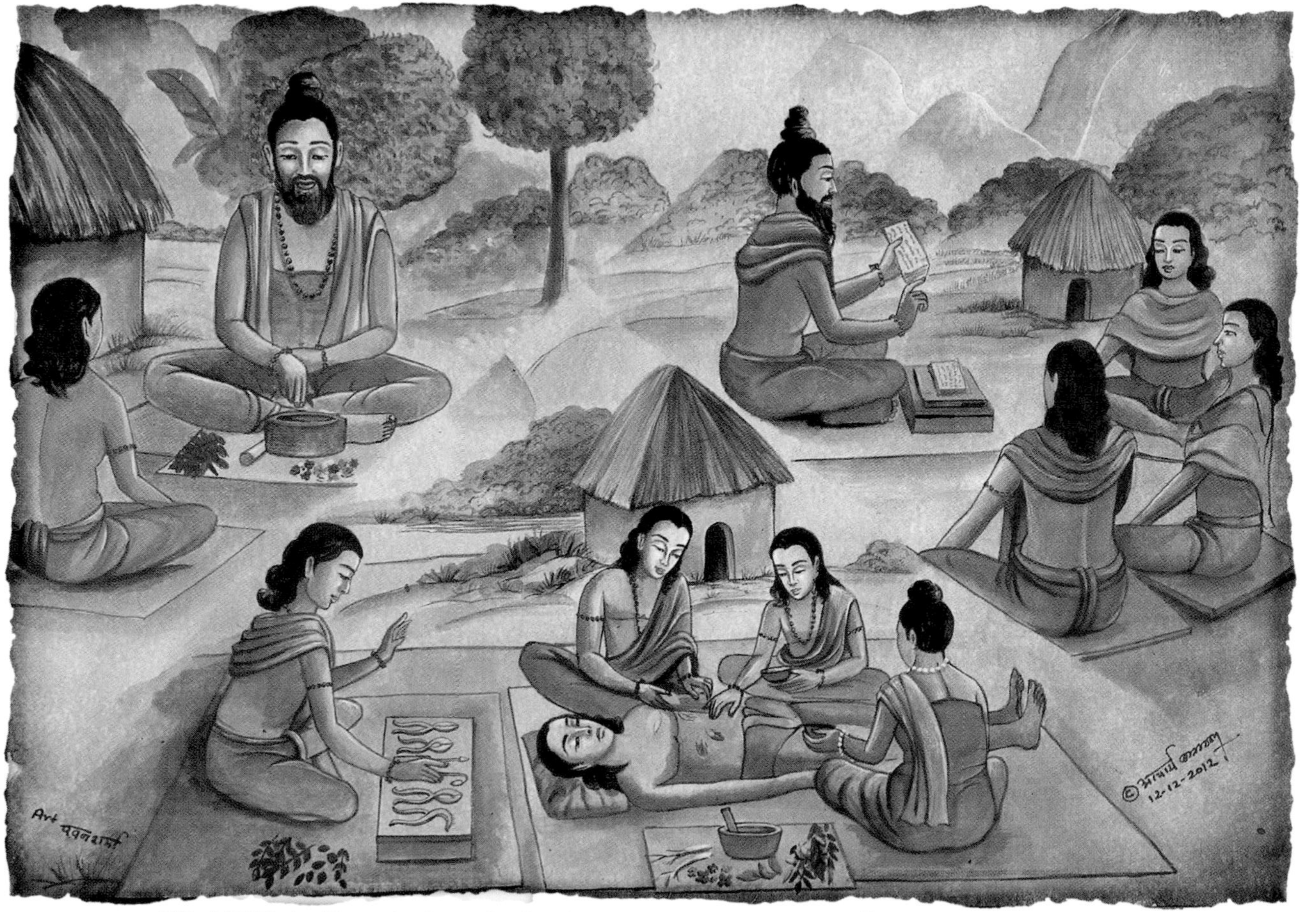

PLATE 1: *Practical methods of teaching and learning Āyurveda in ancient times*

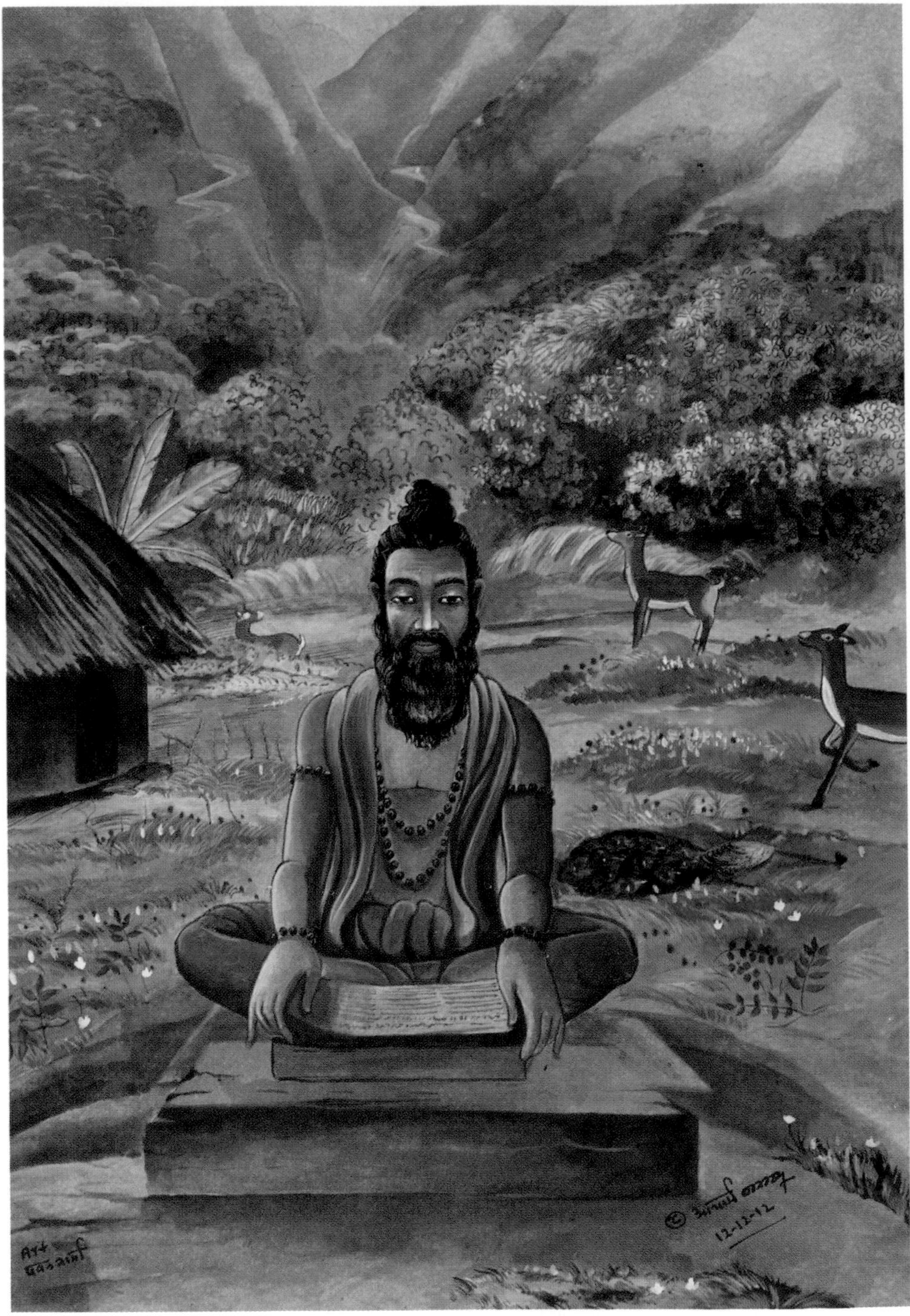

PLATE 2: *An outlook of ancient tradition* : *An Āyurvedic seer*

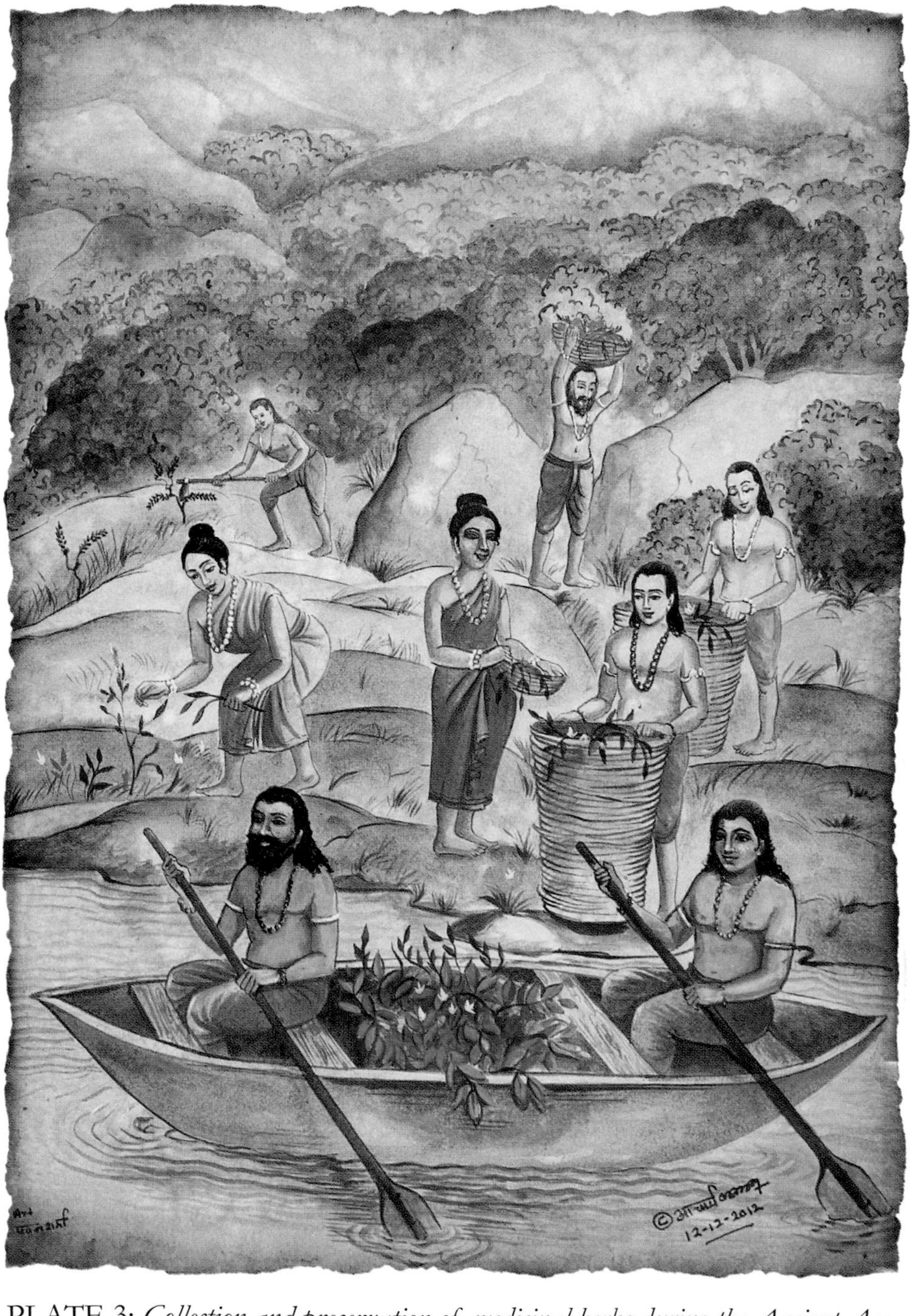

PLATE 3: *Collection and preservation of medicinal herbs during the Ancient Age*

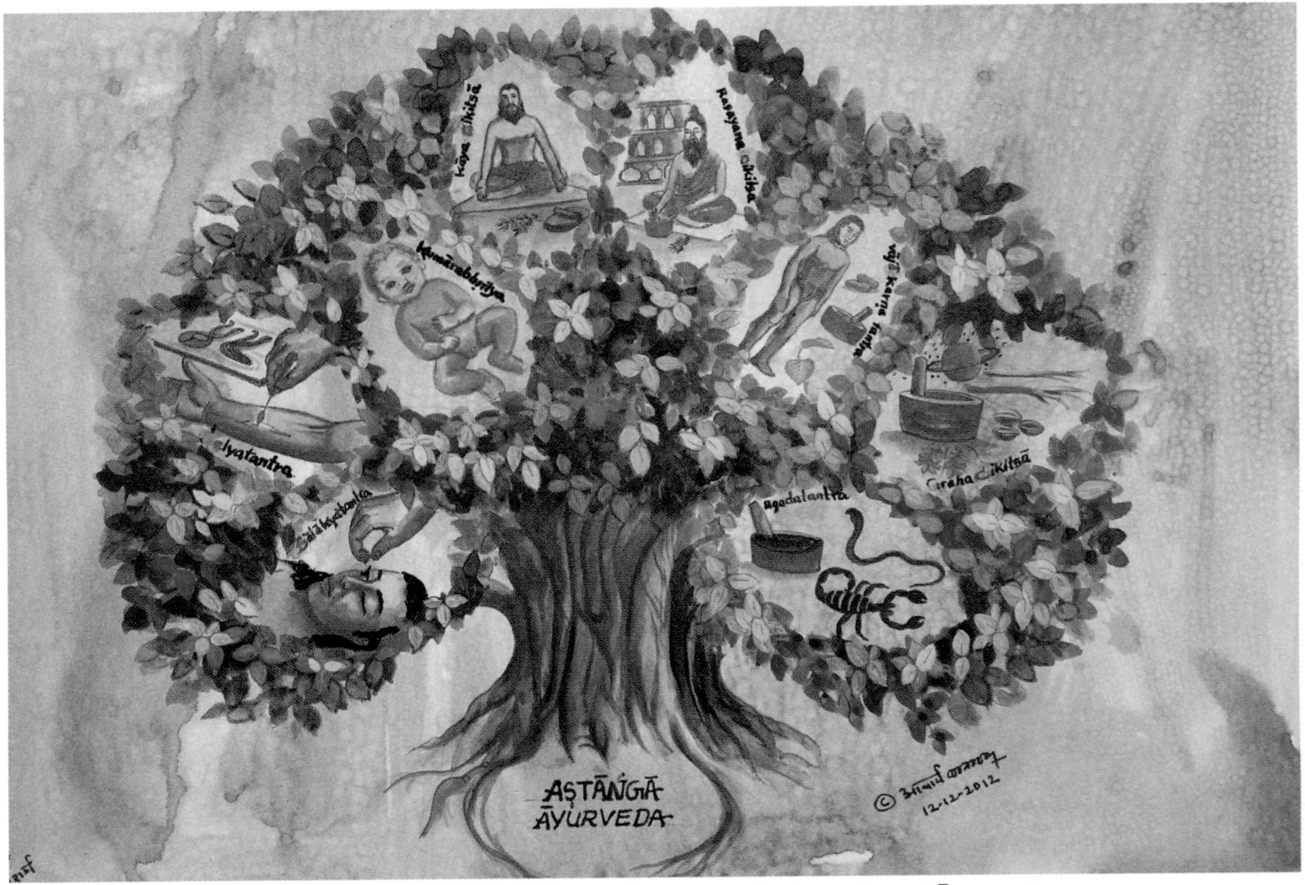

PLATE 4: *Aṣṭanga Āyurveda: The eight branches of Āyurveda*

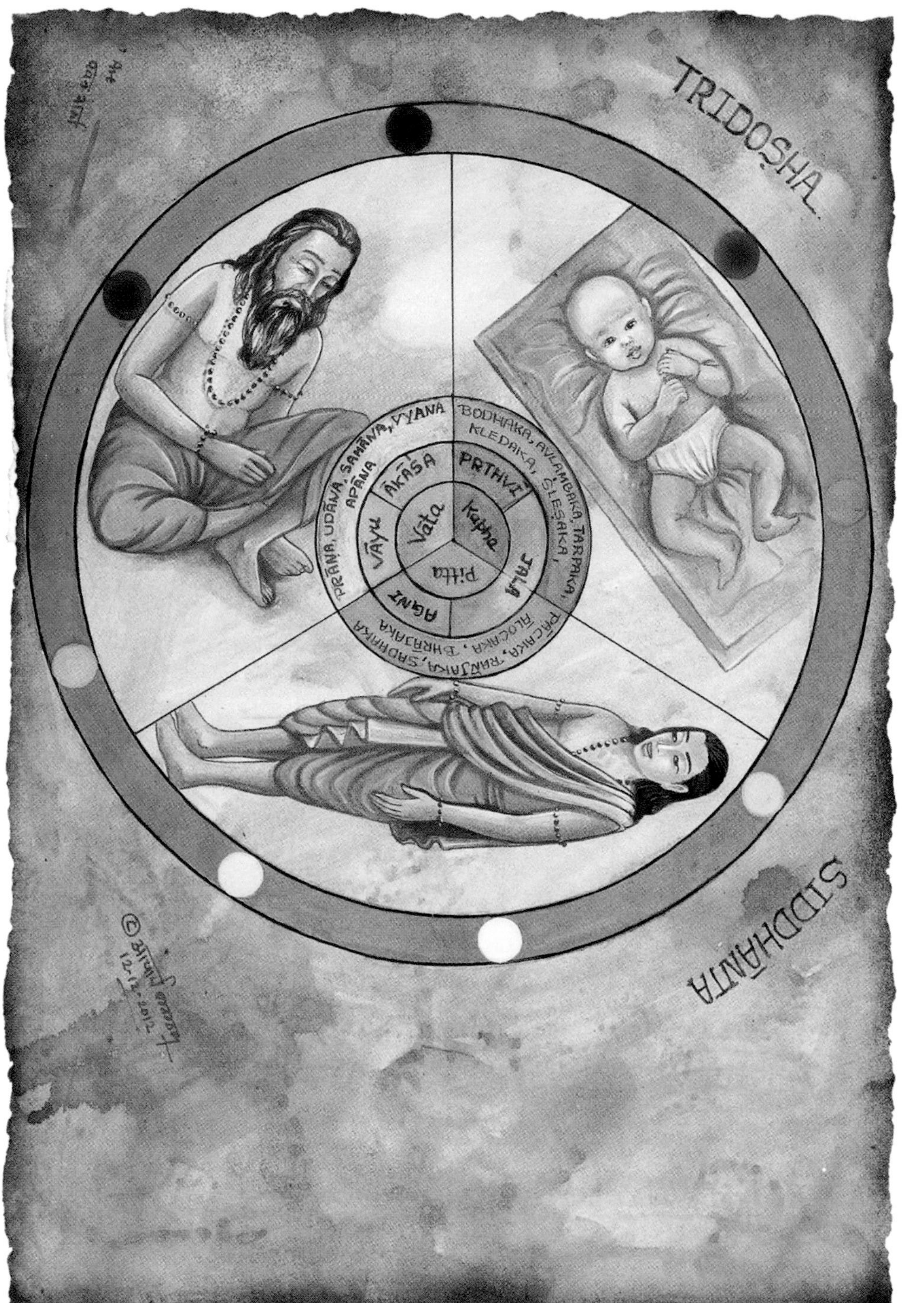

PLATE 5: *The Principle of Tridoṣa*: *The five elements, types of tridoṣa and their role in different ages of life*

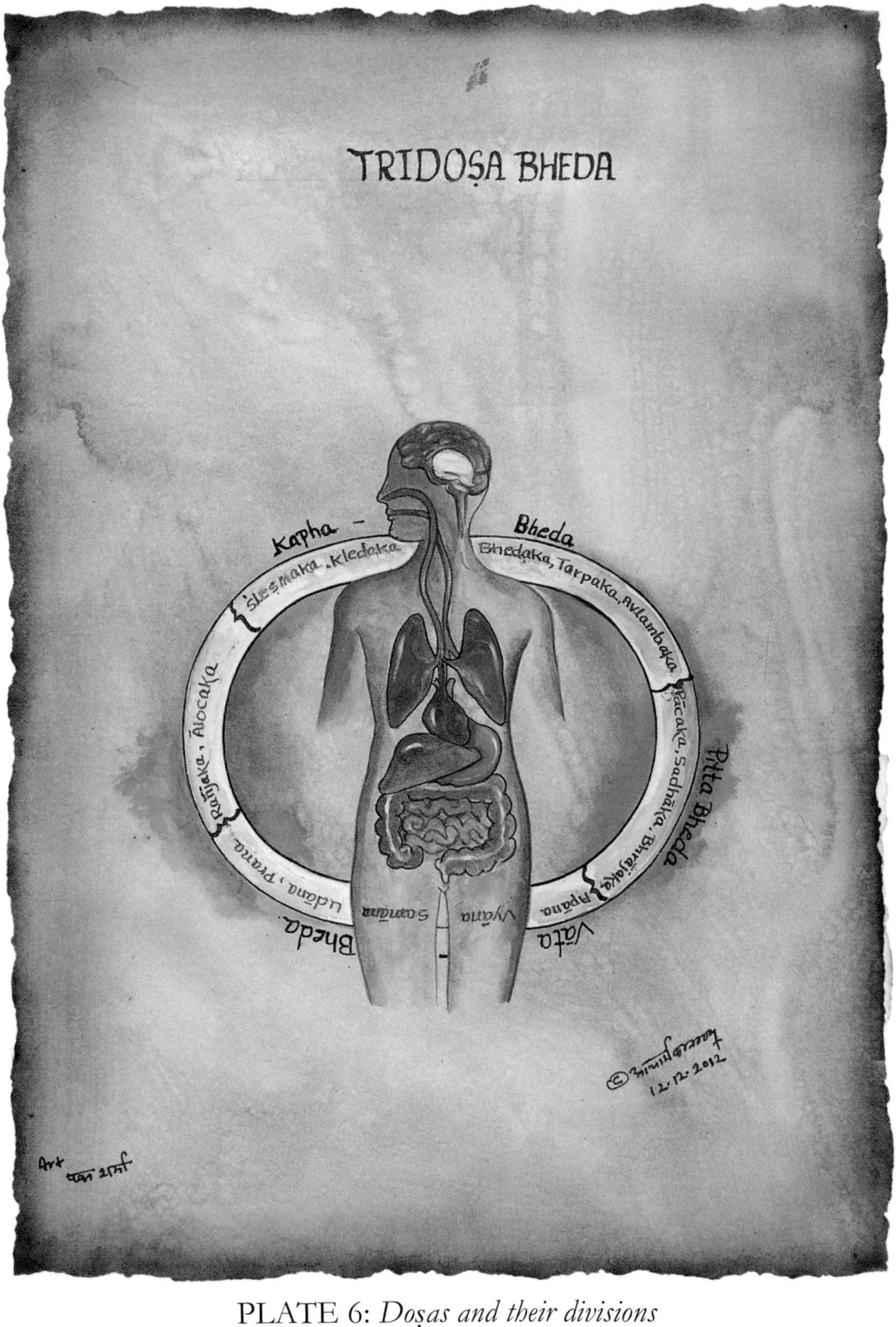

PLATE 6: *Doṣas and their divisions*

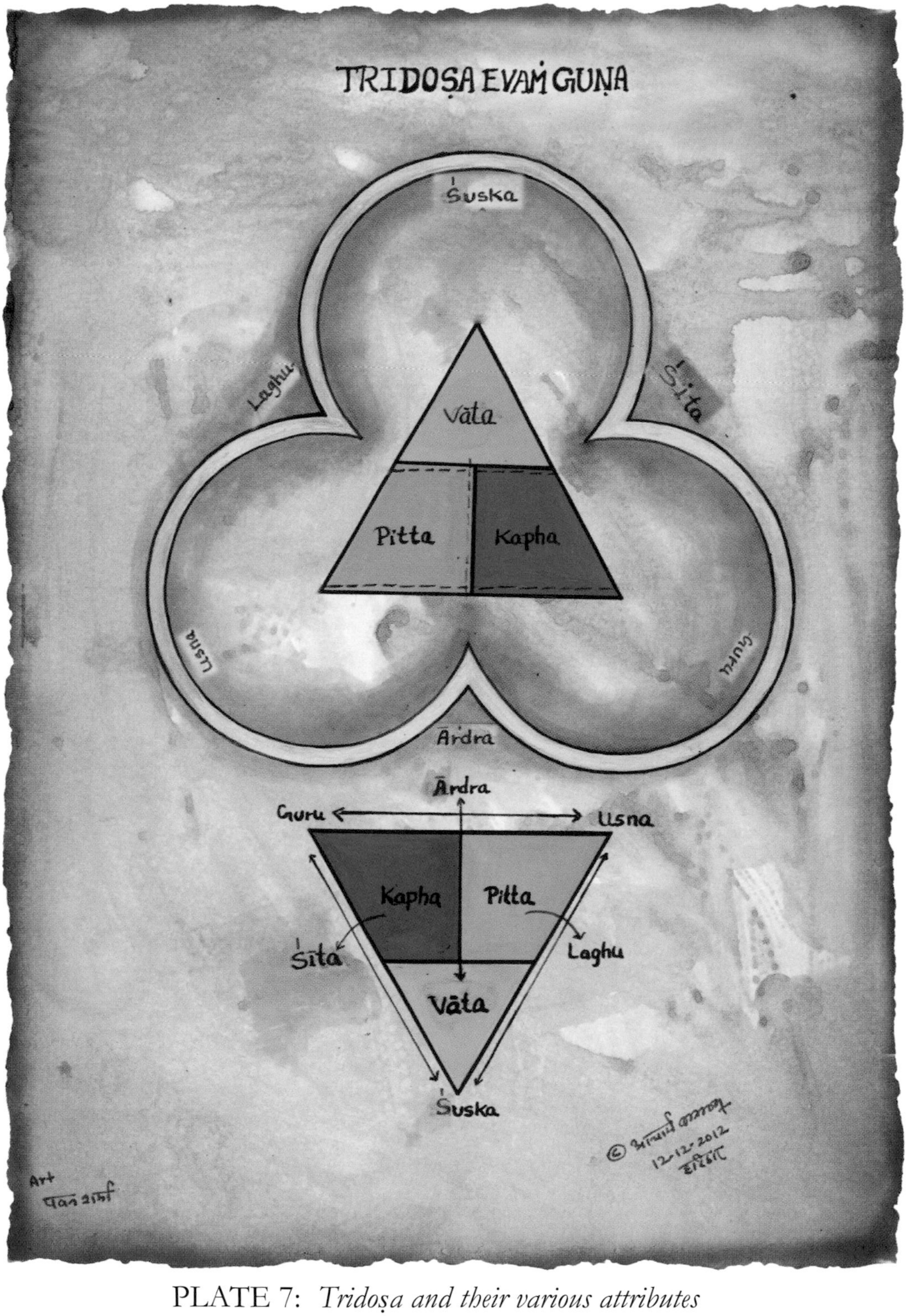

PLATE 7: *Tridoṣa and their various attributes*

Plate 8: *Relationship between Tridoṣa, Triguṇa (Sattva, Rajas, Tamas) and Pañcamahābhūta - their location in the body*

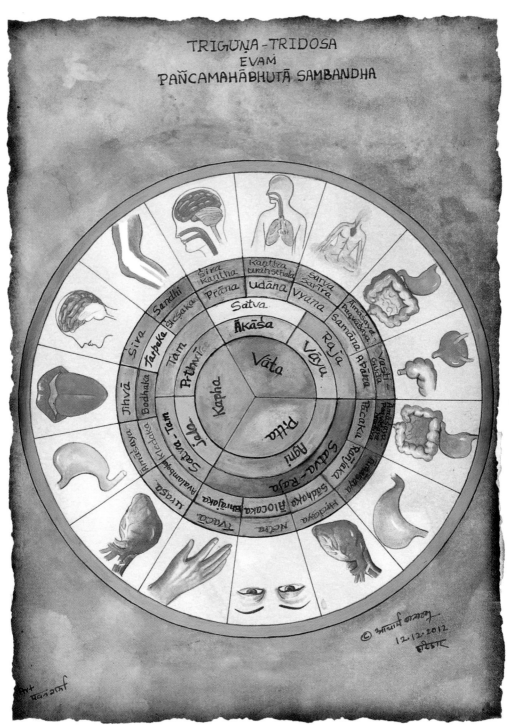

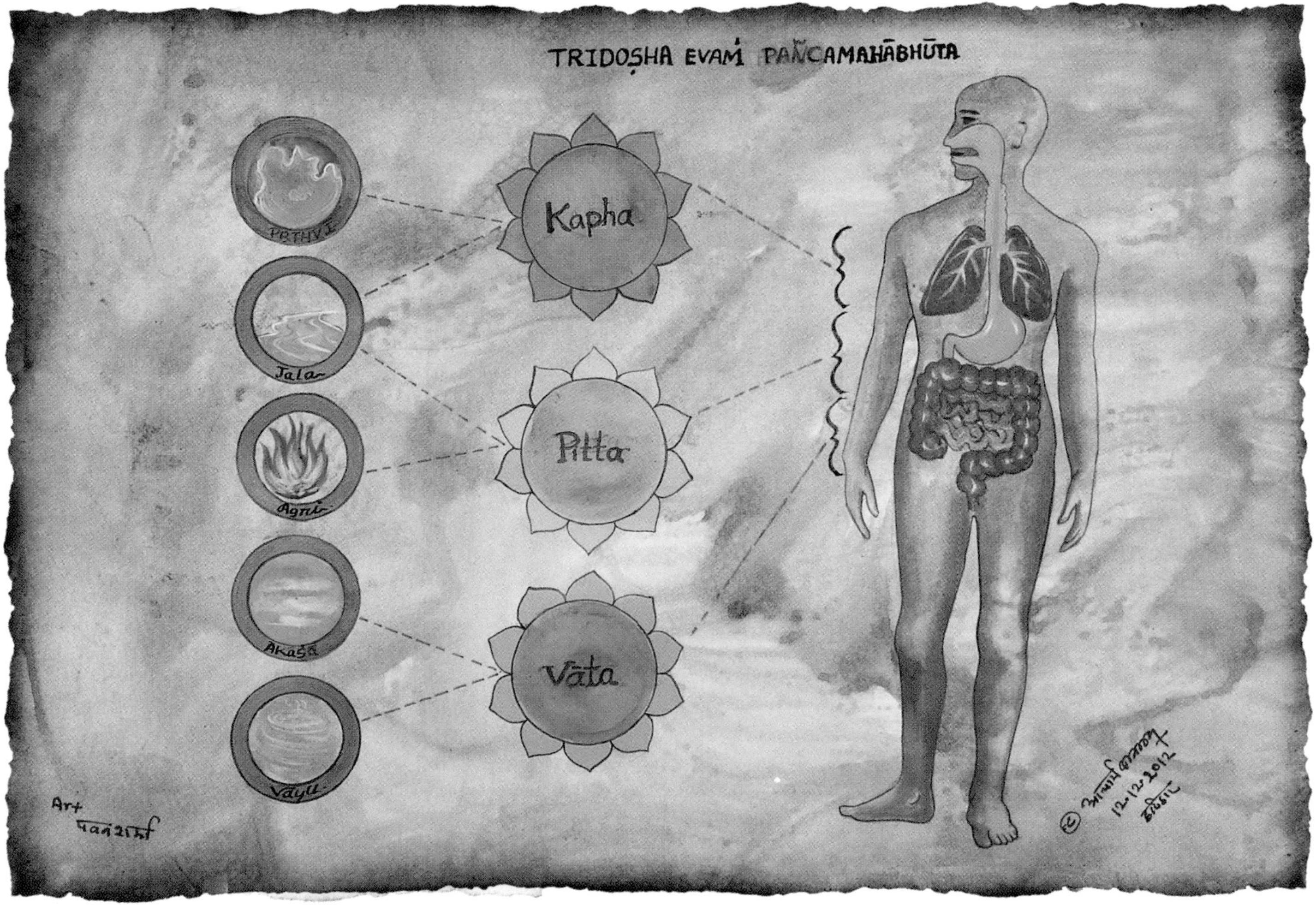

PLATE 9: *Tridoṣa and Pañcamahābhūta* - *their relationship with the human body*

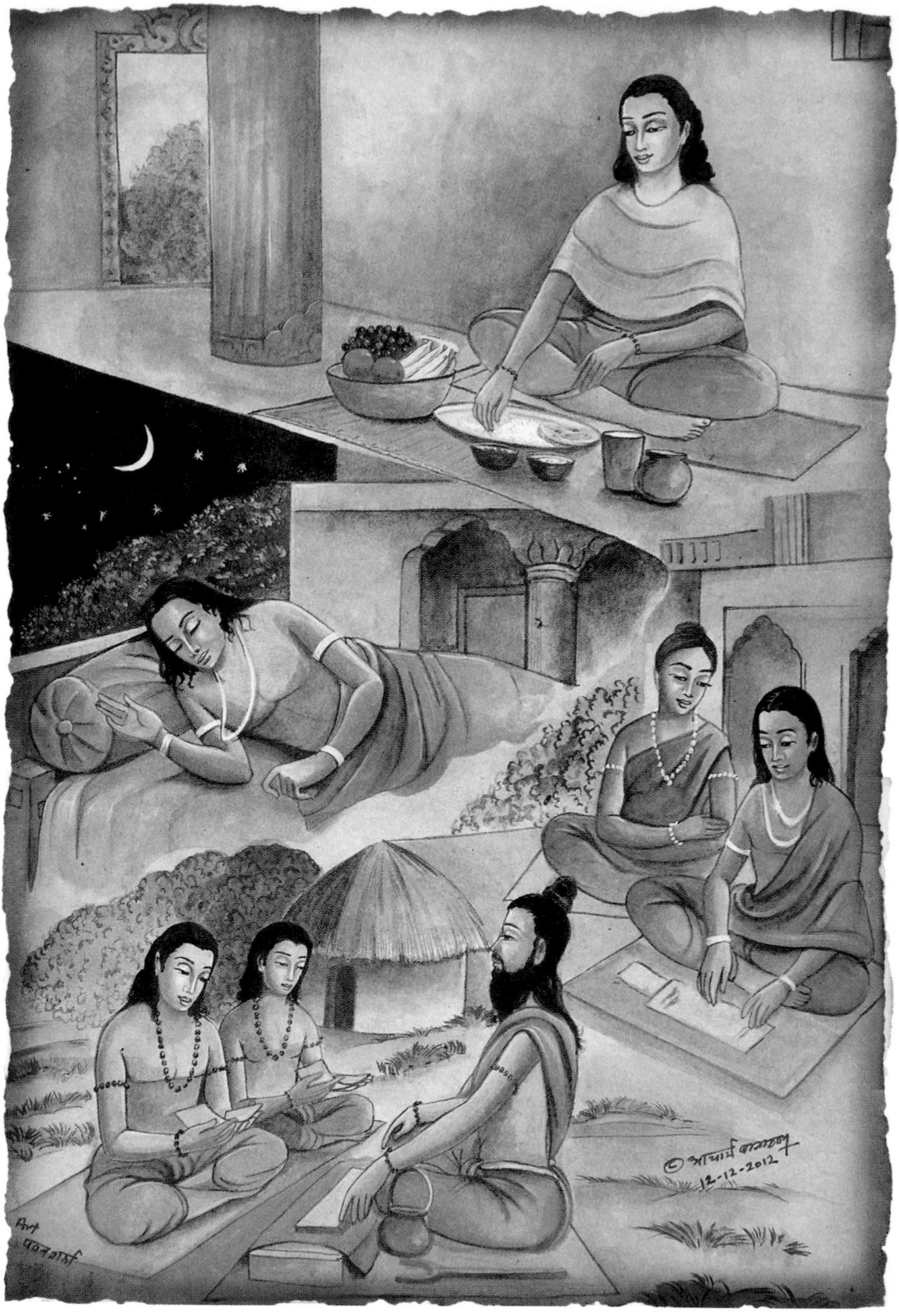

PLATE 10: *Traiyopastambha: The three supporting pillars of the body - food, sleep and celibacy (sexual restraint)*

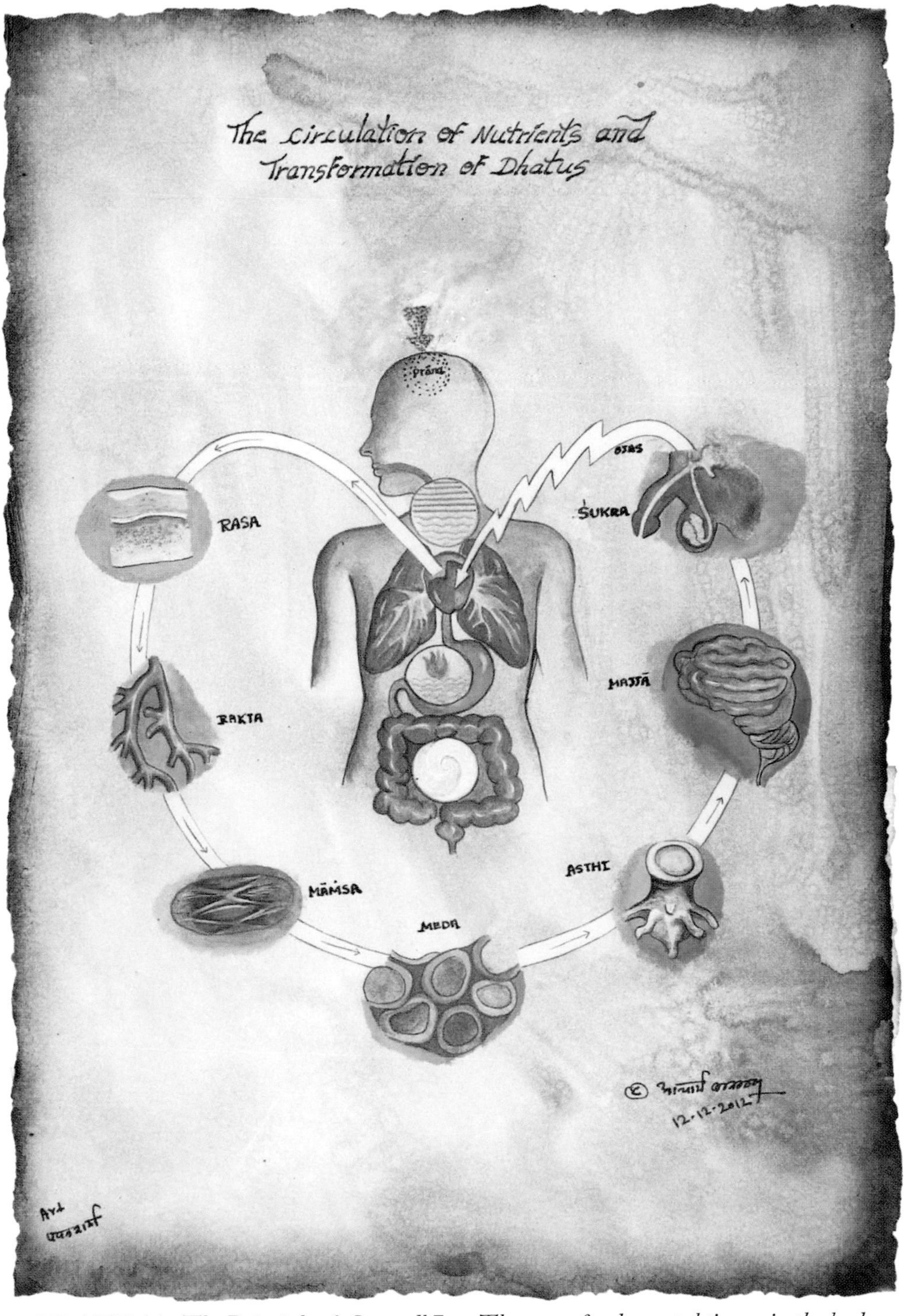

PLATE 11: *The Principle of Saptadhātu: The seven fundamental tissues in the body*

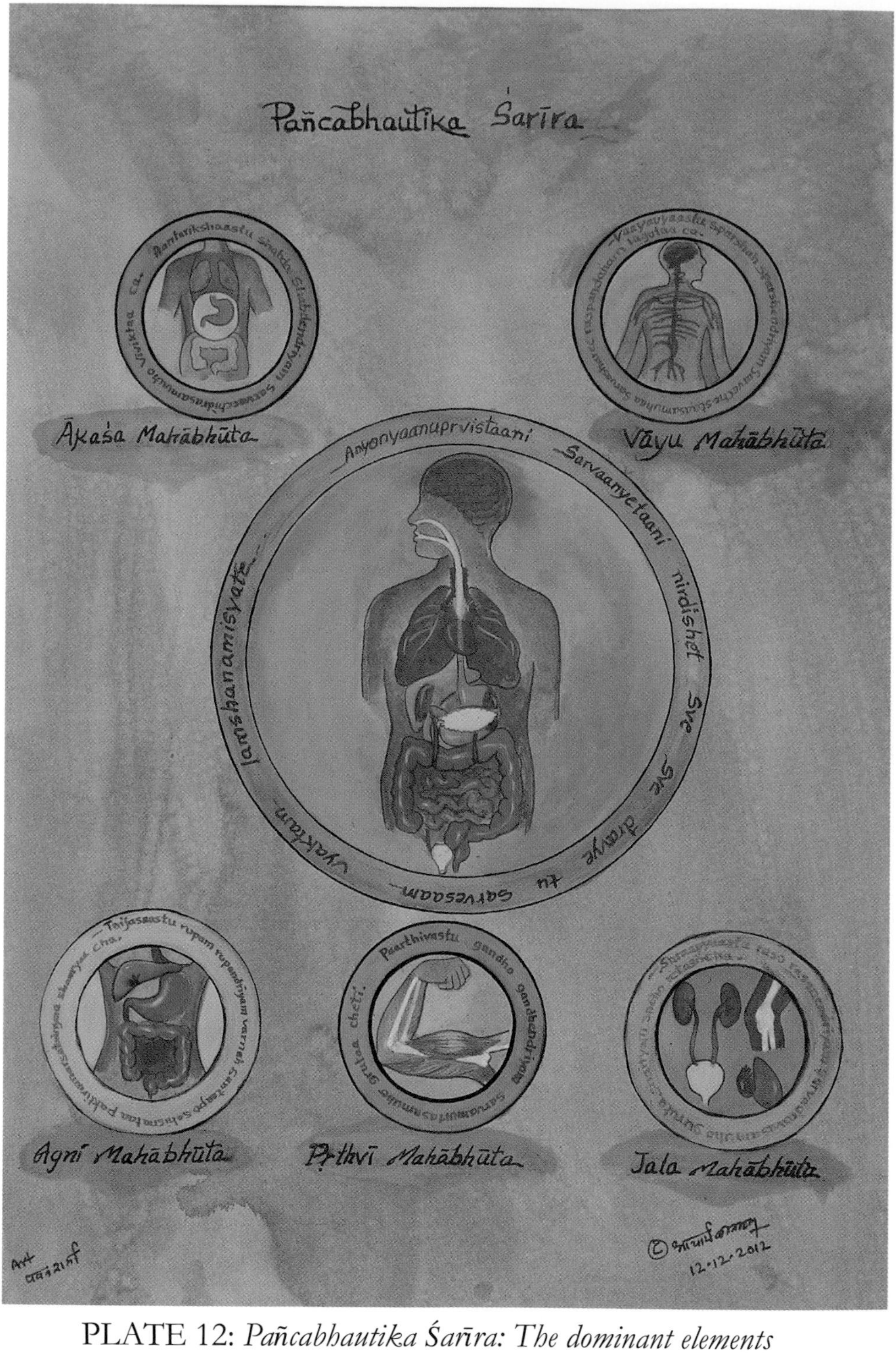

PLATE 12: *Pañcabhautika Śarīra: The dominant elements present in different parts of the body*

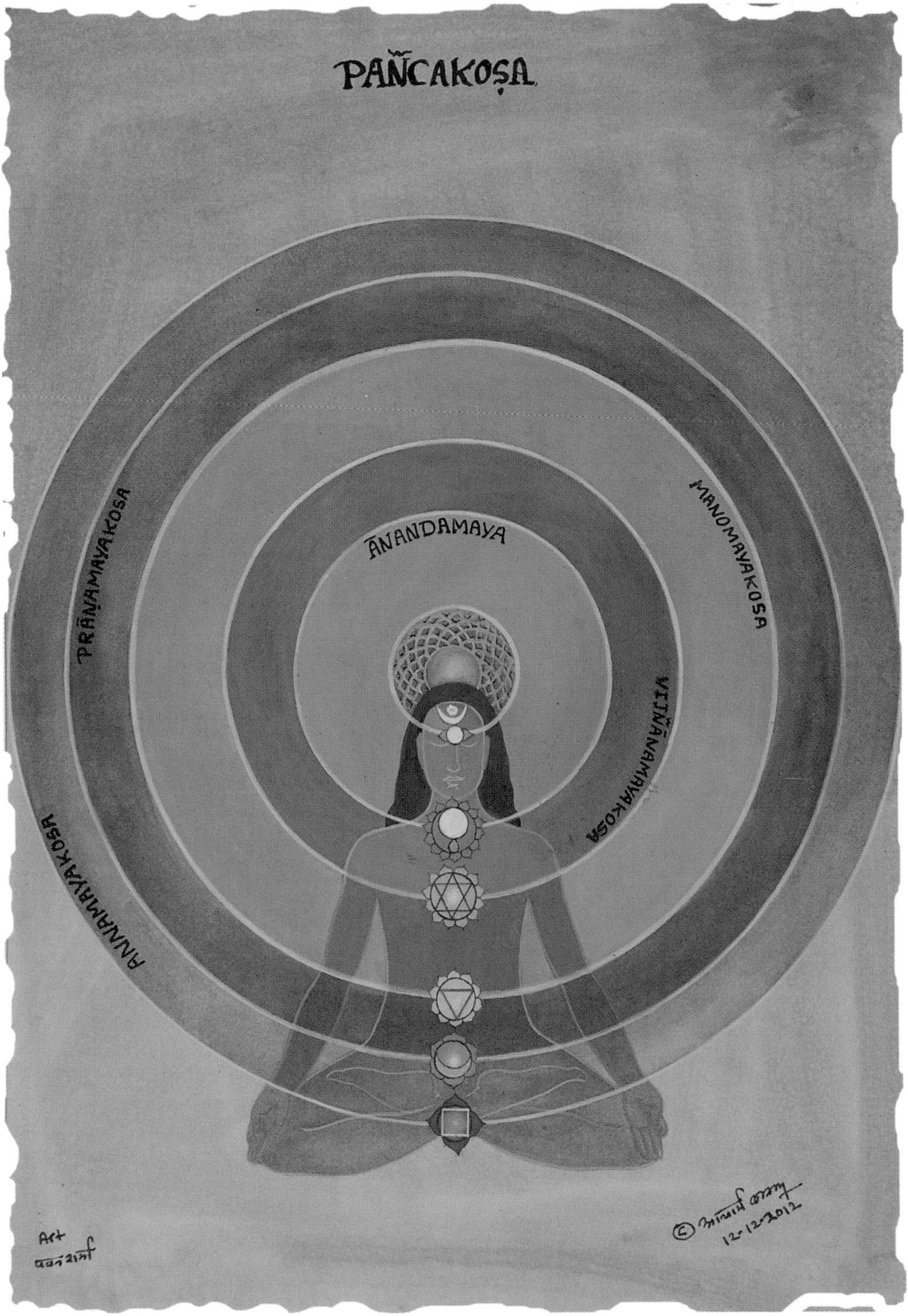

PLATE 13: *Pañcakoṣa: The method to attain subtle knowledge of the body by means of yoga*

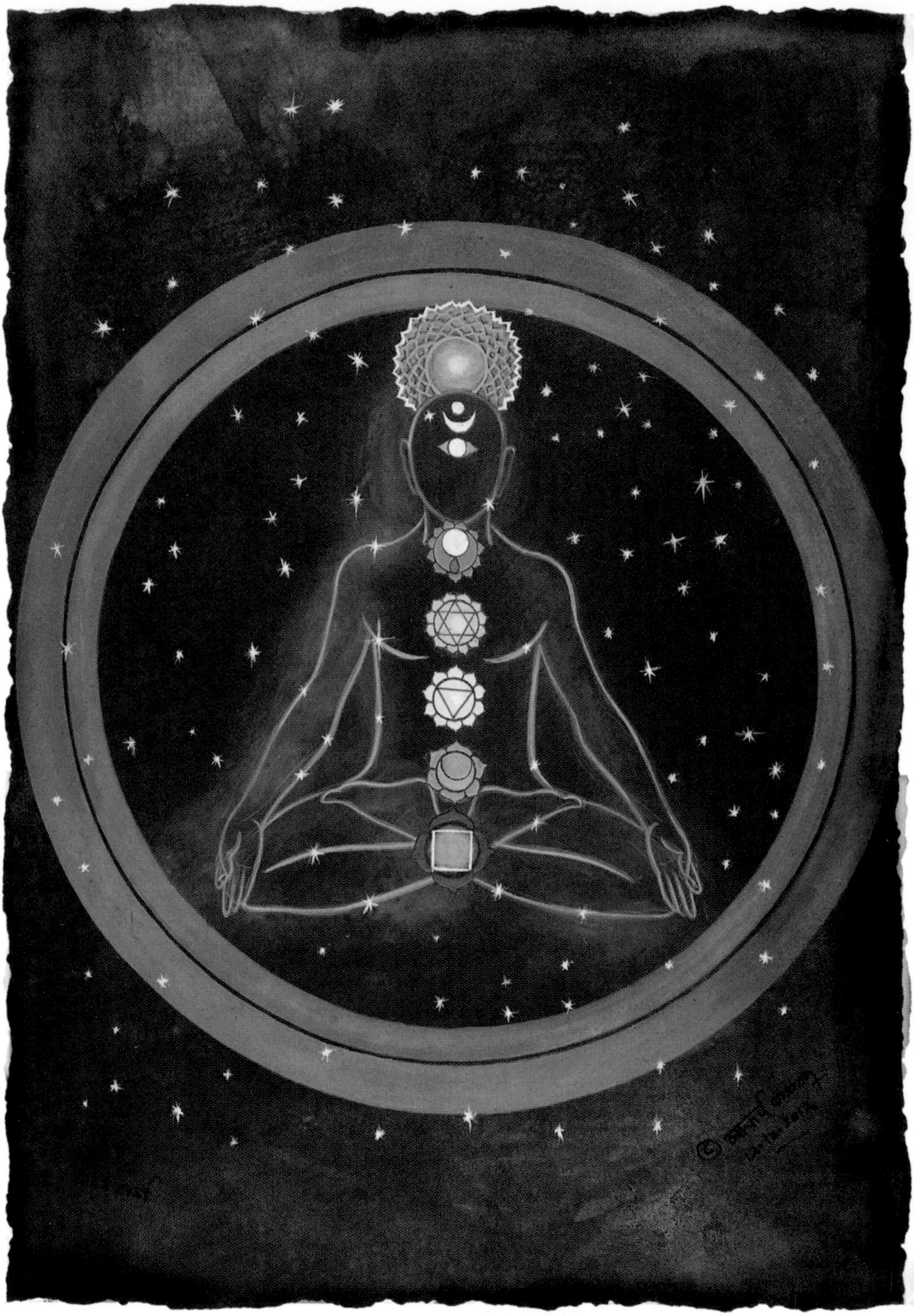

PLATE 14: *Aṣṭacakra - The various energy centers located in the body*

PLATE 15: *Aṣṭacakra and their location in the body*

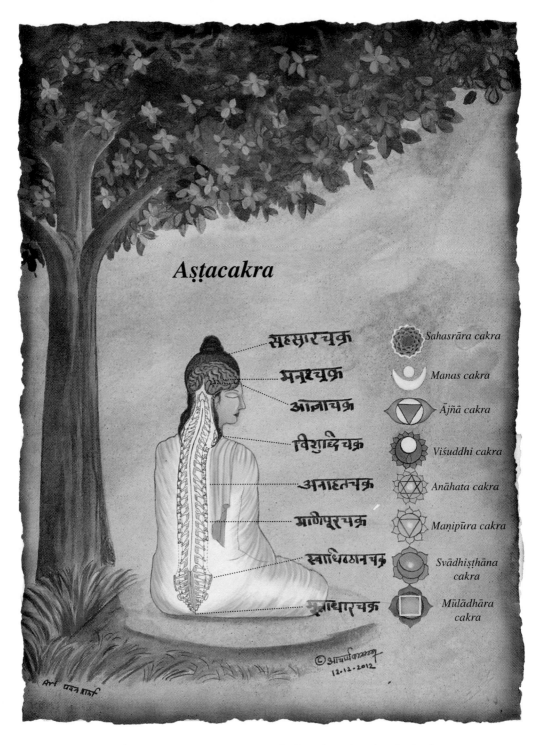

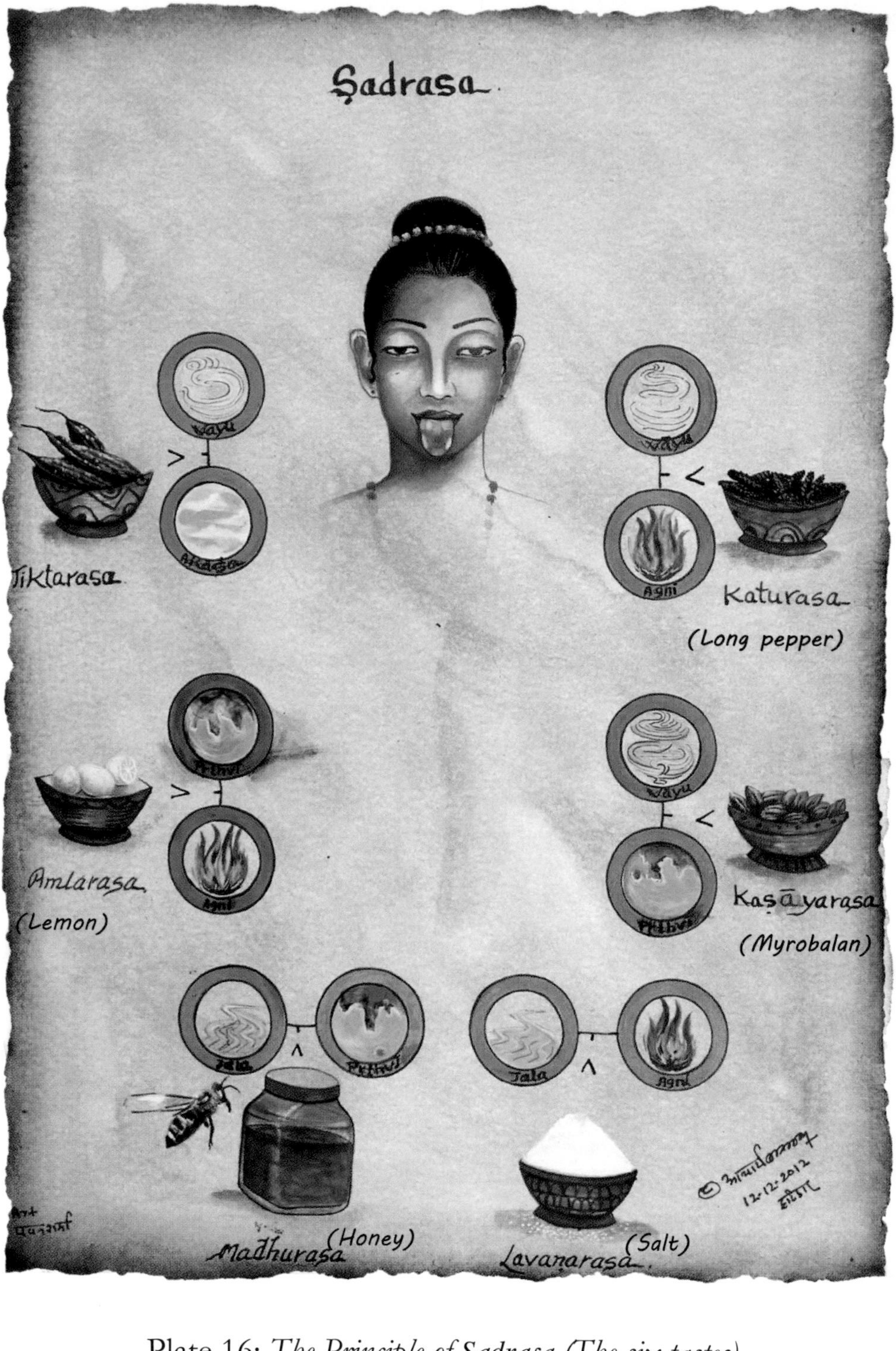

Plate 16: *The Principle of Ṣaḍrasa (The six tastes)*

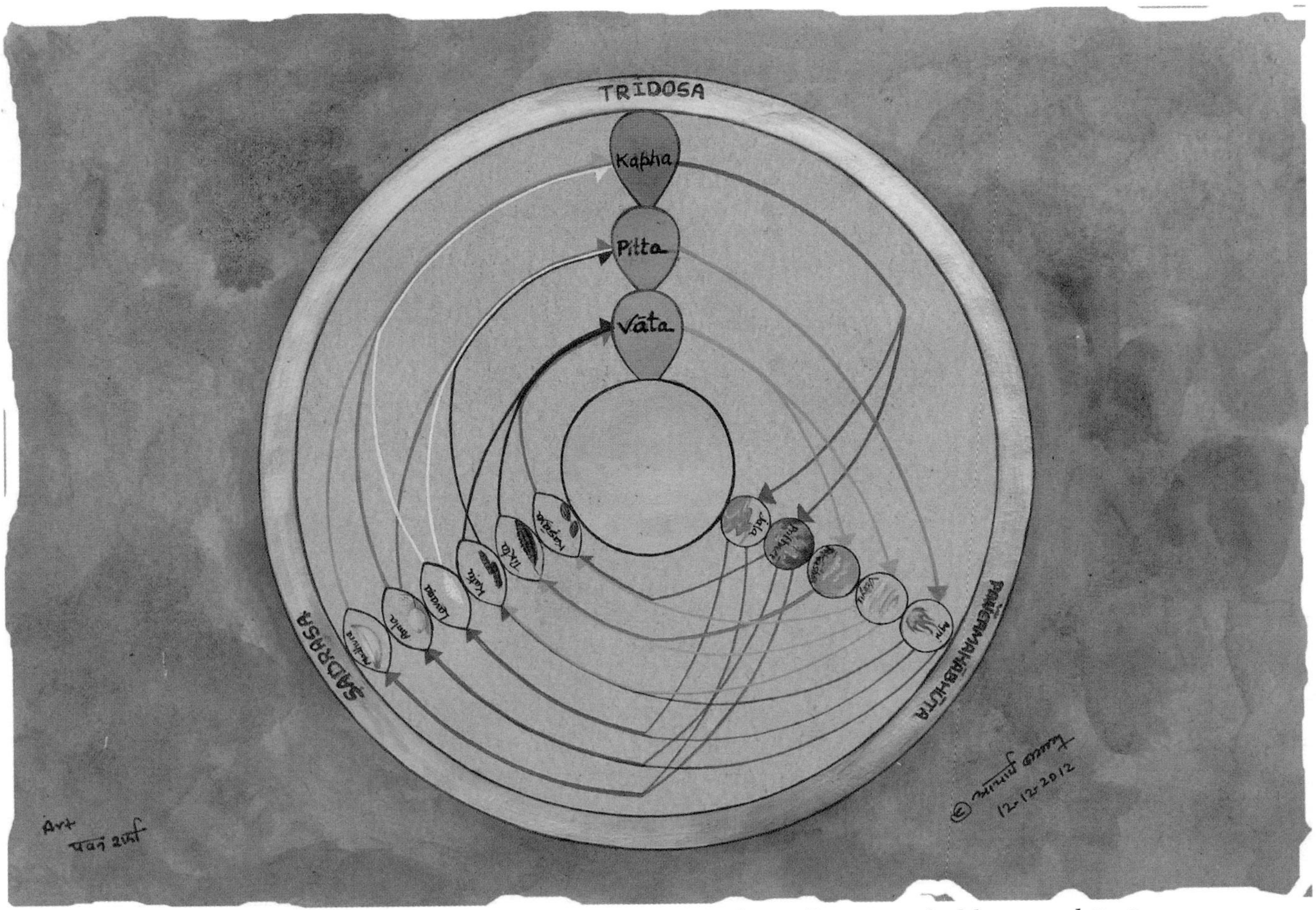

Plate 17: *The mutual relationship between Tridoṣa, Pañcamahābhūta and Ṣaḍrasa*

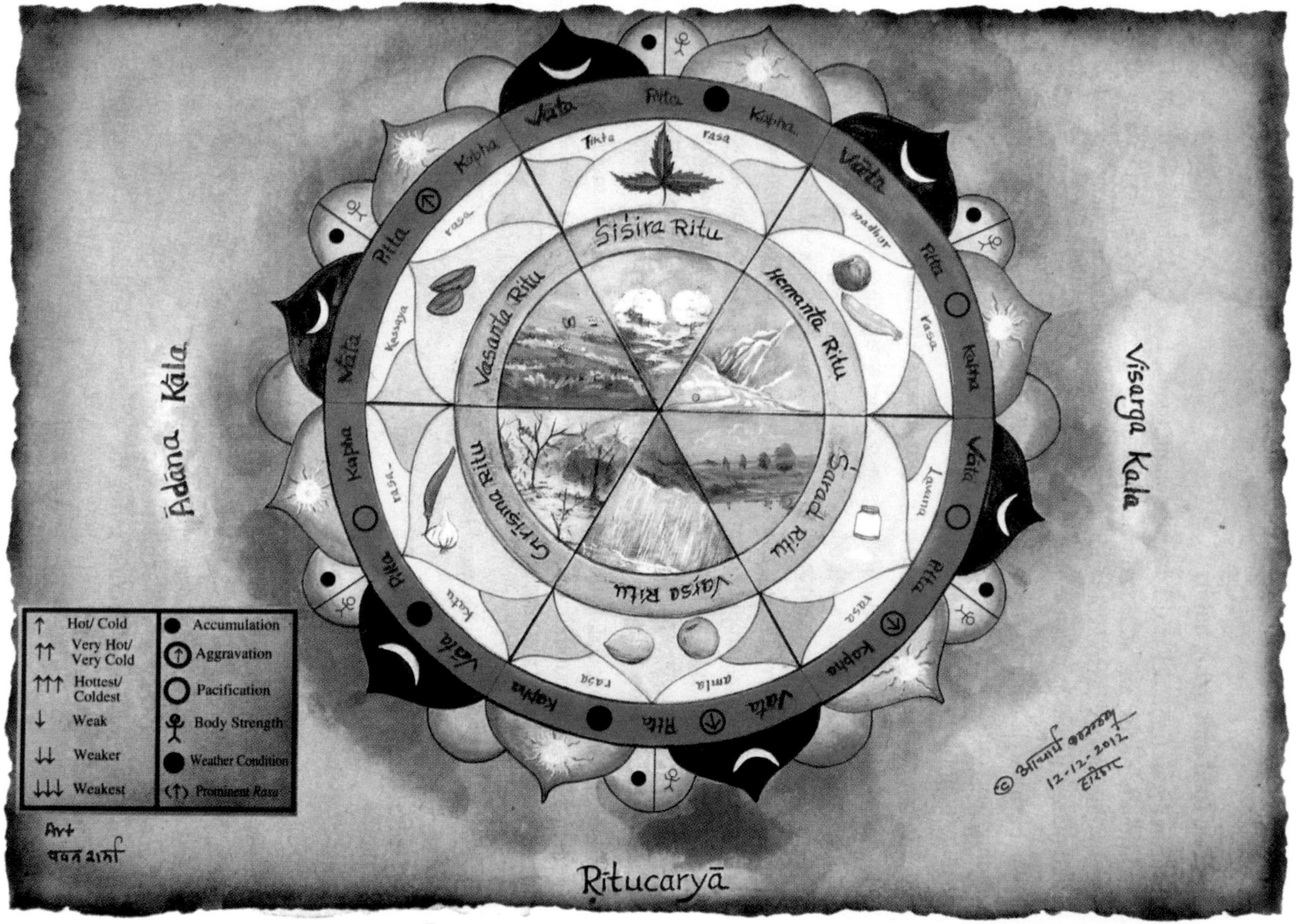

PLATE 18: *The six seasons in Ādāna and Visarga Kāla, condition of the Doṣas and the beneficial taste prominant in each season.*

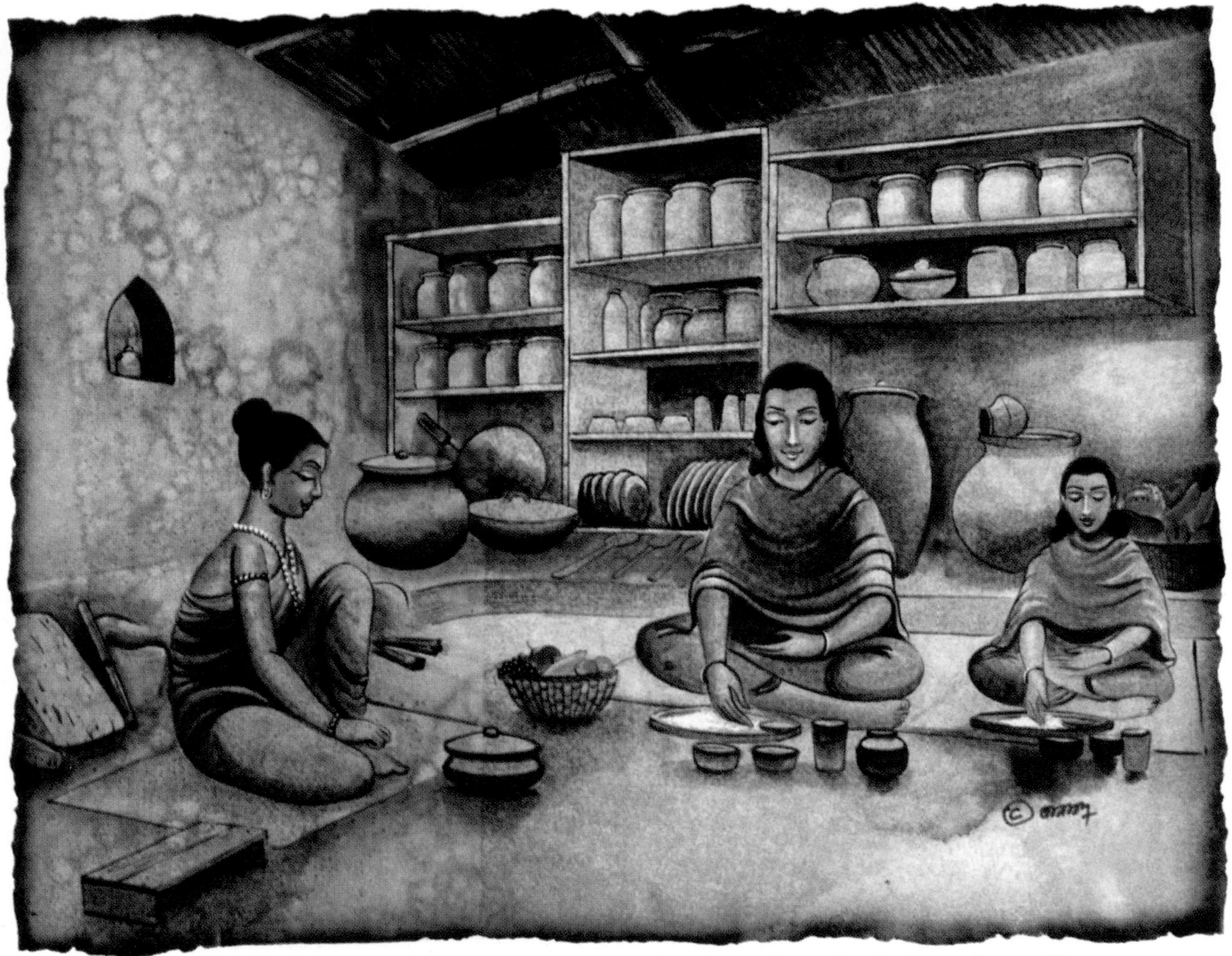

PLATE 19: *An outlook of ancient kitchen: clean, hygienic and sāttvika*

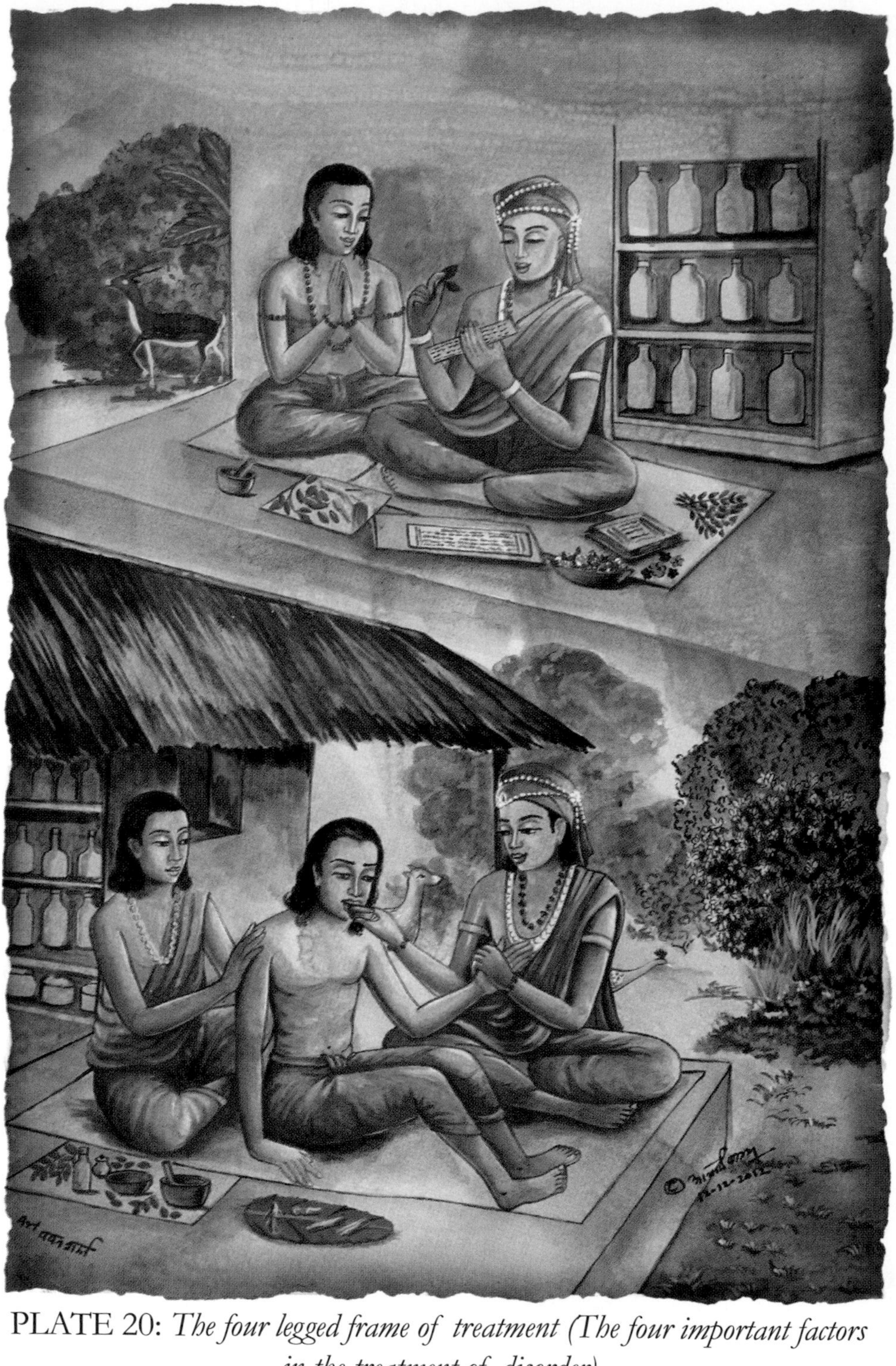

PLATE 20: *The four legged frame of treatment (The four important factors in the treatment of disorder)*

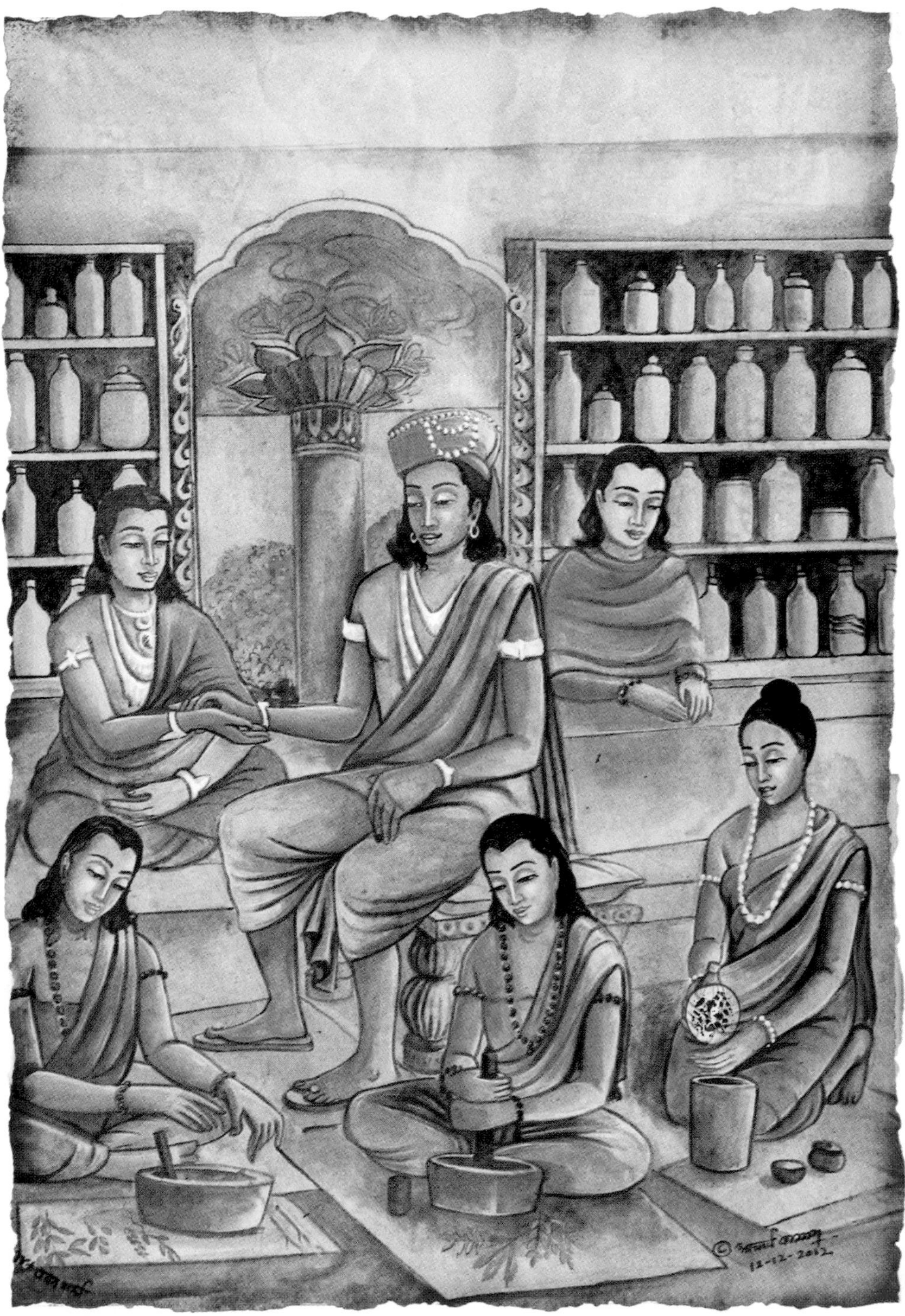

PLATE 21: *Examination of disease and treatment by a skilled physician*

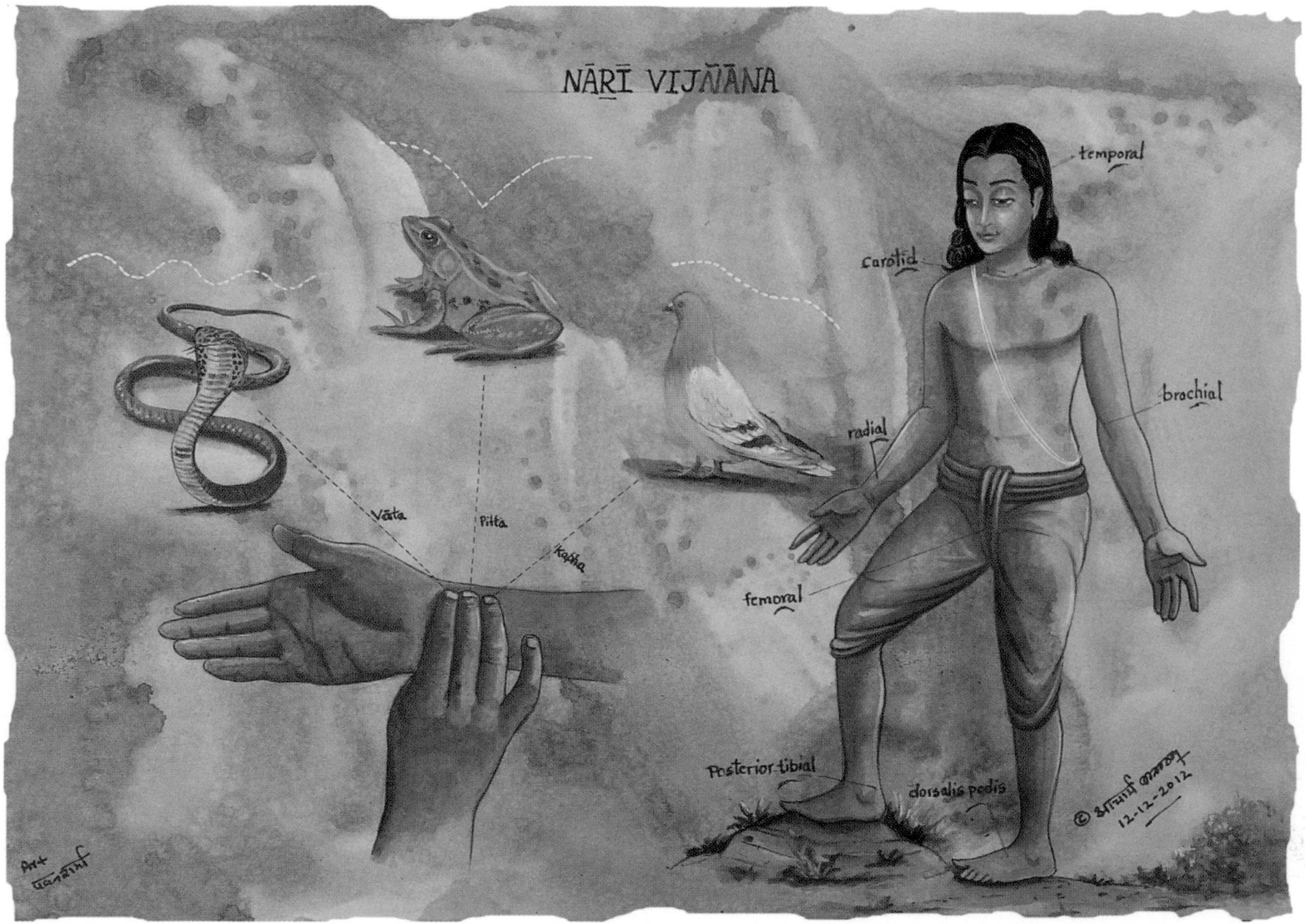

PLATE 22: *The method of pulse examination (nāḍi parīkṣaṇa)*

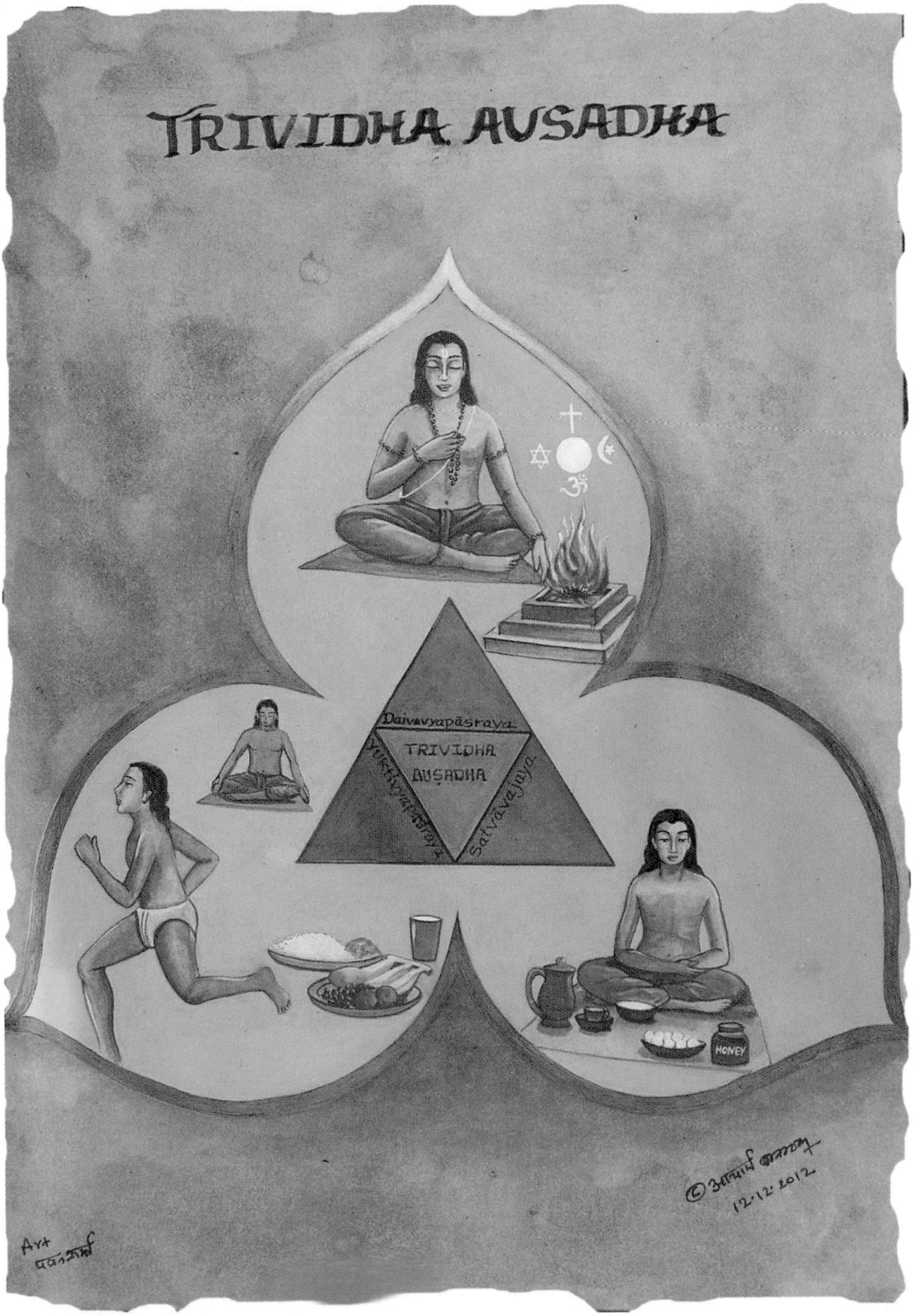

PLATE 23: *The three main types of treatments*

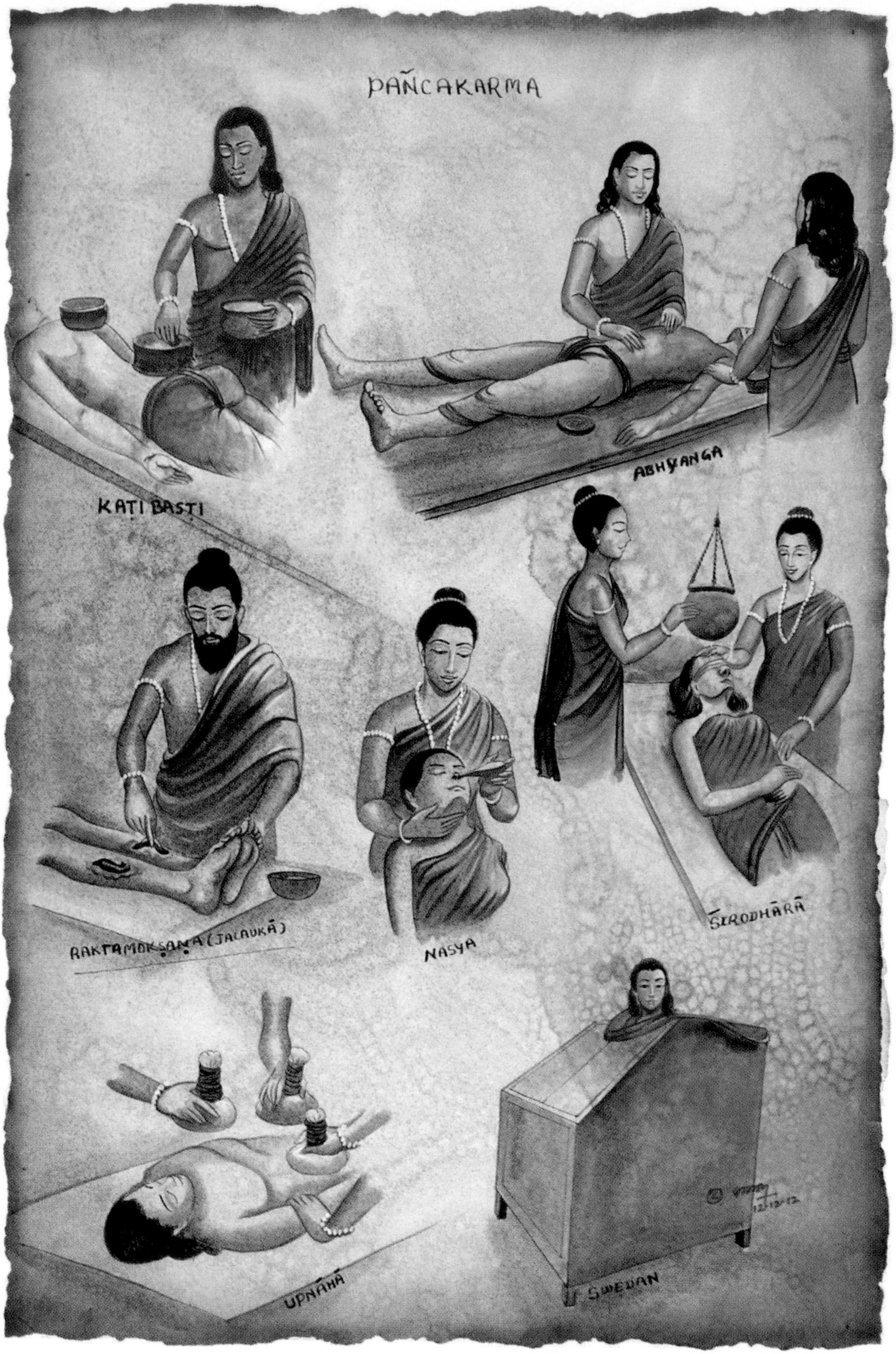

PLATE 24: *Different methods of Pañcakarma*

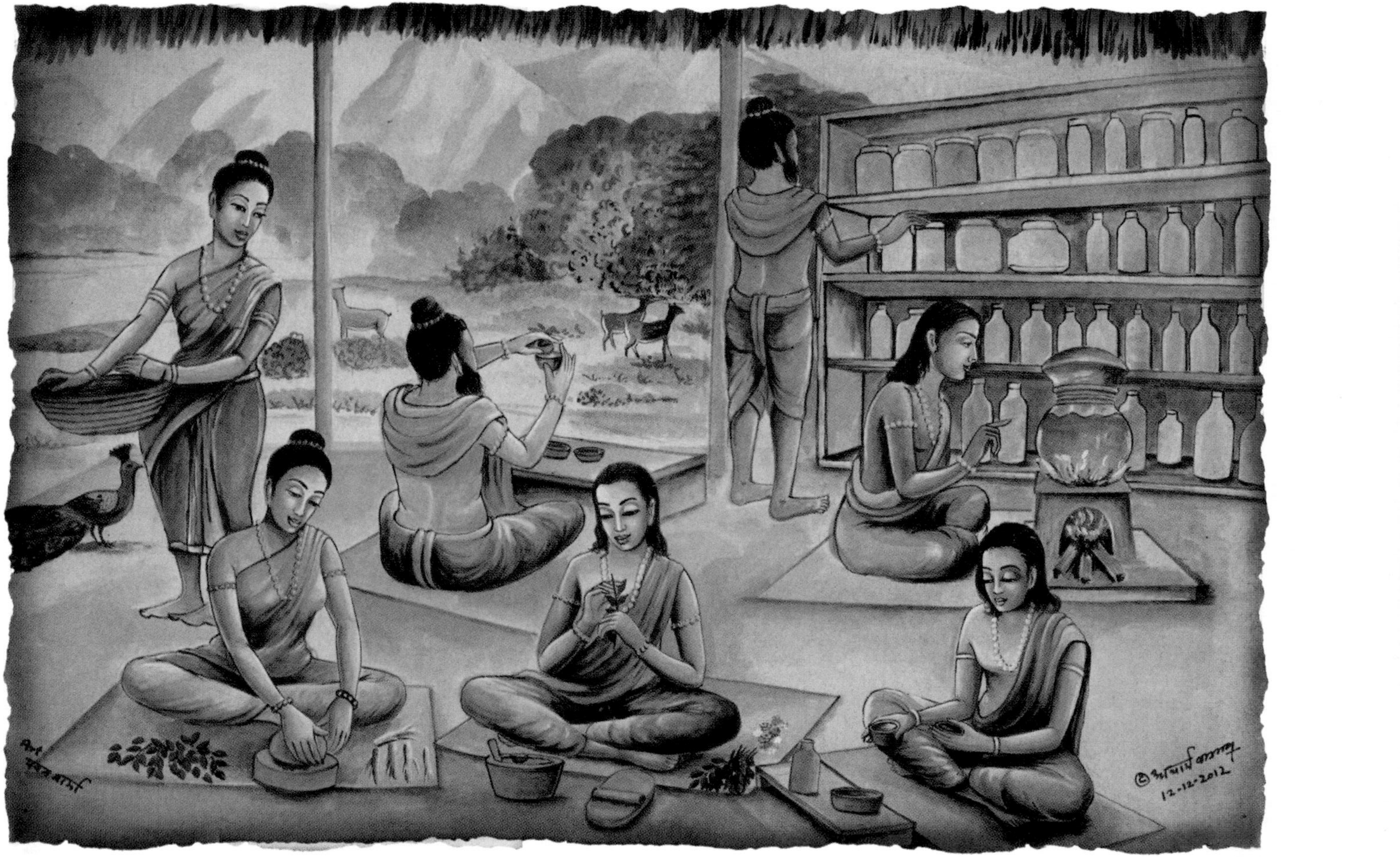

PLATE 25: *A practical approach for preparation and preservation of herbal medicines during ancient ages*

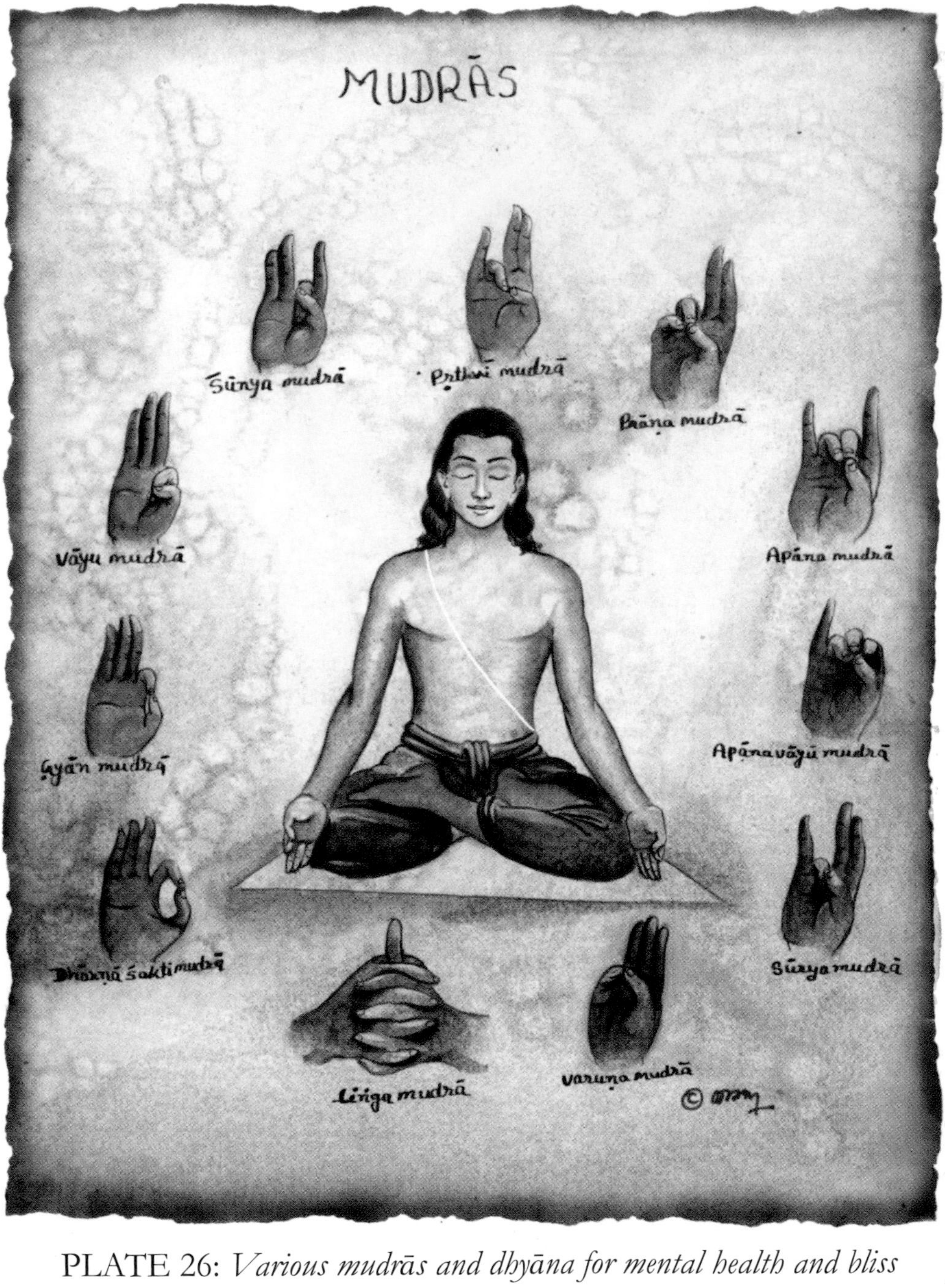

PLATE 26: *Various mudrās and dhyāna for mental health and bliss*

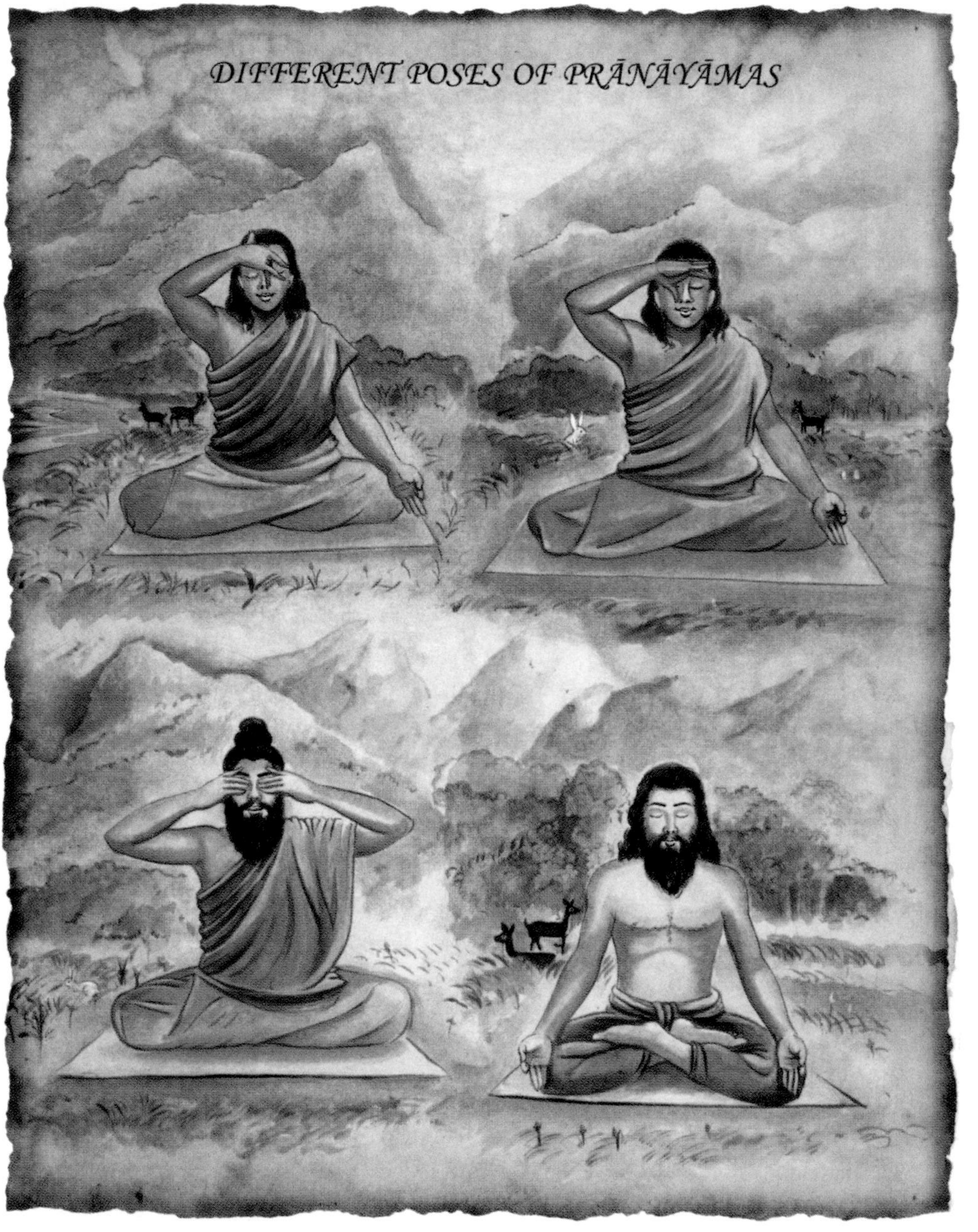

PLATE 27: *Different poses of prāṇāyāmas, at a glance*

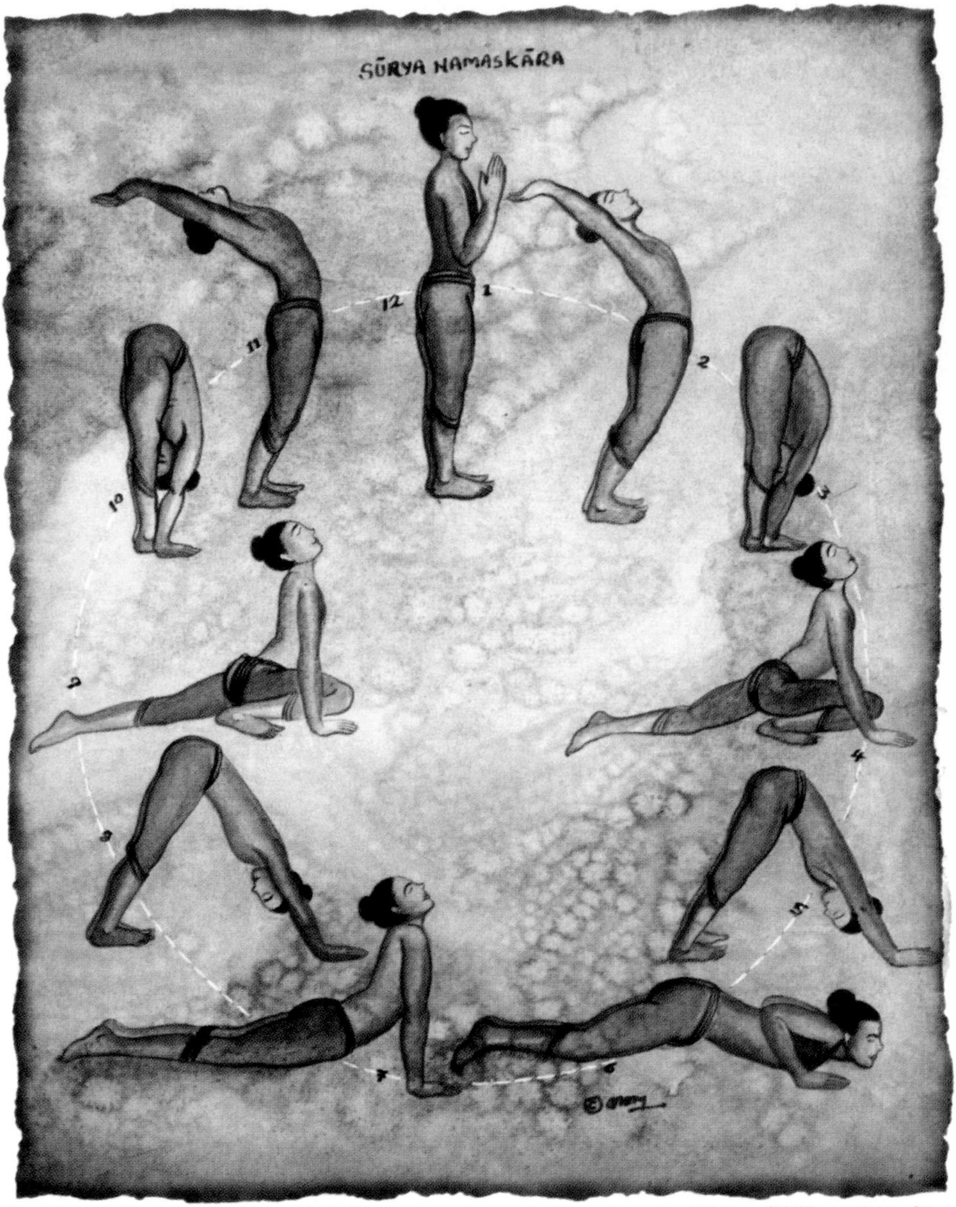

1. Salutation position (*Samasthiti*)
2. Palm tree position (*Tāḍāsana*)
3. Hand to foot postion (*Uttānāsana*)
4. Equestrian position (*Aśwasancalanāsana*)
5. Mountain position (*Adhomukha svānāsana*)
6. Eight limbs position (*Aśṭanga Namaskār*)
7. Cobra position (*Bhujaṅgāsana*)
8. Mountain position (*Adhomukha svānāsana*)
9. Equestrian position (*Aśwasancalanāsana*)
10. Hand to foot postion (*Uttānāsana*)
11. Palm tree position (*Tāḍāsana*)
12. Salutation position (*Samasthiti*)

PLATE 28: *Different steps of Sūrya Namaskar*

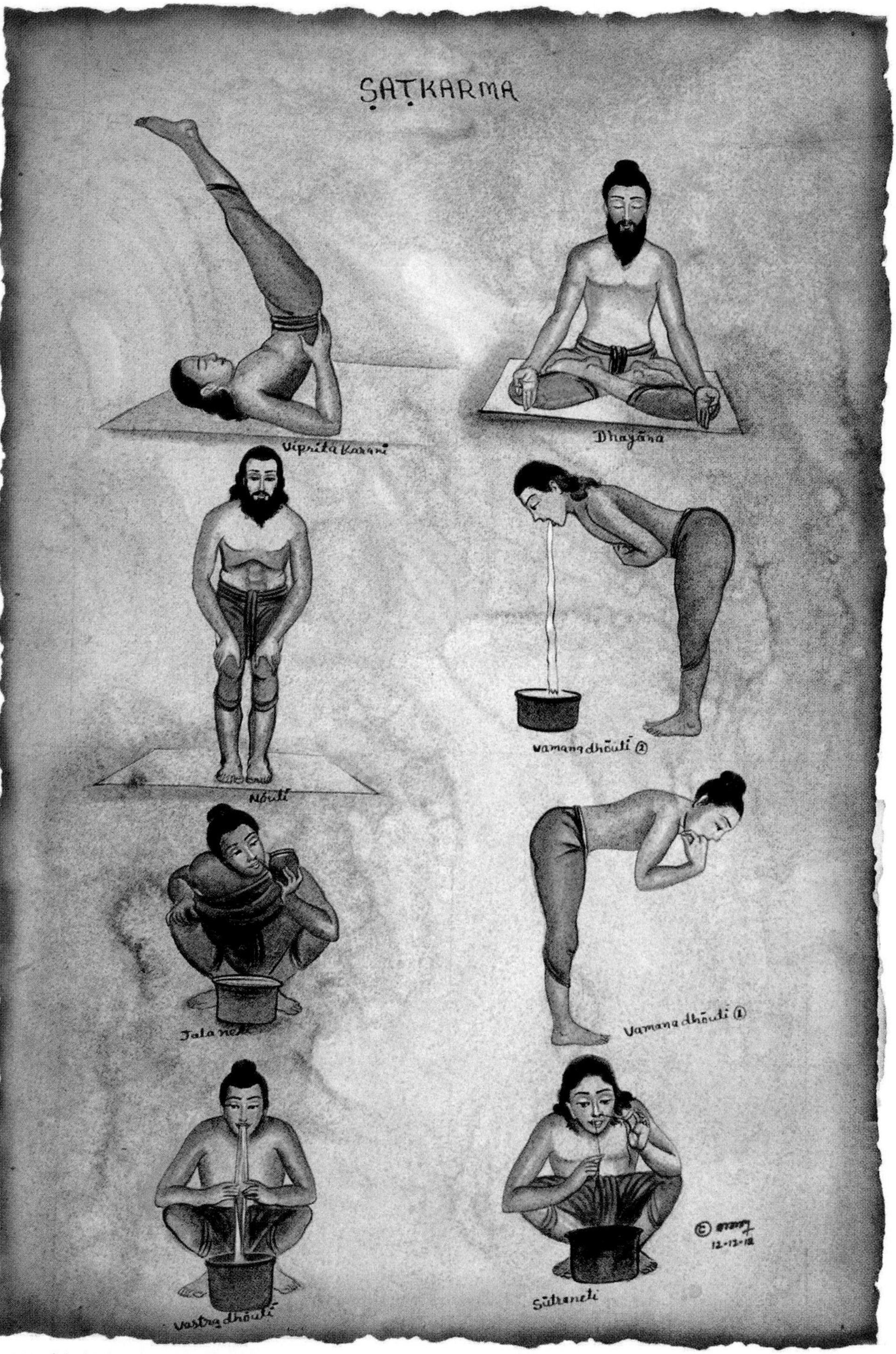

PLATE 29: *Different procedures of Ṣaṭkarma: an ancient and well-know technique for body purification and good health*

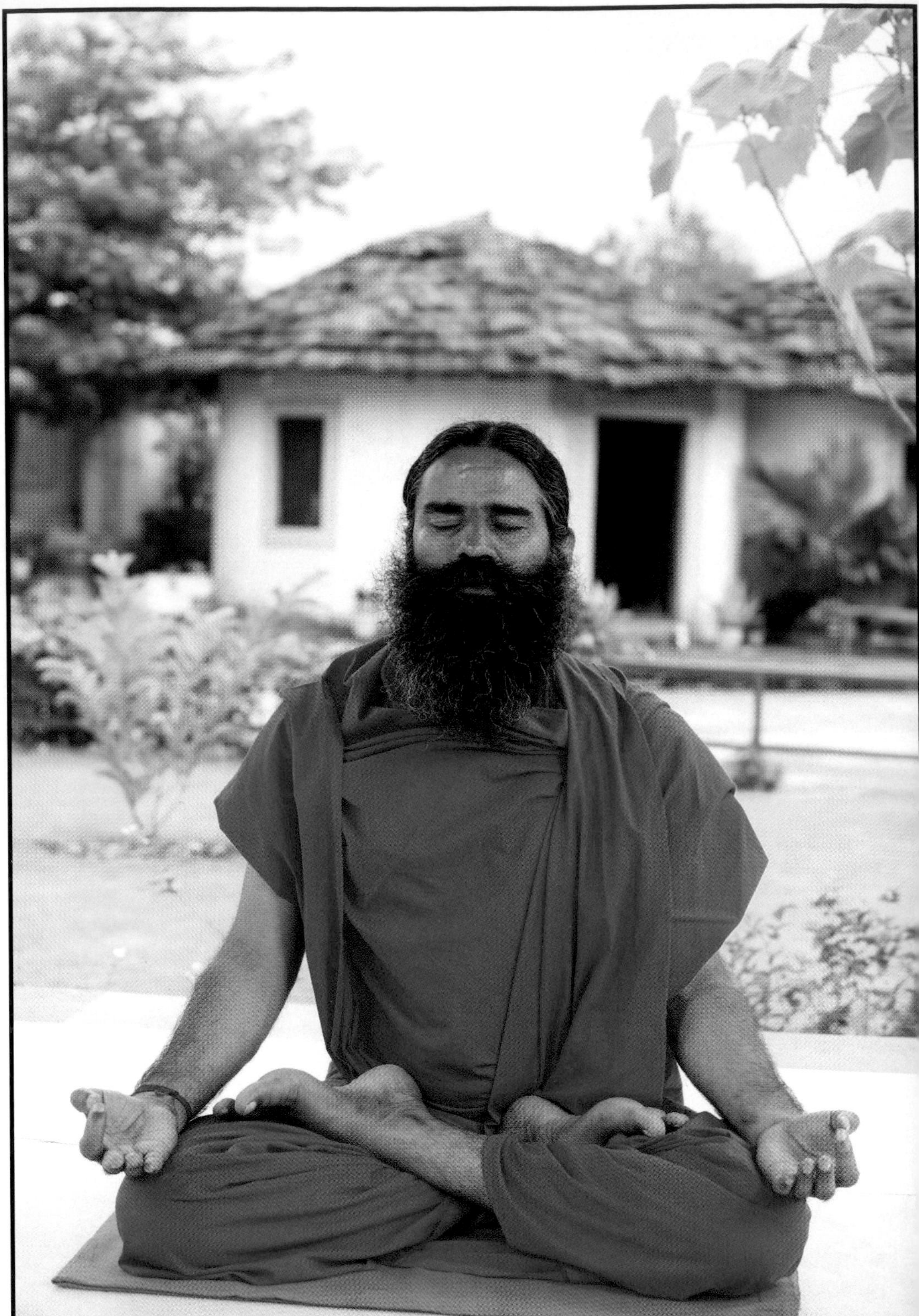

PLATE 30: Swami Ramdev - the *Yoga* guru

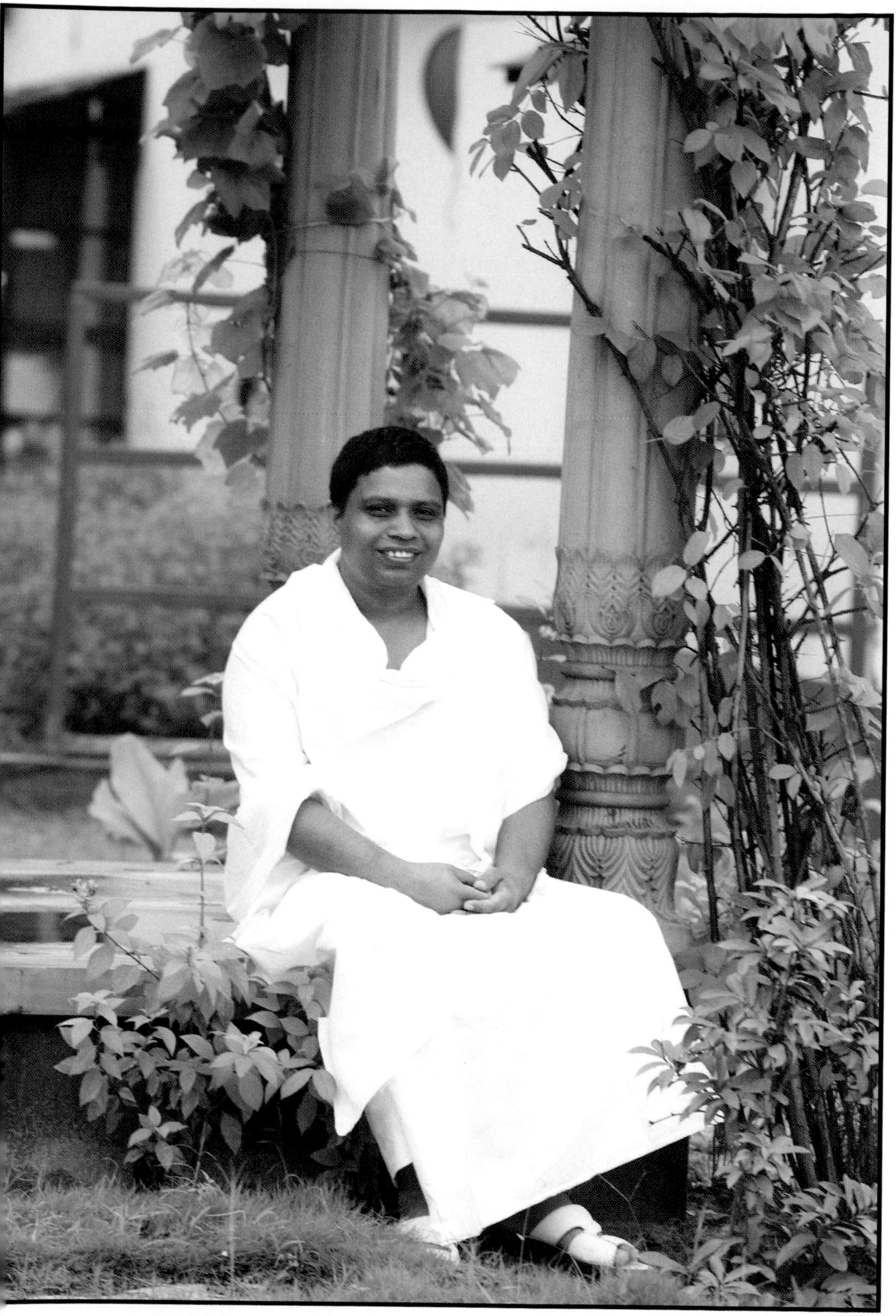

PLATE 31: Acharya Balkrishna - author and *Ayurveda* expert

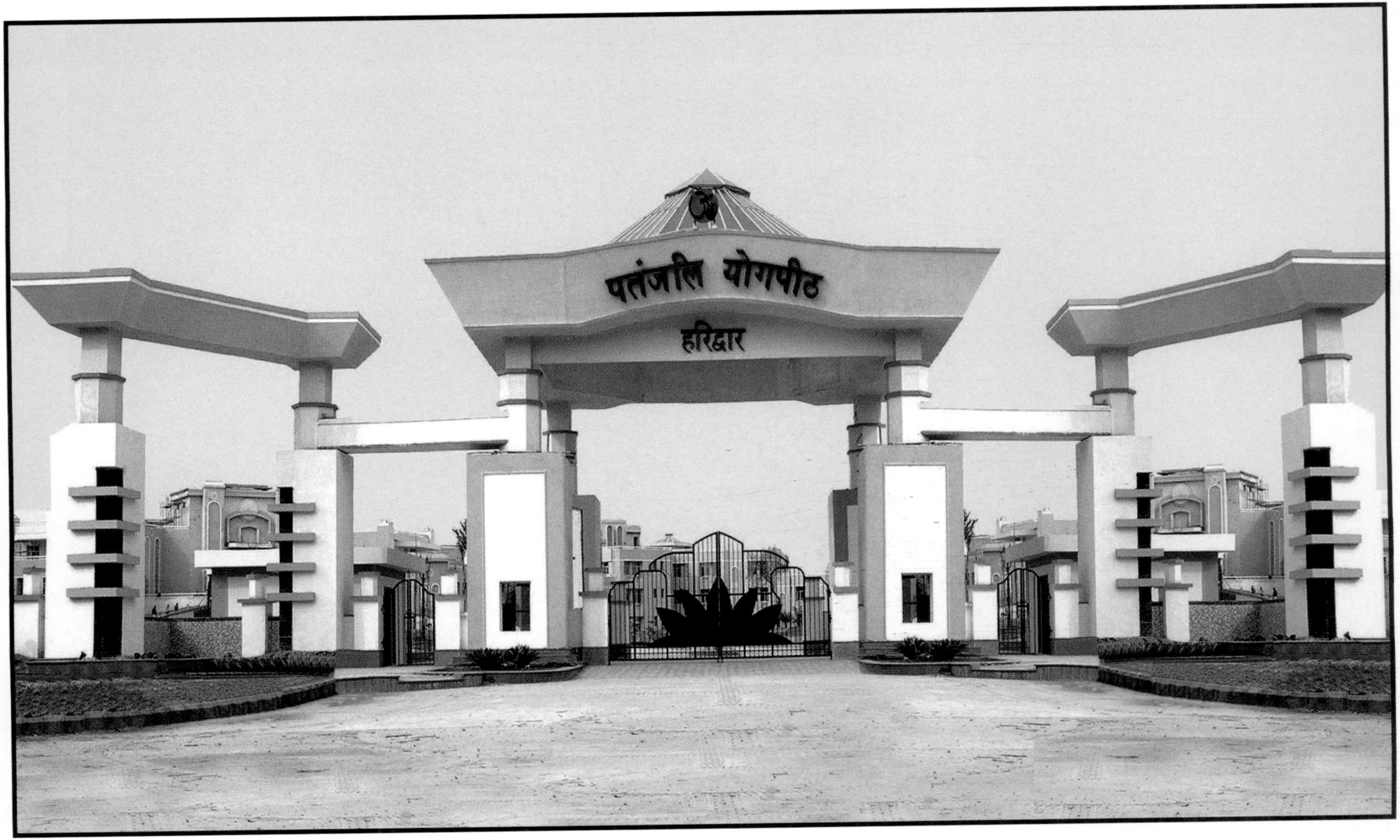

PLATE 32: Patanjali Yogpeeth - founded by Swami Ramdev and Acharya Balkrishna

absence results in problems related to softening of food, which hampers digestion. This way, it may lead to disease development.

Under certain special circumstances, even normal intake of *anupāna* must be avoided. For example, in cough, bronchial asthma, chest injury, excessive salivation, head and neck ailments and sore throat (pharyngitis), intake of water or other adjuvants (drinks) along with food is inappropriate[(4)]. *Āyurveda* recommends different *anupānas* according to foods and illnesses. (Table 21)

Table 21: Types of *Anupāna* (Adjuvants)

Ailments / Substances	*Anupānas* (Adjuvants)
Physiological ailments	
• *Kapha* vitiation	Hot and dry substances
• *Vata* vitiation	Hot and oily substances
• *Pitta* vitiation	Sweet and cool substances
• Bleeding/ Intrinsic hemorrhage	Milk/sugarcane juice
• Poisoning/ Toxic effect	Myrobalan
Physical ailments	
• Fasting, physical exertion, fatigue, weakness due to excessive walking and sexual activity	Milk or clarified butter (*ghee*) or milk with honey. *Āsava* and *ariṣṭa*
• Weakness due to alcohol, emaciation, insomnia, obesity, fatigue, laziness, dizziness	Honey + lemon in warm water
• Cool, heavy and incompatible food; overeating	Warm milk (with added dry ginger powder)
Edible substances	
• With oily substances (*ghee,* oil, butter)	Warm water
• Honey	Water
• Rice, green gram and dishes containing them	Milk
• Black gram pulse	Yogurt, whey, fermented digestive appetizer (*kāñjī*)
• Preparations made from the paste of ground pulses	Oil, soup and fermented digestive appetizer (*kāñjī*)
• Yogurt, rice pudding, dishes of ground grain paste	Cold or normal water

4. *Varjyaṁ turdhvajatrugadaśvāsakāsaprasekahidhmā svarabhedoraḥ kṣatibhirgītabhāṣyaprasaktaiśca.* (*A.saṅ.sū.* 10/55)

Water is the primary *anupāna*(5), being most often used and most easily available. Hence, first of all the necessary information regarding water is quoted here.

1. Water

Pure water is like nectar. It is a vital liquid(6) whose absence can lead to death. Clean and normal water relieves *Pitta* and minimizes toxic effects, relieves dizziness, burning, indigestion, fatigue, syncope, intoxication and vomiting. It also strengthens the heart. *Āyurveda* describes several properties of water, which changes according to its state, on being boiled, cooled, boiled and cooled, warmed and cooled. Keep these properties in mind while using water.

- **Pure and drinkable water**

Rainwater that does not fall on the ground is pure and considered to be the best water if collected properly. Water available from the second rains of the monsoon is considered more pure, as the first rains of the monsoon wash along with it all the impurities and pollutants present in the environment. Due to the mixing of impurities into the rainwater upon reaching the earth°s surface, its purity level changes. It adopts the properties and impurities of the place (rivers, lakes and other such places) being mixed in. Spring water obtained from the earth is another pure form of water after rainwater, but it is not commonly available. Thereafter, water of the falls located at pollution free places is also a natural and pure form of water. Pure water in its natural form is not available for everyone, hence normal water can be used after it has been treated, boiled and cooled. Such water is also as useful as naturally available, pure water. Boiling purifies water which then becomes light, elevates the digestive fire, becomes a good medium for digestion and acquires the ability to calm vitiated *doṣas*.

- **Time, quantity and the method of water intake**

Drinking water at the right time, in the right way and in an appropriate quantity is very important. Excessive water intake weakens the power of digestion, resulting in improper digestion. On the other hand, drinking very little or no water at all also hampers the digestion. It leads to the development of various ailments due to lack of urination and waste elimination, which causes an accumulation of toxic wastes in the body. *Āyurveda* emphasizes drinking a little water at frequent intervals rather than a lot in one go. This fulfills the water requirement of the body and it also boosts digestive power. Water acts like a medicine during bouts of indigestion.

Drinking water after the digestion of food lends strength to the body.

5. *Anupānaṁ tu salilameva śreṣṭhaṁ.*
Sarvarasayonitvātsarvabhūtasātmyatvājjīvanādi guṇayogācca. (*A.saṅ.sū.* 10/42)
6. *Jīvanaṁ tarpaṇaṁ hṛdyaṁ hlādi buddhiprabodhanam.*
Tanvavyaktarasaṁ mṛṣṭaṁ śītaṁ śucyamṛtopamam. (*A.saṅ.sū.* 6/3)

Drinking water before eating weakens the digestive power and results in debility. A few sips of water taken between meals boost digestion and increases the life-span. Water taken an hour after a meal strengthens the body and increases the body mass. Avoid drinking water at least half an hour before a meal. Obese people should drink water between meals and a feeble person after a meal (at least after half an hour). Others should drink water one hour after the meal. Water intake immediately after a meal is harmful for obese and physically strong people. On the other hand, water taken between meals works as nectar. One should consume buttermilk immediately after lunch.

Water intake is beneficial for everyone in all situations, but under certain conditions its quantity should be reduced, such as anorexia, excessive salivation, diabetes, weak digestion, obstinate abdominal ailments (especially ascites), edema, kidney dysfunctioning, chronic cold, tuberculosis, eye ailments, skin diseases such as leprosy and wounds. No water intake also leads to various disorders. If the quantity of water is determined on the basis of circumstances, only then it is advantageous. In *Vāta* and *Kapha* disorders and in obesity, warm water is beneficial, whereas in *Pitta* aggravation cold water is effective. In some conditions warm or hot water is effective and beneficial, whereas in others cold water acts as nectar. Cold water is useful in indigestion and burning in the stomach because it soothes and strengthens digestion, but it is harmful in bronchial asthma, cold and cough. It elevates the problem. Keeping this fact in mind, it becomes necessary to understand the qualities and effects of different types of water.

- **Prohibition of water intake immediately after meal**

Do not drink water immediately after a meal as it obstructs the assimilation of nutrients during digestion and its absorption by different body elements. It is especially not recommended in ailments of the head due to aggravation of *Vāta*, hiccoughs, cough, bronchial asthma and tuberculosis. In head ailments, drinking water after meals causes further aggravation of *Vāta*. Normally, the oil present in the food calms the *Vāta*, but water which is cold in attribute vitiates *Vāta*.

Singers, speakers, teachers or students who have to strain their vocal cords more than usual should avoid drinking water after meals, as it washes off the essential oils taken in with a meal. These oils are soothing and on their removal the throat becomes dry leading to soreness in the throat.

- **Cold water**[7]

Cold water is effective during syncope, dizziness, fatigue, dyspnoea (breathlessness), aggravated *Pitta*, burning sensation, blood vitiation, poisoning, intoxication, vomiting and bleeding, for example from the nose.

7. *Śītaṁ madātyayaglānimūrcchācchardiśramabhramān.*
Tṛṣṇoṣmadāpittāsṛgviṣāṇyambu nihanti tat. (*A.saṅ.sū.* 6/43)

It also boosts digestion. However, cold water aggravates anorexia, distension, flatulence, sprue syndrome, cold (coryza), sore throat, congestion, bronchial asthma, cough, hiccoughs, pain in the ribs, cataract and is detrimental after eating oily foods (clarified butter, oil, butter and other such products).

- **Hot water**[8]

Hot water is light. It boosts the digestive power and alleviates digestive disorders. It pacifies chronic cold, hiccoughs, distension, flatulence and the effects of aggravated *Vāta*. Boiled water is pure and free of all disease-causing elements. Water boiled and reduced to three-fourth of its original quantity acquires properties to pacify *Vāta* and eradicates *Vāta* engendered diseases. Half the original amount of water left after boiling is called *uṣṇa* (hot water). It is always beneficial and rectifies *tridoṣa* (*Vāta*, *Pitta* and *Kapha*) and associated diseases. It purifies urine and is favorable in bronchial asthma, cough, fever and digestive problems. Drinking hot water at night dissolves accumulated *Kapha* and aids in elimination of *Vāta* and excretory problems.

One-fourth of the original quantity of water left after boiling is called *arogyambu*. It is always beneficial, light, easily absorbable and also strengthens digestive fire (*jaṭharāgni*). If taken hot, *ārogyambu* relieves constipation, flatulence, distension in the stomach, severe stomachache, anemia, shooting pain, piles, abdominal swelling, vomiting, colitis, diarrhea, dysentry, fever, edema, rib pain, bronchial asthma, cough, hiccoughs, excessive thirst and *Vāta* and *Kapha* aggravation. It also purifies urine.

Boiled water after cooling is called *śṛtaśīta*. It is effective in diarrhea, intoxication, poisoning, vomiting, dizziness, syncope, excessive thirst, burning sensation, vitiated *Pitta* and blood, *Kapha* and *Vāta* engendered diseases, problems associated with intake of alcoholic substances and simultaneous aggravation of all three *doṣas (sannipāta)*.

Cover the water container after boiling and let it be cool. Such water becomes very light. It does not cause blockage in the *srotas* and alleviates aggravation of all three *doṣas*, worm infestations, excessive thirst and fever.

Boiled water when cooled by transferring it from one container to another is called *dhārāśīta*. It becomes heavy as air flows within it. This water requires time for absorption and may cause constipation. Boiled water becomes heavy if kept for 12 hours or more and is not easily absorbed. It also aggravates all three *doṣas*.

- ***Haṁsodaka* or *aṁsūdaka* water**[9] **(water kept in sunlight and moonlight)**

Water kept in sunlight during the day time and in moonlight at night

8. *Kaphamedo, nilāmaghnaṁ dīpanaṁ bastiśodhanam.*
Śvāsakāsajvaraharaṁ pathyamuṣṇodakaṁ sadā. (*Su.sū.* 45/39)
Pārśvaśūlāmamedaḥ su sadyaḥ śuddhau navajvare.
Dīpanaṁ pācanaṁ kaṇṭhyaṁ laghu basti viśodhanam. (*A.saṅ.sū.* 6/44-45)
9. *Divā sūryāṅśusantaptaṁ niśi candrāṅśuśītalam.*
Kālena pakvaṁ nirdoṣamagasyenāviṣikṛtam.
Hanśodakaṁiti khyātaṁ śāradaṁ vimalaṁ śuci.
Snānapānānavagāheṣu śasyate tadyathā, mṛtam. (*Ca.sū.* 6/46-47)

is called *'haṁsodaka'* or *'aṁsūdaka.'* This water is as beneficial as nectar. Such water becomes smooth and oily and has a calming effect on all three *doṣas*. It is cool and easily digestible, boosts energy and intellect, acts as a rejuvenator and does not obstruct the flow of body fluids in *srotas*. It is free from all the *doṣas*.

- ***Uṣaḥpāna* (water intake in the morning)**

  Drinking water on an empty stomach in the morning prevents sore throat, aggravated cold, bronchial asthma, constipation, edema, and even possibly wrinkles and graying of the hair.

- **Water intake according to the season**

  Summer and autumn: *Ārogyambu*-water boiled to one-fourth of its original quantity.

  Winter, rain and spring: *Uṣṇa*-water reduced to half its original quantity after boiling.

- **Time required for absorption of water**

  Water tthat is not boiled takes three hours, boiled and cooled takes one and a half hour and boiled water that is drunk warm takes 45 minutes to get absorbed. It is clear that unboiled water is the heaviest and boiled and warm water is the lightest. One must choose water according to one°s digestive capacity.

- ***Identification of impure water(10)**

  Water is a carrier of many diseases, so always drink clean and pure water. Easily identifiable impure water contains foreign bodies like mud, slurry, algae, leaves, straw, insects, mosquitoes, flies, their excreta and eggs, several toxic pollutants and industrial wastes. Water that is dirty, has an unpleasant odor or has changed color and taste is also impure. Water that has no access to sunlight and moonlight is also considered impure and unfit for consumption. Water from unexpected, unseasonal rains or water collected from the ground immediately after rains is impure and polluted. Such impure water is unfit for drinking and even for bathing. Water and its impurities are divided into different categories:

1. **Impurity of touch (*sparśa*)**: Water that is rough, harsh or hard (due to added impurities), hot and viscous while drinking.
2. **Visual impurity (*rūpa*)**: Water containing foreign bodies such as leaves, straw, dust and other pollutants and water that has changed color.

10. *Kīṭāhimūtraviṭkothatṛṇajālotkaṭāvilam.Paṅkapaṅkajaśaivālahaṭharṇādisaṁstṛtam.
Sūryendupavanādṛṣṭaṁ juṣṭaṁ ca kṣudrajantubhiḥ. Abhivṛṣṭaṁ vivarṇaṁ ca kaluṣaṁ sthūlaphenilam.
Virasaṁ gandhavat taptaṁ dantagrāhyātiśaityataḥ Anārtavaṁ ca yadidavyamārtavaṁ prathamaṁ ca yat.
Lūtāditantuviṇmūtraviṣasaṁśleṣadūṣitam. Tatkuryāt snānapānābhyāṁ tṛṣṇā,, dhmānodarajvarān.
Kāsāgnisādābhiṣyandakaṇḍūgaṇḍādikānataḥ
Tadvarjayedabhāve vā toyasyānyasya śasyate.* (A.saṅ.sū. 6/21-25)
*Ghanavastraparisrāvaiḥ kṣudrajantvabhirakṣaṇam.
Vyāpannasyāsya tapanamagnyarkāyapiṇḍakaiḥ parṇīmla viṣagranthimuktākatakaśaivalaiḥ.
Vastagomedakābhyāṁ vā kārayettatprasādanam.* (A.saṅ.sū. 6:21-27)

* Even today this discussion is not relevant for millions of people in the world for whom clean and pure water is not available.

3. **Impurity of taste (*rasa*)**:Water with a distinct taste such as salt water.
4. **Impurityof smell (*gandha*)**: Water that has an unpleasant odor.
5. **Impurity of potency (*vīrya*)**: Water which takes time to get absorbed induces thirst even after drinking, causes heaviness and salivation.

Consuming water with these impurities can lead to several types of external problems (boils, pimples, itching, dry and chapped skin, and other skin problems) and internal disorders (digestive disorders, constipation, diarrhea, vomiting, burning in the stomach and so on).

In the absence of clean and pure water, if one is compelled to use impure water, it is necessary to purify the water before consumption. These are the several ways of doing so, exposing it to sunlight, cooling a burning lump of gold, silver, stone in impure water seven times, and straining water through a clean thick piece of cloth or using a filter. This way one can treat impure water and bring into use.

- **Some other useful liquid substances**

There are several other substances that we often use without knowing their qualities, effects and benefits. This chapter describes their qualities, when and how to use them, and in what way. This will help us to choose only those substances that suit us and avoid the ones that are not favorable and also direct us that how to change the potentially harmful substances to suit our body-type.

2. Coconut Water[11]

Nature has also provided us with water within the tender coconut. Coconut water that is naturally available is smooth, sweet, nourishing, cool, strengthening and easily digestible. It relieves excessive thirst; alleviates *Pitta*, *Vāta* and 'heat in the liver'; increases digestive fire; and detoxifies the urinary system. In all seasons, especially in summer, instead of other cold beverages (such as cold drinks and other aerated drinks) drinking coconut water is very advantageous.

Together with water, other liquids like milk, yogurt, clarified butter (*ghee*), oil and so on are also taken regularly in our diet. Not being aware of their properties and effects can lead to several misinterpretations. Hence, here is a brief description of each.

11. *Nārikelodakaṁ snigdhaṁ svādu vṛṣyaṁ himaṁ laghu.*
Tṛṣṇāpittānilaharaṁ dīpanaṁ bastiśodhanam. (*A.saṅ.sū.* 6/51)
Snigdhaṁ svādu himaṁ hṛdyaṁ dīpanaṁ basti śodhanam.
Vṛṣyaṁ pittapipāsāghnaṁ nārikelodakaṁ guru. (*Su.sū.* 45/44)

3. Milk

Milk is believed to be a nectar. In India, cow's milk is one of the best types of milk available, on the basis of the properties of the Indian breeds of cows, followed by goat milk and buffalo milk respectively. From the health point of view, goat's milk alleviates all the three *doṣas*. The milk of a Jersey cow (a breed of cow) is least effective in its properties. Though camel's milk is salty in taste, it boosts the strength. Generally, the taste (*rasa*) of all types of milk is sweet (except camel's milk); its *vipāka* (post-digestive effect) is sweet, oily and heavy; and its *vīrya* (potency) is cool. It alleviates *Pitta* and *Vāta* and increases *Kapha*.

Milk improves the intellect, is an aphrodisiac, provides strength and nourishment, builds *dhātus* and promotes rejuvenation. It has all the qualities of *ojas*, milk replenishes it. Milk is vital, it also adds energy to the life, relieves constipation, stops intrinsic hemorrhages (bleeding), brings smoothness in the body, helps in conception, aids in healing of wounds, enhances the complexion, strengthens the voice and calms the burning effects. It is beneficial in tuberculosis, chronic fever, hyperacidity, stomach ache after meals, stomach disorders, constipation, semen debility and emaciation. It also guards against old-age debilities. Regular intake of milk and *ghee* is particularly nourishing. It is considered to be a very good rejuvenator. Among all types of milk, cow's milk is considered to be the best and sheep's milk the least nourishing.

• Cow's milk[12]

Among Indian breeds of cows, there are about 50 varieties. The milk of those cows is considered best and regarded as heavenly nectar, which graze in the forest on several types of vegetation and medicinal herbs.

Properties

Cow's milk is considered to be the best milk among all types of milk. It is sweet, oily, heavy, cool and nourishing, and it calms *Vāta* and *Pitta doṣa*. Properties of cow's milk varies (according to the different breeds of Indian cows) from cow to cow with differences in the color of the cow and the condition of the cow's uterus. The milk from a young cow is sweet, rejuvenating, nourishing and pacifies all three *doṣas*. Milk from an old cow is not as nourishing. Similarly, milk from a black cow calms *Vāta doṣa* and is better in quality than milk from a yellow or white cow, which calms both *Vāta* and *Pitta doṣa*.

12. *Atra gavyaṁ tu jīvanīyaṁ rasāyanam.Kṣatakṣīnahitaṁ medhyaṁ varṇyaṁ stanyakaraṁ saram. Śramabhramamadālakṣmīśvāsakāsātitṛkṣudhaḥ. Jīrṇa jvaraṁ mūtrakṛcchraṁ raktapittaṁ ca nāśayet.* (A.saṅ.sū. 6/54-55)

Advantages

It boosts the strength and intellect, improves lactation (in nursing women), strengthens the life-force, does not accumulate in *srotas*, works as a laxative, acts as a rejuvenator, minimizes the effects of old-age and is beneficial for people recovering from sickness or injury.

Indications

It is beneficial in cough, chest injuries, excessive thirst, chronic fever, dysuria and intrinsic hemorrhage (bleeding).

- **Buffalo milk**

Buffalo milk is very white and pleasantly smooth. It has a higher total solid fat content than cow's milk, which makes it more creamy and thick.

Properties

Buffalo milk is much cooler, heavier and creamier than cow's milk.

Advantages

It is very good for people with sharp or 'burning' digestive fire. It is considered as one of the best sedative for people suffering from insomnia. Buffalo milk contains a larger quantity of *ghee* compared to cow's milk. However, the quality of *ghee* from cow's milk is said to be better.

Disadvantages

It increases *Vāta,* accumulates in the *srotas* and causes blockages.

- **Goat milk**

Goat milk is not as widely used as cow and buffalo milk, but it is also used medicinally, as it is light to digest. It is very beneficial for infants and patients.

Properties

It is sweet with an astringent flavor, cool and light in attributes. It is anti-diarrheal and absorbs water from the intestines (hence called *grāhī* in *Āyurveda*).

Advantages

Boosts digestion by increasing the digestive fire and strengthens the appetite.

Indications

Goat milk has several medicinal properties. It is beneficial in tuberculosis, fever, bronchial asthma, intrinsic hemorrhage (bleeding), cough, emaciation and poisoning.

Normally unboiled, cold milk has a tendency to accumulate in the *srotas* and is heavy, while boiled thick milk is light and does not accumulate in the *srotas*. Generally, cow milk immediately after extracting, in a natural hot form (*dhāroṣṇa*), buffalo milk that has been cooled after extracting (*dhārāśīta*), and goat milk that has been cooled after boiling (*śṛtaśīta*) are considered best. But, nowadays it is difficult to get freshly extracted milk and also because of microbes present in the environment, it is advisable to drink boiled milk (which then gets Pasteurized and safe from microbes). But according to *Āyurveda*, stale and old milk is not fit to use and is very harmful because after a certain time after Pasteurization, microbial colonization from the external environment may again hamper its quality.

Milk extracted in the morning is heavier and cooler than milk collected in the evening. Milk at night is needed for those who suffer from burning, irritation and acidity caused by food taken during the daytime.

SUGGESTIONS

- Milk boiled without adding water turns heavy and oily. If water is added and then boiled until the water evaporates, it becomes light.
- Adding spices such as long pepper, dry ginger, turmeric and liquorice while boiling, reduces *Kapha* aggravating properties.
- It is believed that one who begins the day with a glass of water, takes diluted yogurt or buttermilk after lunch and drinks a glass of milk before going to bed, remains ever healthy and free of illness.
- Do not use milk if the taste, color and smell of milk is altered or the milk has fermented.
- Do not take salty and sour things with milk. It is an opposite combination and can lead to skin diseases such as dermatitis.

- **Cream of milk** is rich in oil, calms *Vāta* and *Pitta* and is an aphrodisiac (increases semen).
- **Milk of a cow that has recently calved** is heavy, thick, aggravates *Kapha* and is rich in protein. It also has a tendency to accumulate in the *srotas* (channels).
- ***Khoyā*** (dried and condensed whole milk) is heavy, oily, strengthening and an aphrodisiac (semen boosting).
- **Cottage cheese and curdled milk** is strength-providing but is lighter than *khoyā*.
- **Whey** (water left after curdling milk) is very nutritious and strengthening. It is beneficial for people suffering from weak digestion.

4. Yogurt[13]

Yogurt is a very common food that we eat routinely in our day-to-day life. It is one of the most useful foods known in *Āyurveda.* Its digestive properties are well-known. It restores the bacterial balance in the digestive

13. *Rocanaṁ dīpanaṁ vṛṣyaṁ snehanaṁ balavardhanam. Pāke, mlamuṣṇaṁ vātaghnaṁ maṅgalyaṁ bṛṁhaṇaṁ dadhi. Pīnase cātisāre ca śītake viṣamajvare. Arucau mūtrakṛcchre ca karśye ca dadhi śasyate.* (Ca.sū. 27/225-226)
Medaḥ śukrabalaśleṣmaraktapittāgni śophakṛt. Pīnase mūtrakṛcche ca rūkṣaṁ tu grahaṇīgade. (A.saṅ.sū. 6/65-66)

tract. But, there are so many facts that common people do not know about it.

Properties

- Yogurt is heavy and oily, sour in *rasa* (taste) and *vipāka* (post-digestive effect), and is hot in *vīrya* (potency).
- Accumulates and obstructs (block the *srotas*).
- It is anti-diarrheal and absorbs water from the intestines (hence called *grāhī* in *Āyurveda*).
- It mitigates *Vāta* and increases *Kapha* and *Pitta*.

Advantages

- It increases hemoglobin, physical strength and digestive power. It is nourishing and boosts the appetite.
- It acts as an aphrodisiac as it increases the quality and quantity of semen.

Disadvantages

Excessive and improper intake of yogurt may cause swelling (edema), blood disorders, fever, intrinsic hemorrhage (bleeding) and jaundice. It should not be used in diseases where blood is vitiated by *doṣas*.

Indications

It is indicated in abdominal disorders, chronic cold, malaria, debility, dysuria and influenza.

YOGURT: DO'S AND DONT'S

- Do not eat yogurt at night.
- Do not eat yogurt without additives such as *ghee*, honey, sugar, cooked green gram, Indian gooseberry powder, roasted cumin seeds, rock salt and so on. Its properties are enhanced when used with these substances.
- Do not boil or heat it over fire or in sunlight.
- It provocates *Kapha* and *Pitta*, therefore it is not recommended in summer, spring and autumn season.
- Monsoon and winter are the appropriate seasons for yogurt consumption.
- Sweet buttermilk (*lassī*), *rāyatā* (yogurt mixed with chopped fruits or vegetables and seasoned with various condiments) and gram flour (*besana*) + yogurt curry (*kaḍhī*) prepared by diluting yogurt with water can be eaten any time.
- Yogurt should be used only when it is well-set or completely coagulated.

- **Cream of yogurt:** It provides strength, increases semen (aphrodisiac) and is beneficial for hemorrhoids (piles).
- **Yogurt water (whey):** It is light, increases the digestive power, constipating, detoxifies the *srotas*, carminates *Vāta* and other waste products.
- **Butterless yogurt:** It is dry, flatulent, increases *Vāta* and constipation, but is beneficial in colitis or sprue syndrome (*grāhī*).
- **Unset yogurt:** Do not use unset yogurt as it is obstructive in nature, block the *srotas* and hence it is considered very deleterious.

5. Buttermilk

Buttermilk is prepared by diluting yogurt or churning it without water. Depending on the kind of yogurt used, buttermilk can be sweet, sour or very sour. The qualities of buttermilk vary according to the quantity of water and butter in it. Buttermilk made by churning yogurt without adding water is called '*ghola*,' which has one-fourth water is '*takra*,' when the quantity of water and yogurt is equal it is called '*udasvita*.' Buttermilk from which butter has been extracted by churning without adding any water in it is called '*mathita*.' When an adequate amount of water is added to extract butter by churning, the residual liquid is called '*chācha*.' *Chācha* is light, cool, alleviates *Vāta* and *Pitta*, and aggravates *Kapha*. It increases digestion when taken with salt. '*Takra*' with no butter content is very light and beneficial. Buttermilk that is made without extracting any butter content is very heavy, is a strength promoter and aggravates *Kapha*.

Properties of buttermilk[14]

- Buttermilk *(takra)* is light, sweet, sour and astringent, and is sweet in *vipāka* (post-digestive effect). It mitigates *Kapha* and *Vāta*.
- It boosts the appetite, is good for the heart and increases urination.
- It is anti-diarrheal, absorbs water from the intestine and solidifies fecal matter (*grāhī*).
- It is stimulating and scarifying, and purifies *srotas*.

Advantages

Buttermilk is the most potent remedy for *Kapha* and *Vāta* disorders. Buttermilk in different forms is the most suitable treatment for dysentry, colitis, mucus and chronic sprue syndrome.

Disdvantages

Fresh buttermilk (*takra or chācha*) removes accumulated *Kapha* from the abdominal organs, but causes phlegm formation in the throat. Do not use

14. *Takraṁ laghu kaṣāyāmlaṁ dīpanaṁ kaphavātajit. Śophodarārśograhaṇīdoṣamūtra grahārucīḥ. Gulmaplīhaghṛtavyāpadgarapāṇḍvāmayān jayet.* (*A.saṅ.sū.* 6/69-70)

fresh buttermilk in chronic cold, sinus, cough, bronchial asthma and throat problems instead use warm buttermilk. Extra sour buttermilk is harmful. Buttermilk of any kind should be avoided when suffering from chest injury, debility, dizziness, syncope, burning and intrinsic hemorrhage (bleeding). It should also be avoided during the heat generated in rainy season.

Indications

It is beneficial for abdominal disorders, sprue syndrome, abdominal swelling, jaundice, spleen disorders, obesity, dysuria, edema, poisoning and hemorrhoids (piles). It is also beneficial for diseases developed due to excessive intake of clarified butter (ghee) such as obesity. Modern science has confirmed that buttermilk is good for people suffering from obesity-related heart problems.

The effect of buttermilk changes along with different adjuvants added to it.

- Sour buttermilk+dried ginger and rock salt - Advantageous in *Vāta* disorders
- Sweet buttermilk (without any sourness) with added sugar - Beneficial in *Pitta* disorders
- Buttermilk+*trikaṭu* (dry ginger, black pepper, long pepper) and salt of barley (*yavakṣāra*) - Effective in *Kapha* disorders
- Buttermilk+asafoetida+cumin seeds+rock salt - Alleviates *Vāta*; effective in piles, diarrhea, colitis, pain in the bladder and improves digestion
- Buttermilk+jaggery - Beneficial in dysuria and other urinary disorders
- Buttermilk+leadwort *(citraka)* - Beneficial in jaundice

6. Butter

There are two types of butter: (i) made from yogurt, and (ii) made from milk, known as '*navanīta* or *nainū.*'

Properties

- Butter made from yogurt is sweet and astringent when fresh, and is sweet, light and oily in *vipāka* (post-digestive effect) and *śīta vīrya* (cool in potency). It alleviates *Vāta* and *Pitta,* improves the digestive fire, enhances the complexion, acts as a *saṅgrāhī* (anti-diarrheal, binding loose stool), acts as an aphrodisiac and increases semen.
- Butter made from milk is very cool and counters bleeding. It act as a *saṅgrāhī* (anti-diarrheal, binding loose stool).

Advantages

- Butter made from yogurt improves the memory and intellect and lends strength to the heart.

- Butter made from milk is beneficial for the eyes.

Indications

- Butter made from yogurt is beneficial for tuberculosis, emaciation, cough, piles and paralysis.
- Butter made from milk is an excellent medicine for paralysis.

7. *Ghee* (Clarified Butter)

When butter is cooked, its watery portion seperates out and the residual condensed matter prepared from it is known as *ghee* or clarified butter. *Ghee* is the best among all oily substances due to its unique quality of increasing the potency of herbal preparations. Other oily substances do not show this property. *Ghee* made from cow's milk is considered to be the best among all varieties of *ghee.*

Properties

Ghee is heavy, oily and has sweet *vipāka*. It is *śīta vīrya* (cool in potency*)*. It flushes out *doṣas* from *srotas*, clearing and lubricating them, and carminates *Vāta.*

Advantages

Ghee enhances intelligence, memory and sharpens the brain. It increases strength, life-span, semen, vision, fertility, glow, tenderness and voice quality. It is nourishing, lends stability to the body and boosts digestive power. It fortifies the heart and provides nourishment even during old age. It is a good rejuvenator.

Indications

Its medicinal and nourishing properties make it useful for people suffering from mental disturbances and emotional imbalances, fever, burning, inflammation, insanity, tuberculosis, emaciation, wounds, weapon injuries and burns.

Ghee is used in diverse ways: as a part of the diet, with medicinal preparations, for massage, enemas (*anuvāsana basti*) and in *nasya* treatments (nasal inhalation). It can be used for inhalation during bleeding. Massage with old *ghee* is recommended in pain of the ribs, upward circulation of *Vāta (udāvarta)*, emaciation, debility, cough, abortion, diminished vision and chronic fever. Regular intake of milk and *ghee* is the best nourishing and rejuvenating combination.

> According to *Āyurveda* treatises, *ghee* that is 10 years old is called '*purāṇa*'; *ghee* that is 100 years old is called *'kumbhaghṛta'* and *ghee* that have been aged for more than a century is called '*mahāghṛta.*' Despite having a strong odor, old *ghee* eradicates epilepsy, intoxication, syncope, malaria and diminished vision. It also cleans and heals wounds and cures disorders of the head, ears, eyes and female genital organs. It acts as an anti-bacterial and an anti-viral. It alleviates Kapha and is very beneficial in pneumonia.

8. Oil[15]

Oil comes next to *ghee* among the most beneficial oily substances. Traditionally the word 'oil' was used only for sesame oil, but now it is widely used and refers to all types of oils.

Properties

- Oil normally is sweet, astringent and *uṣṇa vīrya* (hot in potency).
- Oil has a peculiar tendency: while it helps a feeble person gain weight, it also helps an obese person to reduce fat. Being liquid, it easily penetrates the *srotas*. The *srotas* of a lean person are contracted or shrivelled. Therefore, oil due to its scarifying and stimulating properties enters these *srotas* and opens them; the *srotas* get dilated making it possible for food to provide wholesome nourishment to the body and thus curing emaciation. On the other hand, being subtle, it penetrates the *srotas* of an obese person and reduces the fat deposited in and around them. In view of modern medical science, the unsaturated fatty acids present in oil does not harm in any way in cases of obesity, diabetes or heart-problems.
- Oil shows another unique quality: it can solidify fecal matter as well as relieve constipation (*grāhī*) because it performs both actions, binds the stool and eliminates the loose stool.
- Old oil becomes more beneficial and these properties increase as it becomes older, whereas the nourishing properties of *ghee* reduce after one year.

Advantages

- It spreads all over the body before being digested, but does not aggravate *Kapha*.
- It provokes *Pitta* and physical strength and nourishes the skin. Oil lends strength, stability and nourishment to the muscles.
- It sharpens intelligence, boosts digestion, binds the stool or fecal matter, reduces frequent urination and clears the vaginal passage for the easy flow of semen.
- Oil is considered the most potent of all *Vāta*-calming substances. Body massages using a variety of oils calms *Vāta* aggravation, relieves fatigue and wards off signs of old age. It clears the vision, brighten and soften the skin, lending it a glow, keep away wrinkles, strengthen the body and bring good sleep.
- When processed with herbs, it acquires their medicinal properties. Hence, oil proves to be a very effective medicinal and curative substance.
- Oiling the hair relieves headache and counters balding, premature graying and hair loss.

15. *Kaṭūṣṇaṁ sārṣapaṁ tailaṁ raktapittapradūṣaṇam.*
Kaphaśukrānilaharaṁ kaṇḍūkoṭhavināśanam. (*Ca.sū.* 27/290)
Kaṭūṣṇaṁ sārṣapaṁ tīkṣṇaṁ kaphaśukrānilapaham.
Laghupittāsrakṛtkoṭhakuṣṭhāśrovraṇajantujit. (*A.saṅ.sū.* 6/104)

Oils extracted from different substances possess the properties of that substance. Oils of sesame, mustard, coconut, groundnut, and linseed are commonly used. They are described here in brief.

- **Sesame oil**

Sesame oil is the best among all oils. It is used both externally for massage and internally as part of a good diet. It can also be used as a cooking medium.

Properties

- It is penetrating and spreads easily throughout the body. It is heavy, hot in potency, cool to touch and nourishing.
- It binds loose fecal matter and acts as a scarifying agent.
- Sesame oil does not increase *Kapha* despite being oily. It calms *Vāta* and also usually calms *Pitta* when used for massage.

Advantages

It lends strength, stability and brings lightness in the body, boosts digestion, sharpens intelligence and purifies the uterus.

Indications

It heals wounds, urinary disorders, frequent urination, *prameha* (urinary abnormalities), headache and ear problems.When taken internally, it is not much beneficial for the skin, hair, heart and eyes, but external use (for massaging) of sesame oil is beneficial for each of these. Sesame oil is also used in sprains, injuries, burns and fractures. It is used for nasal inhalation, fomentation, massage and as an ear drop.

- **Mustard oil**

It is widely used in cooking in Northern India. It has low saturated fat as compared to other cooking oils.

Properties

Pungent, light and hot in potency and in touch; and penetrating. It alleviates *Kapha* and *Vāta* and destroys semen, vitiates *Pitta* and blood, boosts digestion and is stimulating and a scarifying agent.

Advantages

It helps to detoxify the body, makes the immune system strong, stimulates digestion, circulation and the excretory system, and keeps the body warm in winter when used for a body massage.

Indications

The use of mustard oil helps to prevent coronary heart disease, cure rashes, other skin problems, head and ear disorders and destroy worms. It is very beneficial for people suffering from spleen enlargement.

- **Groundnut oil**

It is also known as peanut oil or arachis oil. It is a mild-tasting and a very popular cooking medium these days.

Properties

This oil is hot, heavy and oily. It alleviates *Kapha* and *Vāta*, aggravates *Pitta* and burning. In massage it causes dryness in the skin rather than oiliness.

- **Coconut oil**

It is an edible oil used instead of *ghee* in Southern India.

Properties

It is heavy and cool in its attributes. It alleviates *Vāta-Pitta* and aggravates *Kapha.*

Advantages

It is beneficial for the hair. It is the best natural nutrition for hair, being the best hair oil. It is a very good massage oil for dry skin. It delays wrinkles and skin sagging. Its soothing quality helps in removing stress through gentle massage and gives a cooling effect in summer when massaged on the head.

Indications

It helps in treating various skin problems including psoriasis, dermatitis, eczema and other skin infections. It helps in controlling diabetes and in dissolving kidney stones.

- **Linseed (flax) oil**

It is a colorless to yellowish oil which is dry in nature.

Properties

This oil is sweet-sour, hot in its attribute and pungent in *vipāka*. It vitiates *Kapha, Pitta* and blood, mitigates *Vāta* and causes skin problems.

Indications

It reduces joint inflammation, arthritis, gout and back pain, prevents heart diseases, lowers cholesterol and controls hypertension. It is effective in constipation, hemorrhoids (piles) and gallstones.

9. Honey[16], [17]

Honey is a sweet viscous fluid produced by bees and other insects from the nectar of flowers. There are different types of honey. Though it is typically brown, it can range in color from yellow-tinged to red or even black. In *Āyurveda* honey is considered to positively affect all three primitive material imbalances of the body: *Vāta, Pitta* and *Kapha*. Some learned practitioners like *Suśruta* believed that honey had a calming effect on all three *doṣas*.

"Vātalaṁ guru śītaṁ ca raktapittakaphāpaham.
Sandhātṛcchedanaṁ rūkṣaṁ kaṣāyaṁ madhuraṁ madhu."

Properties

- Sweetness with an astringent after-taste. It is cool, dry and heavy.
- Anti-bacterial properties contribute in treating variety of ailments.
- Anti-oxidant properties strengthen the immune system.
- Being hygroscopic, it absorbs moisture, hydrates the skin and restores damaged skin making it soft, supple and young.
- It is an expulsive substance, reduces cough (*lekhanam*), it helps to expel viscous mucous and catarrh effectively (*chedanam*). It is a soothing agent, very useful in sore throat and cough (*śleṣmahara*).
- It acts as a uniting agent (*sandhānīya*), bringing together the ends of deep wounds or injured parts and cleanses and heals the wounds (*śhodhanam-ropaṇam*).
- Calms *tridoṣa* (*Vāta-Pitta-Kaphaghnam*).
- Natural detoxifying agent (*viṣa praśamana*).
- It is an instant energizer (*bala pradhānam*).
- Improves the appetite and digestive fire (*agnidīpanam*).
- Improves the complexion (*varṇyam*).
- Good for eyes and eyesight (*cakṣuṣyam*).
- Good for the heart (*hṛdya*).
- Quenches thirst (*tṛṭ*) and stop hiccoughs (*hidhmā*).

Newly collected honey is nourishing, increases the body weight, promotes strength and being a mild laxative, relieves constipation. It reduces cough when taken in a small amount. "Old" honey is highly stimulating and scarifying, relieves constipation, helps in metabolism of fat thus reducing fat and cholesterol, and is good for digestion.

Āyurveda explains another special quality of honey which is '*Yogavāhī*,' which means it is an excellent transporter. The substance which has the quality of penetrating the deepest tissue is called '*Yogavāhī*.' When honey is

16. *Madhu tu madhuraṁ kaṣāyānurasaṁ rūkṣaṁ śītamagnidīpanam varṇyaṁ*
Svaryaṁ laghu sukumāraṁ lekhanaṁ hṛdyaṁ vājīkaraṇaṁ
Sandhānaṁ śodhanaṁ ropaṇaṁ cakṣuṣaṁ prasādhanaṁ sūkṣmamārgānusāri
pittaśleṣma medomeha hikkā śvāsakāsa atisāra chardi tṛṣṇā kṛmiviṣapraśa-manaṁ ca, tattu laghutvānt kaphaghnaṁ paicchilyān mādhuryāt
kaṣāyabhāvācca vātapittaghnam. (*Su. sū* 45/32)

17. *Cakṣuṣyaṁ chedi tṛṭ śleṣma viṣahidhmāsrapittanut.*
Mehakuṣṭha kṛmicchardi śvāsakāsa atisārafit.
Vraṇaśodhana sandhānaropaṇaṁ vātalaṁ madhu.
Kūkṣaṁ kaṣāyamadhuraṁ, tattulyā madhuśarkarā. (*A.hr.sū* 5/51-52)

used with other herbal preparations, it acquires and enhances the medicinal qualities of those herbs and also helps them to reach the deeper tissues. Thus honey acts as an excellent transporter and is used frequently with *Āyurvedic* medicines as an adjuvant (vehicle).

Indications

Honey is very beneficial for diseases such as internal bleeding, urinary disorders, *prameha* (urinary abnormalities), dermatitis, bronchial asthma and other pulmonary or respiratory problems, cough, diarrhea, vomiting, toxicity and worm infestation.

IMPORTANT FACTS

- Honey and heat are considered opposing forces.
- Intake of warm honey is not recommended. Hence it should not be taken with hot substances, during summer and in ailments caused due to heat.
- The only condition where warm honey can be used is while administering purgation through vomiting, as the warm honey is eliminated from the body along with the vomit, hence it does not develop any toxic effect.
- Taking honey and *ghee* in equal quantities is not recommended, but consuming the same in small amounts and in different proportions, it becomes nectar.

Chapter 8

The Classification & Examination of Disease

Health is order; disease is disorder. Within the body there is a constant interaction between order and disorder. In *Āyurveda*, the concept of health is fundamental to the understanding of disease, where 'dis' means "deprived of" and 'ease' means "comfort." Therefore, before discussing disease, we must understand the meaning of comfort or health. A state of health exists when: the digestive fire (*agni*) is in a balanced condition, the bodily humors (*Vāta, Pitta* and *Kapha*) are in equilibrium, the three waste products (urine, feces and sweat) are produced in normal amounts and are in balance, the senses are functioning normally, and the body, mind and consciousness are harmoniously working as one. When the balance of any of these systems gets disturbed, a disease cycle begins. Thus, imbalances of the body and mind are responsible for physical and psychological pain and misery.

1. Classification of Diseases

According to *Āyurveda*, a disease can be classified on the basis of its origin - psychological, spiritual or physiological. A disease can also be classified according to the site of manifestation - heart, lungs, liver and so on. Diseases can be further classified on the basis of the causative factors and bodily *doṣas* - *Vāta, Pitta* and *Kapha*. Depending upon the classification a physician prescribes the treatment. The description of various types of classifactions is discussed below.

I) Classification on the basis of *doṣa* and *karma*

1) ***Doṣaja roga***: An unsuitable diet and lifestyle causes vitiation of *Vāta, Pitta* and *Kapha* (increase or decrease) and as a result there are *Vāta, Pitta* and *Kapha* disorders respectively. According to this classification of diseases *doṣaja* ailments are of two types:

a) ***Sāmānyaja roga***: The diseases which are produced due to the vitiation of any *doṣa* are called *sāmānyaja roga* such as fever, diarrhea, abdominal swelling and so on.

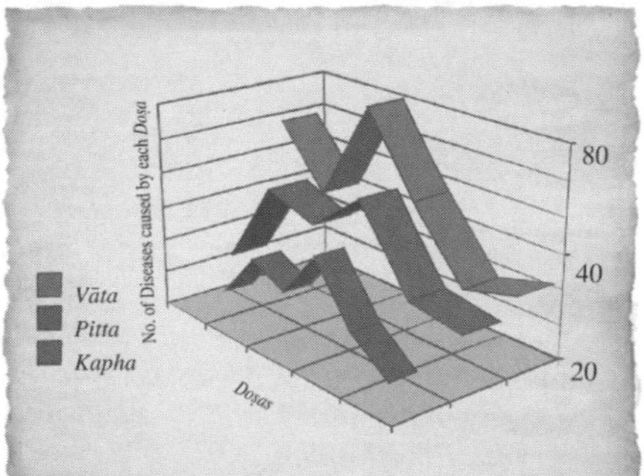

***Doṣas* and Ailments**

b) ***Nānātmaja roga***: The diseases which are produced from a specific *doṣa* and not from any other *doṣa* or their combination are called *nānātmaja roga.* Although no definite counting can be given to such diseases, yet *Āyurvedic* scriptures describe 80 *Vāta* disorders, 40 *Pitta* disorders and 20 *Kapha* disorders.

2) ***Karmaja roga****: The diseases which are believed to be caused as a result of sins of a previous birth or due to wrong deeds performed in this life knowingly and unknowingly are called *karmaja* or *adṛṣṭa karmaja.* In such disorders no specific vitiation of *doṣas* or manifested symptoms occurs, but a patient suffers from diseases which are cured with difficulty.

These diseases emerge suddenly and are difficult to cure in spite of different therapies used. The misery caused by these ailments is only cured by subsiding the effect of evil deeds by noble actions. Such disorders may be alleviated by acts of charity, compassion, service to *brahmins* (holy people), cows, the poor and disabled, and by prayers, meditation and other noble acts.

3) ***Doṣa-Karmaja roga***: The diseases which are produced by the combined effect of *doṣaja* ailments, due to a wrong food regime and lifestyle at the present time plus the sinful deeds of previous births are known as *doṣa-karmaja roga*. As a result, even a mild cause may lead to the occurance of chronic diseases, and at times even a slight increase in the normal level of a *doṣa* may result in more severity of a disease. The treatment is based on the genesis of the disease. The patient will have to tolerate the discomfort which is the repercussion of one's bad conduct in the previous life. Virtuous deeds performed as a therapy help to reduce the effects of the disease.

Classification of Diseases on the Basis of *Doṣas* and *Karmas* (Deeds)

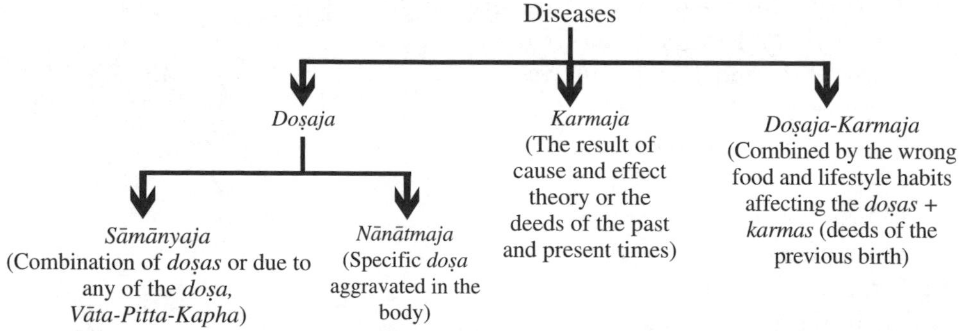

* *Āyurveda* accepts the theory of rebirth and the law of cause and effect (*karma phala*) according to which one recieves the fruits of virtuous and sinful deeds in the form of sorrow or joy, disease or health. Hence, in *Āyurveda,* in context to a healthy approach (*svasthavṛtta*) good conduct, ethics, pious lifestyle, right deeds and virtuous actions are considered most essential for health and happiness.

II) Classification on the basis of treatment

1) **Curable diseases**: The ccurable disease is one which is produced by the vitiation of any one *doṣa* with slow manifestation of preliminary signs and main symptoms. The disease is curable: when the tissues involved are not similar in attribute to those of the vitiated *doṣa*; if a patient's basic constitution is not similar to that of the vitiated *doṣa* (for example, one with a *Vāta*-type body suffering from a *Vāta* disease); if the vitiated *doṣa* is not affected by the season or a particular place; if the disorder is localized and circulated only on a single pathway; if it's a newly generated disorder without any complication; if the body is able to tolerate all treatment therapies (emetic, purgative therapies and so on); if the patient have strong digestive and metabolic powers; and if the four limbs of treatment (physician, patient, drug and attendant) are excellent in their performance. Under such circumstances, the disease can be curable. These diseases are further divided into two types:

   a) **Easily curable**: The diseases with above properties are easily curable diseases.

   b) **Difficult to cure**: The disease is difficult to cure: when the causes, premonitory and main symptoms are moderately manifested; if among the season, constitution and tissues, any one of them is having a similar attribute with a vitiated *doṣa*; if the patient is a pregnant female, child or an aged person; if the ailment is associated with some complications; if the disease originates in vital parts of the body, joints or other sensitive places which are difficult to cure; if the four limbs of treatment are not suitable; if a disease gets aggravated and moves out in another passage from its original one; and if a disease becomes chronic.

Classification of Diseases on the Basis of Treatment

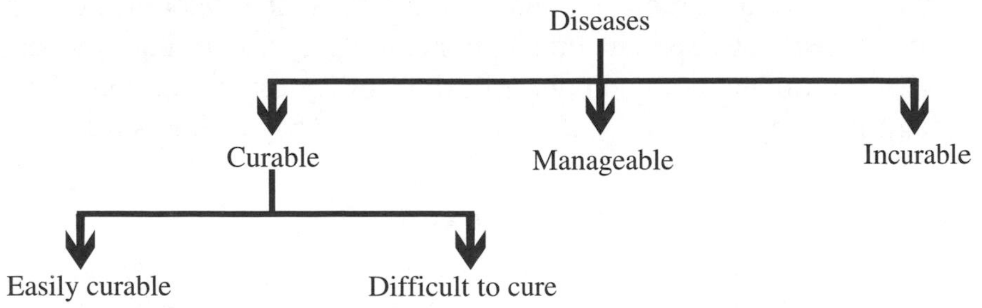

2) **Manageable diseases**: Diseases that get aggravated even under favorable conditions are manageable, not curable diseases. Some diseases get alleviate or subside with medicines or their intensity reduces, but as soon

as the patient stops the medication and with any adverse condition or diet it aggravates again. Such diseases are manageable diseases. Some diseases are manageable as long as one is alive and do not become the cause of death. These include: diseases which are bound to *meda, asthi* and other *dhātus* or those that originate in the vital organs of the body or in the joints; if a diseases is chronic and more than one year old or which reside in the body permanently; and those diseases that result due to vitiation of two *doṣas* comes under this category.

3) **Incurable disease**: Diseases which are not easy to treat in spite of any mode of treatment are called incurable diseases. Such diseases have symptoms similar to manageable diseases and are *tridoṣaja* (emerge due to the aggravation of all three *doṣas*). These diseases are not benefitted by any type of treatment. They are widely diffused throughout the body, and are very complicated, chronic and vicious in nature. The disease is said to be incurable: if the patient suffers from low digestive power and weak will power, feels malaise and is emaciated, is anxious by nature and negative thoughts prevail in the mind, and if the condition appears fatal.

Here, the known fact is that diseases which are considered to be incurable are not always incurable. With the proper diagnosis and new breakthroughs in treatments, they can become curable. For example, tuberculosis and inguinal hernia were incurable in the past, but nowadays these diseases and many such diseases are successfully treated and cured with medication and surgery. Hence, now they are curable diseases. Similarly, *Āyurvedic* treatment aids in the easy recovery of diseases considered incurable in modern medicine.

In this context, do not ignore mild or general ailments because diseases are dangerous like an enemy, poison or fire. Diseases which are common, mild and curable, if not treated in time with proper medication become potent, tough and incurable. For example, the common cold and cough are mild and common diseases, but if they remain untreated for a long time they may cause chronic bronchitis, bronchial asthma and may also result in pneumonia.

III) Primary (root) disease and their complications

Many times diseases are not restricted to their *doṣas, dhātus* and *malas*, but independently produce a new disease or a new disease generate from the primary disease and its related cause. This new disease recovers with the treatment of its root disease.This is known as the complication of a disease. A physician should take this into consideration during the treatment of a disease. Hence, a disease which has its genesis from the beginning and is neither a warning symptom of any disease nor a complication is called a primary or root disease.

IV) Physical and psychological (psycho-somatic) diseases

According to *Āyurveda*, the specific site of all the diseases is either the body or brain. In general, some diseases are produced in the body and others in the mind. Other than that, some diseases are located in both the body and mind. Both are interlinked and can only be treated if they are separated from their root location. Once disease appears in the body, it affects the *psyche* and *vice-versa*. The only difference between them is that at the time of origin, the first sign of distress or any deformity develops at its specific location, i.e., the body or the mind. They are called as either physical and/or psychological diseases, respectively. Besides this, diseases like epilepsy and psychosis are considered to be *ubhayāśṛita*, because they are generated in association with both the body and the mind. When physical and psychological diseases turn chronic, then they merge profoundly (psycho-somatic).

In physical diseases, at first instance *Vāta, Pitta*, *Kapha* and the blood gets vitiated, thereafter it causes discomfort to the mind. In such a condition treatment has to be initiated after the alleviation of the *doṣa*. For example, fever and diarrhea come under physical diseases. In psychological disorders, the first step is to eradicate the main cause of disease caused by the attributes of *Rajas* and *Tamas*. Mental disturbances and emotional imbalances such as desire, anger, fear, over-excitement and other urges come under psychological disorders.

V) Endogenous and Exogenous diseases

The physical and psychological diseases above-mentioned are again of two types, endogenous and exogenous. Some diseases are produced naturally due to disturbance of sleep, thirst or due to aggravation and vitiation of the *doṣas* and other internal causes. These are endogenous diseases. On the contrary, other diseases produced from external injury, trauma, an attack of wild animals (wounds caused by their nails and teeth) are exogenous disorders. These two types of diseases also mutually affect each other because already aggravated endogenous diseases are further vitiated by external factors (bacteria or other microbes and parasites). Simultaneously, in exogenous diseases vitiation of *doṣas* provokes them later and transforms them into endogenous diseases. Hence, in both these diseases, sooner or later, gradually *doṣa* vitiation occurs. Therefore, it is essential that during the treatment, equilibrium of *doṣas* should be maintained. But of course, during the treatment emphasis is laid on the actual cause of the disease at the time of emergence.

As already mentioned, vitiation of *doṣa* is responsible for the origin of disease. These vitiated *doṣas* also weaken and corrupt the *dhātus* and *malas*. Another important factor to be considered is that if any one of the *doṣas* gets aggravated (increase or decrease), it affects the corresponding *doṣa*.

VI) Classification of diseases on the basis of distress

Diseases are again divided into three types based on distress: *ādhyātmika, ādhibhautika* and *ādhidaivika.*

1) **Diseases caused due to psycho-somatic miseries (*ādhyātmika roga*)**: These are the diseases which arise due to mental and physical humors produced in the body. They are further divided into three types:

    (i) **Hereditary diseases (*ādibala or vaṁsaja*)**: Diseases which are due to vitiation of *doṣas* present in the sperm and ovum of the parents at the time of conception, comes under hereditary diseases. Diseases such as thalassemia and bronchial asthma are hereditary. They are further classified into two types:

    a) Maternal diseases (*mātṛja*) – Which originate from the maternal side.

    b) Paternal diseases (*pitṛja*) – Which originate from the paternal side.

    (ii) **Diseases since birth (*janmabalaja or janmajāta*)**: These diseases are due to an incompatible diet, lifestyle and carelessness followed during pregnancy. For example, blindness, muscloskeletal deformities and stunted growth.

    (iii) **Diseases due to potent *doṣas* (*doṣabalaja*)**: These diseases develop from the vitiation of *Vāta* and other *doṣas* due to an incompatible diet, lifestyle and carelessness.They are further classified into two types:

    a) **Diseases originating in the abdominal region (*āmāsayottha*)**: These diseases develop in the abdomen from the stomach to the upper region of the small intestine (duodenum) and include cough, bronchial asthma and liver disorders.

    b) **Diseases originating in the large intestine (*pakvāśayottha*)**: These diseases start from the large intestine and include constipation, flatulence, distention and so on.

2) **Diseases caused by physical miseries (*ādhibhautika roga*)**: These are the pains and discomfort caused by trauma and other external injuries or by antagonistic men, cattle, birds, snakes and other animals. Accordingly they are termed as external diseases (ā*gantuja*) or diseases caused by an antagonistic attack (*saṅghātabalaja*), respectively. They are also further divided into two types :

    (i) **Diseases due to an attack by an animal *(vyālaja)***: Diseases which are produced due to attack and bite of tame and wild animals are termed *vyālaja roga*. These include attacks by animals and injuries by their nails, horns and bites, scorpion stings, snake poison, poisoning from other animals and several bacterial and viral diseases.

(ii) **Diseases due to an attack by a weapon (*śastraja*)**: Wounds produced from instruments, weapons, bomb blasts, shootouts and traumatic injuries come under this category.

3) **Diseases produced by natural calamities (*ādhidaivika roga*)**: Diseases that arise due to natural causes are included here. They are again classified into three types:

(i) **Disorders related to the season (*kālabalaja or ṛtuja*)**: These diseases are due to excessive rain, exposure to heat and cold, and due to mosquitoes and micro-organisms present in the environment during a season. These are air borne and due to heat stroke. They are again divided into two types:

(a) **Diseases due to climate changes *(vayāpanna ṛtu roga)***: Diseases which are produced due to abnormalities in climate (in a particular season at times when it is very hot or cold and at times when it is not as it would have been expected) are *vāyāpanna ṛtu roga*.

(b) **Diseases in normal climatic conditions (*āvayāpanna ṛtu roga)***: Diseases which arise in normal climatic conditions (seasonal diseases) are *āvayapanna ṛtu roga*. When diseases develop due to fluctuations in climate, at first instance treat them with specific medicines and if one does not recover, then use some other therapy. Treat diseases due to seasonal changes with medication suitable to that climate.

ii) **Diseases caused by supernatural agencies (*daivabalaja roga*)**: These are another type of *ādhidaivika roga* which are believed in *Āyurveda* to be caused by divine or supernatural agencies, i.e., by the destruction and outburst of fire, air, space (ether), earth and water elements. Outbreak of diseases as a result of natural calamities come under this category, as does post-traumatic stress disorder, as they occur due to tumultuous disturbances caused by divine power. They are again divided into two types:

(a) **Diseases caused by thunderstorms and fire (*agnija*)**: These diseases are produced by natural calamities related to thunder and fire, include electrocution.

(b) **Outburst of epidemic diseases (*piśācaja*)**:These are diseases that emerge as an epidemic due to the microbes present in the environment. They are also classified in two ways:

1. **Communicable diseases (*saṁsargaja*)**: Diseases due to direct contact or touch.
2. **Air borne (*ākasmika*)**: Diseases which are suddenly generated due to the spread of microbes in the environment.

(iii) **Diseases due to natural needs (*svabhāvabalaja roga*)**: These are the third type of *ādhidaivika roga* which develop due to natural needs of the body such as hunger, thirst, lust, anger, sleep and so on.

According to some treatises and scholars these three types of diseases, psycho-somatic, physical and supernatural, are further classified into seven types. Diseases caused due to: 1. Heredity, 2. Birth-related, 3. *Doṣa* related, 4. Antagonistic attack, 5. Seasonal, 6. Supernatural, and 7. Natural desires of the body.

Classification of Diseases on the Basis of Distress

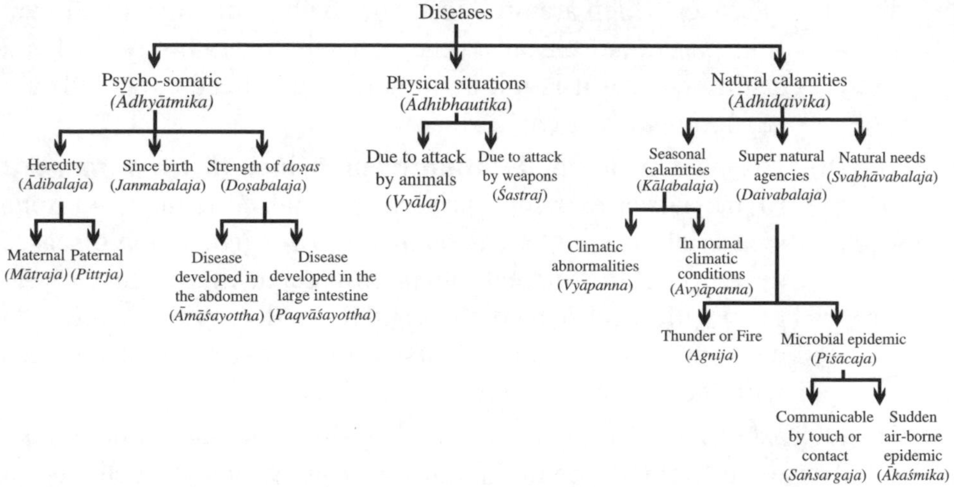

VII) Classification of diseases on the basis of dependency

Disease generated due to the causes mentioned (aggravation of one or more than one *doṣas*) and with clear symptoms of vitiated *doṣa* and which subsides with *doṣa* alleviating treatments, are independent diseases (*svatantra roga*). Contrary to this, the diseases which do not occur independently, but are produced due to causes related to other diseases that are cured with the treatment of the root cause and do not manifest with clear and significant symptoms, are dependent diseases (*paratantra roga*), which are further divided into two types:

1. Preliminary symptoms (*pūrvarūpa*)
2. Complications (*upadrava*)

The minor diseases that are generated before the root disease are said to be preliminary. If the dependent disease does not subside with the treatment for the independent disease, then another line of treatment should be administered to treat the dependent disease, and if complications are more aggressive, then the complication should be treated first before the root disease.

Classification of Diseases on the Basis of Dependency

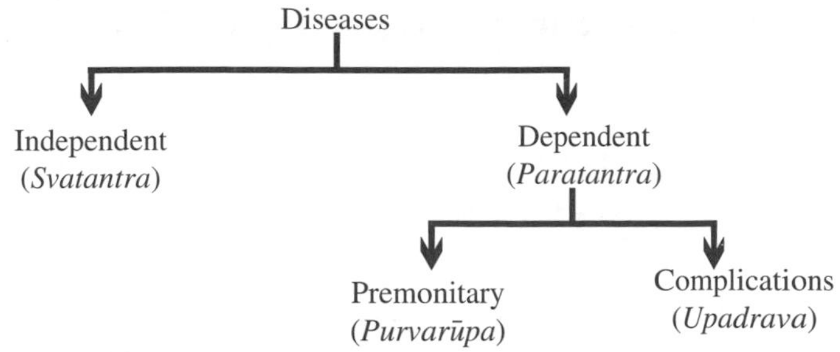

All these diseases are further categorized into different groups. They are named as *rogānīka* or group of diseases. They are as follows:

1. **Classification on the basis of effect (*prabhāva*)**
   (a) Curable diseases: Which can be treated easily.
   (b) Incurable diseases: Which cannot be treated.
2. **Classification on the basis of strength (*bala*)**
   (a) Gentle (*mṛdu*): Easy to cure, less aggressive.
   (b) Vicious (*dāruṇa*): Not easily curable, very aggressive with severe complications
3. **Classification on the basis of location (*adhiṣṭhāna*)**
   (a) Neurological or psychological diseases (*manodhiṣṭhāna*): Diseases evolved from the mind.
   (b) Physical or somatic diseases (*sarīradhiṣṭhāna*): Diseases developed in the body.
4. **Classification on the basis of causative factor (*nimittaja*)**
   (a) Internal causative factors (*svadhātu vaisam nimittaja*): Endogenous diseases which are produced due to vitiation, aggravation and depletion of *doṣas*, *dhātus, updhātus* and *malas* are defined as internal causative factors of disease.
   (b) External causative factors (*āgantunimittaja*): Exogenous diseases which are produced due to injuries, worm infestations and other external causes are defined as external causative factors of disease.

5. **Classification on the basis of residing place**
   (a) Diseases in the abdominal area (*amāśaya samutthaya*): Diseases which are in the abdomen and originate from there such as *Pitta* and *Kapha* disorders.
   (b) Diseases in the large intestine (*pakvāsaya samutthaya*): Diseases which are in the large intestine and originate from there such as *Vāta* disorders.

Before the examination of a patient or disease and before selecting the specific line of treatment, a physician should have knowledge of all types of diseases.

2. Four Legged Frame of Treatment (Four Important Factors in the Treatment of Disorders)

In *Āyurveda* for a complete, systematic and successful treatment of any disease, four components or parts are essential[(1), (2)]:

(I) A knowledgeable physician

(II) Drugs and medicines

(III) Nurse including attendant

(IV) A patient

These four components are the four legs of treatment. A leg is that part of the body by whose support a person stands. A person without a leg is called lame. Exactly the same condition is applied to the field of treatment. In the absence of any one of the components or due to lack of qualities, successful treatment is not possible. In each of these four components, fourfold qualities are essential. [PLATE 20]

(I) **Qualities of a physician**: The one who treats the patient or the disease is the physician. A good physician must have four qualities.These are expertise, thorough knowledge of *Āyurvedic* scriptures, practical experience, and honesty and dedication (a pious mind and body)[(3), (4)]. In brief, a physician must be learned, an expert, pure and benevolent. These are the fourfold

1. *Bhiṣgdravyāṇyupasthātā rogīpādacatuṣṭayam.*
   Guṇavat kāraṇaṁ jñeyaṁ vikāravyupaśāntaye. (*Ca.sū.*9:3)
2. *Bhiṣg dravyāṇyupasthātā rogī pādacatuṣṭayam.*
   Cikitsitasya nirdiṣṭaṁ pratyekaṁ taccaturguṇam. (*Aṣṭ.saṅ.sū.* 2:22)
3. *Dakṣastīrthāttaśāstrārtho dṛṣṭakarmā śucirbhiṣak.* (*Aṣṭ. saṅ. sū.* 2:23)
4. *Śrute paryavadātatvaṁ bahuśo dṛṣṭakarmatā.*
   Dākṣyuaṁ śaucamiti jñeyaṁ vaidye guṇacatuṣṭayam. (*Ca.sū.* 9:6)

characteristics of a skilled physician. A good physician is one whose utmost aim is the well-being of a patient, selflessly.

Suśruta mentioned some other qualities of a good physician, such as being self- experienced, one who can competently and firmly handle the medical procedure, brave, one who possesses all drugs and equipment, intelligent, one who makes a good decision on time, one who is laborious and progressive, and one who follows the path of truth and virtuous duties.

Many times, without proper medical qualifications some people start practicing as a physician. When innocent and needy people come to them, the result can be hazardous. One should be aware of such physicians. *Caraka Saṁhitā* describes the three types of physicians:

(a) **Pseudo physicians**: One who is not properly qualified and is unaware of medical science yet may have consulted some medicinal books and studied about the use of some medicines and acts as a physician. They advertise themselves as skilled and eminent physicians, but actually are unskilled, spurious imposters.

(b) **Fake physicians**: Such persons are closely associated with rich, reputed and learned practitioners or they use their family prestige and fame associated with a reputed and skilled medical professional already present in the family. Being associated with a skilled practitioner and having gathered the superficial knowledge, they start an individual practice and advertise themselves as an eminent physician, in reality they are not true physicians. People who belong to this category are fake physicians. One should be careful when undergoing treatment from these two types of physicians.

(c) **Genuine physicians**: An expert, skillful and capable physician is one who saves the life of a patient suffering from a severe disease and gives new life to the patient. Such physicians have thorough knowledge of medicines and different treatment systems. They are successful in the field of medicine and provide relief to the patient. In brief, they have adequate knowledge about causes or etiology, signs and symptoms, and about treatment and prevention of disease recurrence. A skilled and genuine physician is well-educated, has a pious mind and soul, has a self-controlled lifestyle, is well acquainted with social affairs, has expertize, has adequate equipment for treatment, has strong and healthy sensory organs, has knowledge of disease occurence through manifested signs, is an expert in surgery, is one who can give proper direction to the patient for the use of medicines, and is one who can take an immediate and right decision at the time of distress. Such a physician provides new life to the patient and relief from the ailment. These physicians have adequate knowledge of human anatomy, physiology and embryology. They are experienced and can easily detect the causes, preliminary signs and main symptoms for the diagnosis of disease and its nature, and knows whether it is curable or incurable. They are confident and free of ambiguity or any sort of doubt while selecting the specific treatment therapy associated with the disease.

(II) **Qualities of a drug**: Easily available (in quantity and approach) and in multiple formulations (such as tonics, decoctions, tablets, powders, etc.). They have multiple properties and can treat several diseases. They are enriched with attributes such as *rasa-guna-virya-vipaka*, and are suitable and beneficial for the patient. These four qualities are essential in a good drug[5], [6]. Selection of an appropriate drug, in proper doses is possible only by an expert physician. Therefore, in *Āyurveda* it is of utmost importance that a physician, along with the treatment procedure, should also possess knowledge of the properties of the substances and production methods of the medicines.

(III) **Qualities of an attendant**: An attendant should be trained enough to take care of the patient. This helps the patient to recover soon. An attendant should possess following qualities: be loving and compassionate towards a patient, be clean and calm, be skilled in his/her work (to give proper medicine at proper time), and have a good knowledge of nursing, and be intelligent and wise so as to make the right decision at the right time, without losing patience[7], [8].

(IV) **Qualities in a patient**: For successful and quick treatment, a patient should follow the instructions of his physician, be capable of expressing his symptoms; must have strong will-power, and be tolerant so that he can easily bear the effects of medicines and the misery of a disease[9], [10]. Besides these, treatment becomes easier if a patient is young, brave, can keep a check on taste and control over the mind, and is financially sound and resourceful.

For a successful treatment all four participants are essential, but among them physician is most important[11]. For example, if cooking vessels, hot plate (fire work) and food ingredients are all available, but a good cook

5. *Bahukalpaṁ bahuguṇaṁ sampannaṁ yogyamauṣadham.* (*Aṣṭa.saṅ.sū.* 2:23)
6. *Bahutā tatra yogyavatvamanekavidhakalpanā.*
Sampacceti catuṣko, yaṁ dravyāṇāṁ guṇa ucyate. (*Ca.sū.* 9:7)
7. *Anuraktaḥ śicordalṣo buddhimān paricārakaḥ.* (*Aṣṭ.saṅ.sū.* 2:24)
8. *Upacārajñatā dākṣyamanurāgaśca bhartari.*
Śaucaṁ ceti catuṣko, yaṁ guṇaḥ paricare jane. (*Ca.sū.* 9:8)
9. *Smṛtirnirdeśakāritvamabhīrutvamathāpi ca.*
Jñāpakatvaṁ ca ragāṇāmāturasya guṇāḥ smṛtāḥ. (*Ca.sū.*9:9)
10. *Āḍhyo rogī bhiṣagvaśyo jñāpakaḥ satvavānapi.* (*Aṣṭa. saṅ. sū.*2:24)
11. *Kāraṇaṁ ṣoḍaśaguṇaṁ siddhau pādacatuṣṭayaṁ.*
Vijñātā śāsitā yoktā pradhānaṁ bhiṣagatra tu. (*Ca.sū.* 9:10)

is unavailable, then preparation of food is difficult. Similarly, if a skilled physician is not available but a good attendant, patient and drugs are all available, treatment is not possible.

3. Methods to Assay the Cause of a Disease

Before starting an *Āyurvedic* treatment, the first step taken by a practitioner is to examine a disease while considering the mentioned facts. The following methods help to examine a disease:

(A) *Pramāṇa*: The Means of Valid Knowledge

The means of gaining experience or practical and true knowledge is known as *pramāṇa*. This knowledge or *pramāṇa* is used while examining a patient and a disease. In *Āyurveda* classics mainly the following *pramāṇas* are considered useful while examining a disease:

(i) *Āptopadeśa* (Authoritative Testimony)

(ii) *Pratyakṣa* (Perception or Direct Observation)

(iii) *Anumāna* (Hypothesis or Inference)

(iv) *Yukti* (Reason)[12]

(i) ***Āptopadeśa* (Authoritative Testimony)**: One who is free of doubts, enmity, fear, arrogance, indignity, self-importance, ignorance and who has gained certainty, complete and practical knowledge of his subject, one who is able to express the subject knowledge for the well-being of humans, such persons are called '*āpta*' or '*śiṣṭa*' (authorized or reliable). *Caraka* says "those who are free from '*rajas*' and '*tamas*' ('*rajas*' is the root cause of attachment and aversion, while '*tamas*' is the covering of ignorance; these defects make a person unfit for being in a position of authority) and endowed with strength of penance and knowledge; whose knowledge is flawless, always uncontradicted are known as '*āpta*' (having acquired the knowledge) or '*śiṣṭa*' (expert in the discipline)." They are free from ambiguity or doubt, which is true as they are devoid of '*rajas*' and '*tamas.*' '*Śiṣṭa*' means 'with knowledge of the scriptures'as well as 'of noble conduct.' Thus '*āpta*' or '*śiṣṭa*' are credible persons, devoid of doubts, acquisition, attachment and aversion. The discourse, sermon or scriptual testimony of such learned persons is termed '*āptopdeśa*' or '*śabda pramāṇa*[13]' (authoritative statement of those having acquired perfect knowledge). Usually, knowledge obtained by such a person in each subject is the first step in examining a disease, followed by direct observation and inference, which further verifies a disease.

12. *Dvividhameva khalu sarvaṁ saccāsacca, tasya caturvidhā parīkṣā- Aptopadeśaḥ, pratyakṣam, Anumānaṁ yuktiśceti.* (*Ca.sū.* 11:17)
13. *Rajastamobhyāṁ nirmuktāstapojñānabalena ye. Āptāḥ śiṣṭā vibuddhāste teṣāṁ vākya masaṁśayam. Satyaṁ vakṣyanti te kasmādasatyaṁ nīrajastamāh.*(*Ca.sū.* 11:19)

According to *Āyurveda*, a physician who has not gathered knowledge about diseases by āptopdeśa can not determine a disease by observation and inference.

Caraka Saṁhitā, *Suśruta Saṁhitā*, *Aṣṭāṅga Hṛdaya* and other treatises are the scriptual testimony (*āptopadeśa*) in *Āyurveda*. By means of these, a practitioner can gather knowledge regarding a specific disease, its causes or diagnosis, imbalance of *doṣas* and vitiated tissues, the form and type of a disease (whether physical, mental, internal cause, external injury and others), location of a disease, the spreading path of a disease, preliminary signs, symptoms, diagnostic symptoms, category of a disease; whether curable, incurable or which can relapse, complications of a disease, name of the disease, type of treatment required, and compatible and incompatible diet for a patient. An appropriate knowledge of these facts and other such types of useful information are not possible without *āptopadeśa*. Hence, *āptopadeśa* is an important method to assay a disease.

(ii) *Pratyakṣa* (Perception or Direct Observation): Perception is the knowledge acquired by interaction of the sensory organs (eyes, ears and so on) with their subjects. The clear knowledge (indisputable and complete) that arises by mutual association of self (soul), mind, sensory organs and their subjects is termed as *pratyakṣa*[14] (perception or observation). In brief, the information obtained by self-recognition with the help of the subjects by the sensory organs and its perception by the mind is termed as '*pratyakṣa*.'

This definitive information in the form of perception is obtained by mutual connection with the soul, and essentially requires a definite sequential order. This involves, the connection established between the soul and mind, mind to sensory organs and sensory organs with their concerned subjects through the stimuli received from the external environment.

With the help of observation and perception, except for the tongue, the remaining sense organs (eyes, ears, nose and skin) and their concerned actions (visualization, hearing, smell and touch) are essential for examining a disease. A disease is diagnosed by visualizing the color of the skin of a patient; shape, measurements and constitution of the body; brightness and glow in the body and eyes; natural or abnormal expression of the body; color of the wound; inflammation and its types; substances eliminated in the stool, urine, phlegm, blood and vomit; menstrual blood, pus discharge from wounds and so on. For the assay of disease, auditory perceptions help

14. *Ātmendriyamano, rthānāṁ sannikarśāta pravartate.*
Vyaktā tadātve yā buddhiḥ pratyakṣaṁ sā nirucyate. (*Ca.sū.* 11: 20)

to analyze the gurgling sound produced by the stomach and intestines; the cracking sound produced by the flexion of knee and finger joints; heartbeats and sound perception from lungs and other organs; and the voice of a patient. Olfactory perceptions help to detect the patient's body smell and smell in the feces, urine, phlegm, blood, sweat and wounds for disease examination. Fever, edema, body temperature and heat generated on the surface of the abscess or wounds, coolness, softness, hardness, roughness, smoothness, dryness, pulse and other perceptions can be examined by touch. All these sensory analyses are included in the perception or observation (*pratyakṣa*).

In modern days, different types of equipments and techniques are available for the assay of disease like the stethoscope for heartbeats, the thermometer for temperature and the sphygmomanometer for blood pressure. In modern medical science, whichever technique being used for the diagnosis of a disease, be it different blood examinations, ultrasound, X-rays, CT Scan, MRI, angiography and endoscopy, comes under direct observation or perception establishing the cause of a disease.

(iii) *Anumāna* (Hypothesis or Inference): The word '*anumāna*' is derived from two words '*anu*' + '*māna*.' To derive an actual fact about related incidence by visualizing its signs is '*anumāna*' (hypothesis or inference). Inference is the knowledge of a signee (disease) on prior perception of the sign. At first, the sign is perceived; thereafter the knowledge of the signee (disease) arises with the application of invariable concommitance. Just as one on seeing smoke infers about a hidden fire and establish a confirmation, similarly smoke rising far in the sky helps to infer about a fire somewhere near. A conclusion based on facts is '*anumāna*.' According to *Charak*, '*anumāna*' is the fact that expects experimental confirmation. In simple words, '*anumāna*' is to know the unknown subject or event consequent upon the union of two or more causative factors[(15), (16)].

It is not possible to examine many diseases and their symptoms by the valid knowledge of perception. Therefore, to examine these diseases, inference or hypothesis is required. Examination of taste (*rasa*) of a patient cannot be obtained by the knowledge of perception; hence, it can only be examined by inference. For example, on the basis of digestion and metabolism of food, one can analyze the strength and work done by the digestive fire in a patient's body, and exercise helps to analyze the body strength and efficacy of a patient.

Knowledge of auto-immune diseases can be gathered only through hypothesis or inference. Sometimes it is difficult to identify a disease by direct observation or by authoritative or scriptual testimony and the fact that

15. *Pratyakṣapūrvaṁ trividhaṁ trikālaṁ cānumīyate.*
Vahninirgūḍhodhūmena maithunaṁ garbha darśanāt. (*Ca.sū.*11:21)
16. *Evaṁ vyavasyantyatītaṁ bījāt phalamanāgatam.*
Dṛṣṭvā bījāt phalaṁ jātamihaiva sadṛśaṁ budhāḥ. (*Ca.sū.*11:22)

the patient is suffering from a difficult situation. At such time, a hypothesis or inference is helpful to identify the disease.

(iv) *Yukti* (Reason): *'Yukti'* means intellect or reason or understanding of an object. It is an experimental confirmation. It is defined as the knowledge of intellectual perceptions or understanding of an object or event which sees the things produced as a consequence of a combination of multiple causative factors, valid in the three known time phases (past, present and future) and is also helpful to achieve the three objects or goals of life (virtue, wealth and lust) is known as '*yukti*' (reasoning)[17]. Just as the growth of crops depends on the combination of several factors such as water, ploughing, seed and season, so is yukti (reason) a rational and fruitful combination of all constituent factors[18]. These four means of *pramāṇa* (gain in knowledge), based on *yukti* (reasoning) helps to alleviate diseases if combined and used rationally. The essential factor in the successful treatment of a disease is '*yukti*' (reasoning).

(B) Examination by Interrogation

If physicians do not get accurate information through inference, then they can gather the information from the patient by questioning. It is known as examination by interrogation. The following information can be obtained by taking the history of a patient: their likes and dislikes of food, favourite food according to taste; types of dreams in sleep, type of sleep; nature of bowel movements (mild, medium or hard); causes of disease, location of pain, increasing or decreasing time of disease intensity, favorable or unfavorable conditions, information about excretion of feces, urine, flatus; age and birth place of a patient.

On the basis of these *pramāṇa*, a physician can examine the patient rationally. If a physician is not able to examine the patient properly, if he is unable to gather perceptions by sensory organs, and if he gets wrong answers while interrogating, then as a result, due to improper reasoning, a physician is unable to rationally confirm the disease.When all these facts do not allow the physician to define the nature of a disease, the physician gets confused. Due to a wrong diagnosis, the treatment of a disease can be misguided and not ascertained.

The examinations involved in the above perception, inference and so on can briefly be divided into the following six ways[19].

1. **Ausculatory examination by means of ears (The act of hearing)**: To ausculcate the gurgling sound of the intestines, heartbeat and so on.

17.*Buddhiḥ paśyati yā bhāvān bahukāraṇayogajān.*
Yuktististrikālā sā jñeyā trivargaḥ sādhyate yathā. (Ca.sū.11:25)
18.*Jala karṣaṇa bijartusaṁyogāt sasyasambhavaḥ.*
Yuktiḥ śaḍdhātusaṁyogād garbhāṇāṁ sambhavastathā. (Ca.sū.11:23)
19.*Pratyakṣatastu khalu rogatatvaṁ bubhutsuḥ sarvairindriyaiḥ.*
Sarvānindriyayārthānāturaśarīragatān parīkṣet, anyatra rasajñānāt,
todyayathā āntrakūjanaṁ, sandhisphuṭanamaṅgulīparvaṇāṁ ca,
svaraviśeṣāṁśca,........................iti pratyakṣato,
numānādupadeśataśca parīkṣaṇamuktam. (Ca.vi. 4:7)

2. **Tactile examination by means of skin (The act of touch)**: From coolness, warmth, hardness, touching the wounds, acne and by pulse examination, a physician can obtain the knowledge of disease.
3. **Ophthalmic examination by means of eyes (The act of vision)**: Examining the disease by observing patients body color, complexion, splendour, sustenance, weakness or emaciation.
4. **Gustatory examination by means of tongue (The act of taste)**: Examining the taste through inference or hypothesis.
5. **Olfactory examination by means of nose (The act of smell)**: By the odor of the body and different organs, odor from wounds or abscesses. For example, body odor or pungent smell from sweat helps to examine the disease.
6. **Disease examination by interrogation**: By asking questions to the patient or family and taking the history of a patient.

By means of these *pramāṇas* (valid knowledge), a physician can completely examine and diagnose a disease and can prescribe an effective treatment and can attain success in his work. [PLATE 21]

4. Different Methods of Disease Examination

Besides examining the disease on the basis of '*pramāṇa*', *Āyurveda* describes different methods for appropriate and accurate diagnosis, including[20]:

(A) ***Nidāna Pañcaka* (The Five Signs of Diagnosis)**: This includes the etiology, preliminary symptoms, manifested symptoms, exploratory therapy and pathogenesis.

(B) ***Ṣaṭkriyākāla* (The Six Stages of Manifestation of Disease)**: Due to different seasons and varying climatic conditions throughout the world, diseases occur due to the vitiation of *doṣas*. For the correct diagnosis and right treatment of the disease cycle, proper understanding of the stages of disease manifestation is necessary. These six stages, which include accumulation, aggravation, dissemination of *doṣa*, site of manifestation, symptom manifestation and differentiation and chronicity of a disease require specific management of the disorder.

(C) ***Aṣṭavidha Parīkṣā* (The Eight *Āyurvedic* Methods of Disease Examination)**: The diagnosis of a disease on the basis of *doṣa*,

20. *Tasyopalabhirnidānapūrvarūpaliṅgapaśayasamprāptitaḥ* (*Ca.ni.*1.6)

identification of the nature of disease, whether curable or incurable, including pulse examination and other examination methods is *Aṣṭavidha Parīkṣā*.

They are elaborated as follows:

(A) *Nidāna Pañcaka*: The Five Signs of Diagnosis

On the basis of '*Pramāṇa,*' a physician examines a disease and gathers knowledge about its nature. If a physician acquires accurate information regarding the nature of the disease, its type and the cause of aggravation or the place of origin (*doṣas, dhātus, malas, srotas* and *agni*), then the acquired knowledge is more than enough for the appropriate line of treatment at the first instance based on *Āyurvedic* norms. After this information, a physician needs to examine the following factors.

(i) Etiology (Causes of disease)

(ii) Preliminary symptoms (Those that occur before the onset of a disease)

(iii) Manifest signs and symptoms (Actual signs of a disease)

(iv) Exploratory therapy or Therapeutic suitability (Using medicines, a diet and lifestyle that oppose the disease and its causes)

(v) Pathogenesis (Appearance of a disease)

These are collectively termed '*Nidāna Pañcaka*'- a group of five signs for the diagnosis of a disease.

At the initial stage, none of the diseases become clearly apparent. First of all, there is a deep relationship between the cause of the disease and the body. Later on, as a result of these causes, some preliminary signs or changes are manifest, by which a skilled physician can infer about a disease that will occur. Then steadily, specific symptoms of the disease are manifest differently. At this stage, disease spreads in different ways throughout the body. On this basis, information about the disease is obtained. A brief introduction of these is as follows:

(i) **Etiology (Cause of a disease)**: In *Āyurveda* several *Sanskrit* words like *hetu, nimitta, kartā, kāraṇa, yoni* and *mūla* are used in place of '*nidāna*' (etiology) as synonyms for the cause. Inappropriate food habits, lifestyle and other external factors that cause disequilibrium (increase/decrease) in *doṣas* (*Vāta, Pitta* and *Kapha*), *dhātus* (plasma, blood and others), *malas* (fecal matter, urine and other *malas*) and mental attributes - *rajas* (action or passion) and *tamas* (ignorance or inertia) - are the internal causes that result in endogenous diseases and external factors such as poison, weapons, fire, microbes, trauma and so on are the external causes (which do not vitiate the *doṣas* and *dhātus*) that results in exogenous diseases. These reasons or causes are termed '*nidāna*' (etiology)[21]. These causes are divided into four categories.

(a) ***Sannikṛṣṭa kāraṇa*** **(Precipitating causes)**: These are the factors responsible for the sudden aggravation of the *doṣas* without the stage of accumulation. It also hastens the process of disease evolution, e.g., exposure to the cold produces a severe cold.

(b) ***Viprakṛṣṭa kāraṇa*** **(Causes of longer duration or distant causes)**: *Doṣas* accumulate in the body over a period of time and subsequently produces disease. In such conditions, the cause may be present, but the expression of disease takes a longer time. For example, frequent travelling, irregular eating habits and exposure to cold are all responsible for *Vāta* vitiation over a period of time.

(c) ***Vyabhicārī kāraṇa*** **(Feeble causes)**: These are the weak causes, unable to produce the disease, but act as a carrier. When a favorable situation arises for the manifestation of disease, the disease arises. They are not the direct causes of the disease.They do not produce a disease unless their strength is increased by certain favorable factors such as a stressful environment, incompatible diet and a *doṣa* aggravating lifestyle, which does not produce disease immediately, but with a favorable environment, they result in outburst of disease.

(d) ***Prādhānika kāraṇa*** **(Fulminating causes)**: These are the causes which react instantly and produce disease quickly, e.g., toxins, poisons and accidents.These causes are again divided into two groups.

- **Exogenous factors**: This includes unfavorable food habits, lifestyle and seasonal adaptability.
- **Endogenous factors**: These factors provoke the *doṣas* and *dhātus* (tissues) towards disequilibrium, resulting in disease development.

Etiology or the specific causes of the diseases also include:

(1) **Intellectual blasphemy (*Prajñāparādha*)**: The intentional violation of socio-religious code of conduct. It may lead to indisposition, impairment or misuse of intellect or mental activities, patience, composure and memory, which further results in undesirable activities wherein one gets struck in stress, depression and other stress-related psycho-somatic disorders. Such persons are the victims of intellectual blasphemy. In this condition all the three types of *doṣas* are aggravated.

(2) **Incompatibility of sense organs**: This is caused by the connection of the senses with unfavorable and incompatible subjects, which include

21. *Tatra nidānaṁ kāraṇamityuktamagre.* (*Ca.ni.* 1:7)

all those actions that are considered to be the cause of overuse, underuse and misuse of the eyes and other sense organs with their subjects.

(3) **Unfavorable season and time**: If in a specific season adverse climatic conditions occur, then that season is considered to be unfavorable. For example, excessive heat in summer or extreme cold in winter or heavy rains in the monsoon are the extremeties of the season. If the effect of these conditions is less in certain seasons, then it is a moderation of the season. If in a certain season opposite conditions are produced (like rain in winter, cold in summer) then it is called an altered state of season. When a person faces unfavorable seasons and harsh conditions, he may become victimized by many diseases.

(ii) **Premonitory signs and symptoms**: When accumulated *doṣas* get aggravated due to different reasons, this leads to vitiation in the *dhātus* (tissues of the body), *agni* (digestive fire) and *srotas* (channels), which will naturally produce a disease. For the manifestation of disease, *doṣas* have to pass through many levels before the actual onset of the disease (This will be described under the stages of disease manifestation).

In this sequence, accumulated and aggravated *doṣa* spread throughout the body and ultimately localize at a specific place. During accumulation at a specific location, some premonitary symptoms develop. On this basis, a physician infers about the disease that will evolve. These signs are preliminary or premonitory signs and symptoms[22]. For example, preliminary signs of fever are fatigue, discomfort, change in skin and complexion, lacrimation, pain and heaviness in the body, yawning, anorexia, cold, blackouts, tasteless tongue and so on. These signs indicate the emergence of fever. There are two types of premonitory symptoms:

(a) **Generalized symptoms**: Those preliminary signs that inform only about the general nature of a disease are called generalized preliminary signs. For example, fatigue is a preliminary sign of fever.

(b) **Specific symptoms**: Those preliminary signs that give definite and exact information about the nature of disease are called specific preliminary symptoms.

(iii) **Manifest signs and symptoms**: Symptoms that indicate the actual onset of the manifestation process, indicate the specific features of a disease and also vitiated *doṣas* and condition of *āma* are *rūpa*[23] (sign or symptom). In *Āyurveda*, this is also known by other terms such as *liṅga, cinha, lakṣaṇa* and so on. When a disease becomes more pronounced and is at its peak, specific and clearly defined symptoms appear. For example, high temperature in fever, watery stool in diarrhea, coughing in bronchitis.

(iv) **Exploratory therapy or therapeutic suitability**: This is a method to diagnose a disease through many types of treament systems. When a physician

22. *Pūrvarūpaṁ prāgutpattilakṣaṇaṁ vyādheḥ.* (Ca.ni.1:8)
23. *Prādurbhūtalakṣaṇaṁ punarliṅgam. Tatra liṅgamākṛtirlakṣaṇaṁ cinhaṁ saṁsthānaṁ vyañjanaṁ rūpamityanarthāntaram.* (Ca.ni.1:9)

is not able to diagnose a disease on the basis of preliminary signs and specific symptoms, then exploratory therapy[24] is required. For the confirmation of disease, therapeutic pathology tests are performed. This therapy also includes suitable trials with drugs, diet and daily regimen, which may be contrary to the etiology of disease or which produce effects contrary to both the etiology and disease or producing specific effects by acting directly or indirectly against the causative factor (*hetu*) or the disease (*vyādhi*). There are two categories on whose basis these treatments are of 18 types.

I) *Viparīta*: These include trials with medicine, diet and daily regimen which are opposite to the etiology (*hetu*) and disease (*vyādhi*), or both of them.

II) *Viparītārtttakārī*: These include trials with medicine, diet and daily regimen that produces the opposite effect, though not entirely opposite to either etiology (*hetu*) or disease (*vyādhi*), or both of them.

These two categories are further divided into 18 types.

(1) Cause opposite medicine	(10) Cause *Viparītārthakārī* medicine
(2) Cause opposite diet	(11) Cause *Viparītārhākārī* diet
(3) Cause opposite daily regimen	(12) Cause *Viparītārtakārī* daily regimen
(4) Disease opposite medicine	(13) Disease *Viparītārthhakārī* medicine
(5) Disease opposite diet	(14) Disease *Viparītārthakārī* diet
(6) Disease opposite daily regimen	(15) Disease *Viparītārtakārī* daily regimen
(7) Cause-Disease opposite medicine	(16) Cause-Disease *Viparītārthakārī* medicine
(8) Cause-Disease opposite diet	(17) Cause-Disease *Viparītārthakārī* diet
(9) Cause-Disease opposite daily regimen	(18) Cause-Disease *Viparitārthakārī* daily regimen

(v) **Pathogenesis:** The complete sequence of occurence of disease is called pathogenesis[25].It starts from the accumulation of *doṣas* to aggravation of either one, two or all three *doṣas*, spreads (circulation of *doṣas* in the entire body or at some particular location in the colon, stomach, liver, spleen, uterus, skin and so on), localizes at specific sites (combination of *doṣas* and *dhātus* (tissue) vitiated by the *doṣa*) and then manifests (emergence of a disease). Thus, it is the process of emergence of disease by the provoked *doṣas* which

24. *Upaśayaḥ punarhetuvyādhiviparītānāṁ viprītārthakāriṇāṁ causạdhāhāravihārāṇāmupayogaḥ sukhāmubandhaḥ.* (*Ca.ni.*1:10)
25. *Samprāptirjātirāgatirityanarthāntaraṁ vyādheḥ.* (*Ca.ni.*1:11)

are circulating all over the body. Pathogenesis is of six types(26). In *Āyurveda*, pathogenesis or '*samprāpti*' is also denoted by terms like '*jāti*' and '*āgati.*' Origin or birth of a disease is *'jāti'* and the velocity of spreading the disease is '*āgati.*' Through pathogenesis we obtain an accurate knowledge for the diagnose of a disease.

Diseases are mainly of two types: Endogenous and Exogenous

- **Endogenous disease**: When immunity of the body gets defeated from the causative factors of a disease, then endogenous diseases occur. If *āma* (undigested food) blocks the *srotas* (channels), it results in the provocation of the *doṣas*. This way, in all endogenous diseases a combination of undigested food and provoked *doṣas* (either as the main cause or present due to the effect of each other) are the causative agents of deformity in *srotas* (channels) and *dhātus* (tissues), which causes a disease.
- **Exogenous disease**: Exogenous factors of a disease (such as trauma, mosquito bites, snake and scorpion poisoning and other wild animal attacks), first of all cause affliction with pain caused by injury or wounds and poisoning, later they get associated with the *doṣa* in them. Afterwards as a result of *āma doṣa* (a combination of undigested food and *doṣa*) vitiation in *dhātus* (tissues) and *srotas* (channels) develops in a combination. In endogenous diseases, firstly a combination and interaction between *doṣa* and *dhātu* (tissues) occur, followed by manifestation and pathogenesis.

(B) *Ṣaṭkriyākāla*: The Six Stages of Manifestation of Disease

As a result of seasonal changes, all three *doṣas* (*Vāta, Pitta* and *Kapha*) keep getting provoked and pacified naturally. For example, *Vāta doṣa* accumulates in summer; gets aggravated during the monsoon; and gets balanced to come back to its normal condition in autumn. *Pitta doṣa* accumulates in the monsoon, gets provoked in autumn and gets back into equilibrium during winter. Similarly, *Kapha doṣa* accumulates in winter; gets aggravated in spring; and is normalized in summer.

At all places and in all countries, seasonal conditions are not the same. Due to this variation, the time and process of accumulation, aggravation and alleviation (to get back to equilibrium) of *doṣas* also varies. If this disequilibrium of *doṣas* is within limits, then the body is able to tolerate this imbalance with its immunity and is protected from disease. But, if the accumulation and provocation of *doṣas* exceeds its limit, then the body's immunity is unable to fight with the disease and one contracts a disease.

26. *Sā saṅkhyāprādhānyavidhivikalpabalakālaviśeṣairbhidyate.* (*Ca.ni.*1:12)

Besides seasonal changes, many other causes such as inappropriate food and lifestyle also vitiate the *doṣas* and provoke disease. For the manifestation of a disease, *doṣas* have to pass through several stages. These phases are called *kriyākāla* (stages) in *Āyurveda*. They are six in number. If imbalance of *doṣa* is controlled in an initial phase, then further stages do not appear, and as a result disease does not occur; but if it does, then after diagnosis of a disease in a primary stage, it can be easily controlled and managed by means of treatment and knowledge. This is only possible by means of *Āyurveda*. Hence, to make the world disease-free, basic knowledge of *Āyurveda* is essential for every individual. Then the onslaught of many diseases can be controlled before the genesis of disease. These six stages of disease manifestation are (i) accumulation, (ii) aggravation, (iii) dissemination, (iv) localization or site of manifestation, (v) symptom manifestation, and (vi) differentiation or chronicity of a disease[27].

(i) **Accumulation**: If the intake of food and adoption of lifestyle and seasonal changes are in accordance with the action, properties and effect of the corresponding *doṣa*, then the affected *doṣas* increase at its specific location. These *doṣas* accumulate at those locations and are unable to circulate all over the body. This phase is the accumulation phase, the phase of disease genesis.

The accumulation period is the first opportunity provided for treatment. If in this phase accumulated *doṣas* are expelled then further phases and disease will not occur.

(ii) **Aggravation (Provocation)**: If *doṣas* do not subside in the accumulation phase, then the aggravation phase starts. Just as butter melts with a little heat, in such a way availability of favorable food and lifestyle causes accumulated *doṣas* to gets aggravated. *Vāta* aggravation causes pain in the abdomen and flatulence. Provoked *Pitta* results in heartburn, acidity, increased thirst and a burning sensation. In provocation of *Kapha*, anorexia, nausea and other symptoms develop. It is the second stage where treatment is possible.

(iii) **Dissemination (Spreading)**: If treatment is not given in the provocation period, then the dissemination or spreading phase starts. Just as butter at high temperature not only melts, but flows out from the vessel, in such a way *doṣas* provoked by unfavorable food, lifestyle and season move away from their specific location and spread in other organs of the body. *Pitta* and *Kapha* themselves are inactive, but with the help of *Vāta*, they also speed

27. *Sañcayaṁ ca prakopaṁ ca prasaraṁ sthānasaṁśrayam.*
Vyaktiṁ bhedaṁ ca yo vetti doṣāṇāṁ sa bhavedbhiṣak. (*Su.sū.* 21:36)

up and spread. When these aggravated *doṣas* spread to different organs by induced *Vāta*, diseases also originate in those organs. This way, disease can emerge all over the body or in any one organ or in any one part of that organ. Circulation of these *doṣas* occurs through lymphatics. Those *doṣas* that are not much aggravated remain suppressed in the *srota* (channels) of the body, even if they are not treated.

(iv) **Site of manifestation (Localization)**: If *doṣas* are not treated in the spreading phase, then the manifestation phase starts. In this condition *doṣas* are disseminated throughout the body through lymphatics and locates at a particular place due to the blockage of channels and therefore localizing the *doṣa* to one place. These disseminated *doṣas* localize in those organs which have low immunity and are weak, and where these dispersed *doṣas* get a positive or favorable environment.

These *doṣas* pollute one or more than one tissue (plasma, blood and other tissues) and waste matter (feces, urine, sweat) at that particular site or organ, and along with them, produces the disease according to that place. This stage of combination of *doṣa* and *dūṣya* (*dhātus* and *malas*) is called the manifestation phase or the site of manifestation. In this phase, preliminary signs and symptoms are developed. For example, if the tissues of the lungs, musculature of the bronchial tubes and synovial membranes are weak in a person, then *Kapha* disseminates from the stomach and accumulates in the lungs or respiratory channels. As a result, cough, cold and sneezing emerge as a preliminary sign which may be an indication of bronchial asthma. In a similar manner, when *Vāta doṣa* accumulates in the abdomen, it leads to abdominal swelling, abscess and distention in the abdomen; when it accumulates in the urinary bladder, it causes calculi, *prameha* (urinary abnormality) and obstruction in urination; and when it accumulates throughout the body, there develops preliminary signs and symptoms of *Vāta* diseases, emaciation, anemia and so on. It requires the fourth phase of treatment.

(v) **Symptom manifestation**: If treatment is not given in the fourth phase, then clearly differentiated specific symptoms of a disease emerge. This phase is symptom manifestation. For example, high temperature during fever, watery and frequent passing of feces in diarrhea, difficulty in breathing in bronchial asthma, yellow color in jaundice, acute abdominal pain in cholera and so on. It requires the fifth phase of treatment.

(vi) **Differentiation or chronicity of a disease**: It is the last and sixth stage of a disease cycle. If symptoms persist, yet the disease is not treated, then fever, diarrhea and other manifestations become vicious and reach the chronic stage. In the case of edema and abscess, abscess bursts and develops into a wound or ulcer. It is the phase of differentiation. It is the sixth stage of treatment. If in this phase disease is not treated, then it becomes incurable.

The first five phases come under the stage of pathogenesis of a disease, differentiation is a later stage. For a skilled physician, it is very essential to know these six stages, because if the *doṣas* are treated at the very first stage of accumulation, then provocation and other stages of the disease cycle will not emerge.

(C) *Aṣṭavidha Parīkṣā*: The Eight *Āyurvedic* Methods of Disease Examination

Other tthan the above-said examinations (on the basis of *doṣa*, etc.), eight other types of examinations are also conducted to know the constitution (*prakṛti*), curability and/or incurability of the diseases. These examinations are known as *Aṣṭavidha parīkṣā*[28]. They are as follows:

(i) *Nādī parīkṣā* (Pulse examination)

(ii) *Mūtra parīkṣā* (Urine examination)

(iii) *Mala parīkṣā* (Fecal examination)

(iv) *Netra parīkṣā* (Ophthalmic examination)

(v) *Jihvā parīkṣā* (Tongue examination)

(vi) *Svara parīkṣā* (Voice examination)

(vii) *Sparśa parīkṣā* (Tactile examination)

(viii) *Ākṛti parīkṣā* (General appearance and nature examination)

All these examinations are based on the fundamental principles of *Āyurveda*. Apparently, *Āyurveda Nāḍī Parīkṣā* (pulse examination) does not resemble the pulse examination in the modern medical science. The former technique is absolutely different from the latter. The *Sāttvika* feeling of a physician is very important to attain the deeper insight of pulse examination. Also proximity of a skillful teacher/ practioner is very important to teach this knowledge. Hence this knowledge can be gained by a worthy disciple from a skillful preceptor. Diagnosis through pulse examination is a blessing or divine knowledge provided by the *Āyurvedic* seers as a gift. Brief explanation of all these examinations is as follows:

28. *Rogākrāntaśarīrasya sthānānyaṣṭau nirīkṣayet.*
Nārī mūtraṁ malaṁ jihvā śabdaṁ sparśadṛgākṛtī. (*Yo.Ra.Nāḍīparīkṣā-1*)

(i) *Nāḍī parīkṣā* (Pulse examination)

Pulse examination[29] is one of the most important methods to know about the patient and the nature of disease, because healthiness or unhealthiness affect the heart rate and its palpitations, which simultaneously affects the arterial pulsation. A suitable time for pulse examination is with an empty stomach in the morning, as the pulse rate becomes erratice and inconstant after eating, massage and physical exertion. Therefore, immediately after these activities, the correct diagnosis of a disease by means of pulse examination is difficult. In the same way the accurate pulse rate cannot be checked if the patient is hungry or thirsty. The pulse is examined at the radial artery approximately half an inch below the thumb of the hand. The pulse is examined in the right hand of a male and left hand of a female[30]. At times, for the clarity of the pulse, the radial arteries of both hands of males and females are examined. Patients should keep the arm straight and flexible and loosen the hand for pulse examination. The fingers and thumb should also be kept straight and spread. A physician should carry out pulse examination with the right hand. The pulse is felt with the first three fingers, the index, middle and ring fingers. It is important in pulse examination to keep all three fingers on the radial artery. The index finger is kept on the root of the thumb. Mild and equal pressure is given with the finger tips to feel the throbbing of the pulse and finger pressure is increased and decreased slightly, again and again, to know the accurate and definite pulse rate and also to sense the varying movements of the pulse. In this way, the nature of disease is determined on the basis of pressure felt on a particular fingertip. The pressure felt on the index finger denotes the pulse of *Vāta*, middle finger denotes the pulse of *Pitta*, and pressure felt on the ring finger indicates the pulse of *Kapha doṣa*.

Identification of pulse

Vāta: Index finger placement denotes the pulse of *Vāta*. The pulse feels like the movement of a snake, quick and slithery. The pulse is fast, narrow, feeble, cool and irregular.

Pitta: Middle finger placement denotes the pulse of *Pitta*. The pulse feels like the movement of a frog, active and jumpy. The pulse is excited, prominent, jumping, hot, moderate and regular.

Kapha: Ring finger placement denotes the pulse of *Kapha*. The pulse feels like the movement of a floating pigeon or a swan or a peacock. The pulse is slow, strong, steady, soft, broad, regular and warm.

29. *Doṣakope ghane, lpe ca pūrvaṁ nāḍīṁ parīkṣya ca.*
Ante cādau sthitistasyā vijñeyā bhiṣajā sphuṭam. (*Yo.Ra.Nāḍīparīkṣā.*1)

30. *Nāḍīmaṅguṣṭhamūlādhaḥ spṛśeddakṣiṇage kare.*
Jñānārthaṁ rogiṇo vaidyo nijadakṣiṇapāṇinā. (*Yo.Ra.Nāḍīparīkṣā*-1)

However to know the proper nature of a disease, a physician should be acquainted with the type of movement of the pulse. If movement of the pulse is like that of a snake (wave-like motion), it denotes the predominance of *Vāta doṣa*(31). If movement resembles a frog (active and exciting pulse with jumping movement), it represents *Pitta doṣa*(32). If the pulse moves like a pigeon (strong and floating), it denotes the prominency of *Kapha doṣa*(33), (34).

If the pulse throbs 30 times at the normal rate, it means the disease is curable and the patient will survive, but if obstruction occurs in between, it means that if immediate treatment is not provided, the patient may die soon. In fever, the pulse felt is hot and its movement is also fast. In the same way, pulse movement is fast in case of lust and anger, and slow in anxiety and fear. The feel of the pulse is very mild in dyspepsia (weak digestive fire) and during loss of tissue elements. In the same way, the pulse felt is light, but rapid in persons with strong digestive power and is heavy in case of *āma* (if the food is undigested).

By means of pulse examinations a physician gains insight about three *doṣas* and can ascertain the status of seven *dhātus*, thirteen *agnis*, *ojas* and *srotas*. Not only physiological disorders, but the knowledge of *tridoṣa* gathered by means of pulse examination also helps to diagnose the psychological condition of the patient. Though the pulse mainly denotes *tridoṣa* status, the complete body physiology is reflected in *tridoṣa*, because *tridoṣa* is the basic principle of existence of the body. [PLATE 22]

- **Incurable pulse according to *Āyurveda***

A skilled physician through pulse examination is able to determine whether the disease is curable or incurable and whether the patient will survive or not. A pulse with many different movements slow, weak, unstable, obstructive and mild is known as *sannipātika* (suffering from vitiation of all three *doṣas*). It is incurable and causes death.

When the movements of the pulse resembles with *Pitta, Vāta* and *Kapha* types, respectively and then revolves like a fast moving wheel, with high frequency and volume rhythm and then suddenly falls down from its normal speed and gets slows. This also denotes that the disease is incurable. A pulse

31. *Vātānmale tu dṛḍhatā śuṣkatā cāpi jātate.*
Pītatā jāyate pittācchuktatā śleṣmato bhavet. (*Yo.Ra.Malaparīkṣā*.1)
32. *Sarpahaṁsagatiṁ tadvadvātaśleṣmavatīṁ vadet.*
Harihaṁsagatiṁ dhatte pittaśleṣmānvitā dharā. (*Yo.Ra.Nāḍīparīkṣā*-17)
33. *Muhuḥ sarpagatiṁ nāḍīṁ muhurbhekagatiṁ tathā.*
Vātapittasamubhūtāṁ tāṁ vadanti vicakṣaṇāḥ. (*Yo.Ra.nāḍīparīkṣā*-16)
34. *Rājahaṁsamayārāṇāṁ pārāvatakapatayaḥ.*
Kukkuṭasya gatiṁ dhatte dhamanī kaphasaṁginī. (*Yo.Ra.Nāḍīparīkṣā*-15)

which is feeble with high pulse rate and cold also denotes that the disease is incurable and life is at an end.

- **Health indicative pulse or curative pulse**

The patient with a pulse throbbing like that of a swan and with a cheerful face denotes that the patient is healthy. In this way, precise explanation of pulse movement is elaborated in *Āyurveda*. On this basis, a skilled physician can easily determine the causes of disease, diagnosis of disease, curability, incurability, birth and mortality of the patient, and can prescribe a suitable treatment at a right time.

(ii) ***Mūtra parīkṣā* (Urine examination)**

For urine examination in *Āyurveda,* the first sample of urine is collected at an ambrosial hour (*Bhrama muhūrta*) or after rising from the bed. Urine is collected in a clean glass or transparent vessel. Avoid the first stream of urine. Thereafter the mouth of the vessel is closed and the urine is examined at the time of sunrise.

On the basis of the color of urine, one can determine the nature of the patient and the disease. If the urine is pale yellow in color, it means patient is V*āta* dominated. If the urine is white in color and with foam, it means *Kapha doṣa* predominates.Yellow or orangish-red color in the urine is an indication of *Pitta doṣa*. In the same way, if urine is dusky and lukewarm, it is an indication of *Pitta* and *Vāta* vitiation. If urine is white in color with effervescence, it means *Vāta* and K*apha doṣas* predominates. If urine is red in color with haziness like clouds, it is an indication of *Kapha* and *Pitta* aggravation. In chronic fever, urine is red like blood and yellow in color. If urine is transparent and black, it means patient suffers with *sannipātika roga* (provocation of all three *doṣas*). Urine examination is also based on the theory of *tridoṣa*, in a similar manner to pulse examination.

(iii) ***Mala parīkṣā* (Fecal examination)**

In *Āyurveda*, examination of the stool is a diagnostic tool used to understand the disease. The color of the stool is also helpful in determining the nature of disease. If the stool is thick with a bluish black color, it emphasizes a predominance of *Vāta doṣa*[35], [36]. In this condition the stool is hard and dry. If the patient is constipated, he/she will excrete rough, frothy stool in small and dry pieces. An excess of *Pitta doṣa* gives the stool a green or yellow color and it is liquid in form. A white color indicates a *Kapha* disorder. In such patients, the stool is cool, generally well-formed, in sufficient quantity and lined with mucus. If the stool is thick and bluish black with whiteness,

35. *Sannipāte ca sarvāṇi lakṣaṇāni bhavanti hi.*
Truṭitaṁ phenilaṁ rūkṣaṁ dhūpanaṁ vātakopataḥ. (*Yo.Ra.Malaparīkṣā.*2)
36. *Rūkṣā dhūmrā tathā raudrā calā cāṇtarjvalatyapi.*
Dṛṣṭiryadā tadā vātarogaṁ rogavido jaguḥ. (*Yo.Ra.Dṛk parīkṣā.*1)

it indicates *Vāta* and *Kapha doṣas*. If the stool is yellowish and well-formed but excreted in small pieces, it is an indication of *Vāta* and *Pitta doṣas* being aggravated.

If digestion and absorption are functioning normally, the stool is well-formed and will float in water. But if digestion is improper, the stool sinks and can be sticky and slimy, containing undigested food and with a bad odor. This is an indication of *āma* and toxins within the system.

If the stool is white and has severe unpleasant smell, it denotes the onset of ascites. If the stool is black or bluish-black with a severe purulent smell and immediate treatment is not available, then the patient will not survive and death is definite. So an *Āyurvedic* physician can determine the nature, curability and incurability of the disease on the basis of color, form and smell of the stool.

(iv) ***Netra parīkṣā* (Ophthalmic examination)**

By observing the color of the eyes and other conditions, a physician can determine the nature of disease. *Vāta* predominant eyes are small, dusty, dry, sunken and nervous[37] with drooping eyelids, dry and with scanty lashes, and with unsteady pupils and burning sensation in the eyes.

In *Pitta doṣa*, the eyes are moderate in size, sharp, lustrous and sensitive to light (photophobia) with burning sensation. The lashes are scanty and oily and the iris is yellow or red in color. According to *Āyurveda*, eyes derive their energy from the basic fire element. The fiery energy in the retina results in sensitivity to light. Thus, people of *Pitta* constitution, having an abundance of fire in the body, often have eyes that are hypersensitive to light. An excess of *Kapha doṣa* gives white color to the eyes. The eyes are large, beautiful and moist with long, thick and oily eyelashes with excessive discharge, lusterless and sleepy with heaviness in the eyelids and unsteady pupil.

A combination of symptoms appears in the eyes of the patient if any two *doṣas* provocate. If the eyes are bluish-black in color in *sannipātika doṣa* (all three *doṣas* get aggravated together) and vision is stable, then the eyes look sleepy. If the eyes are red or black in color and look fearful, then the patient is incurable. Ophthalmic examination thus plays an important role in knowing the cause, curability and incurability of the disease.

(v) ***Jihvā parīkṣā* (Tongue examination)**

The tongue is an organ of taste and speech. Besides, it is a sensory organ, hence observation of the tongue is an important part of the examination.

37. *Jihā śītā kharasparśā sphuṭitā mārute, dhike.*
Raktā śyāmā bhavetpitte kapheśubhrā, tipicchilā. (*Yo.Ra.jihvāparīkṣā.*1)

Tongue examination also helps a physician to determine the condition of a patient. If the tongue is cold, numb, dry, rough and with crevices, it indicates that *Vāta doṣa* is predominant. If it is red or blue in color with a burning sensation and prickliness, it indicates predominancy of *Pitta doṣa*. In *Kapha* vitiation, the tongue is white in color, wet, cool, slimy, heavy and thickly coated. If the tongue is black in color, dry, rough, bitter, with crevices, burning and prickliness, it indicates aggravation of *sannipātika doṣa*.

A coating covering the tongue indicates toxins in the stomach, small intestine or large intestine. If only the posterior part is coated, toxins are present in the large intestine. If the middle part of the tongue is coated, toxins are present in the stomach and small intestine. Examination of the tongue is also helpful to know about the condition of fever, curability and incurability of a disease.

(vi) ***Svara parīkṣā* (Voice examination)**

If the voice becomes rough and hoarse, it indicates predominance of *Vāta doṣa*. If the voice is clear and loud, it denotes *Pitta doṣa*. If the voice becomes heavy and hoarse, it indicates that *Kapha doṣa* is predominant.

(vii) ***Sparśa parīkṣā* (Tactile examination)**

Vāta aggravated skin is coarse, rough and dry with below normal temperature giving a sensation of coolness. *Pitta* influenced skin has a high temperature. If the skin becomes oily, cold and moist, it indicates that *Kapha doṣa* is predominant.

(viii) ***Ākṛti parīkṣā* (General appearance and nature examination)**

Besides the above-said examinations, some other points are also helpful for a physician to know the nature of the disease.

In the *Vāta* aggravated individual: The appearance of skin and hair is rough and dry, the skin is cracked and the hair has split ends. Their nature is not amicable; they lack patience, memory and intellect; they are very talkative; and their liking is for cold substances.

In the *Pitta* aggravated individual: The appearance of the skin is yellowish and hot; the palms, soles of the feet and face resemble the color of copper; they have less bodily hair; and the hair are golden in color. Their nature is short-tempered and egoistical.

In the *Kapha* aggravated individual: The appearance of the skin is white, and they have well-formed joints, bones and muscles. According to their nature, such individuals are not much affected by hunger, thirst, grief and pain.

Other than the above-mentioned eight examinations, some physicians also diagnose the causes of disease by examination of the mouth and nails too.

- ***Āsya (mukh) parīkṣā*** **(Oral cavity (mouth) examination)**

Aggravation of *Vāta doṣa* is indicated by a sweet taste in the mouth. Aggravation of *Pitta doṣa* is indicated by a bitter taste. A sweet-sour taste denotes the provocation of *Kapha doṣa*. If taste is of mixed type, this is an indication of provocation of *tridoṣa*. Indigestion is reflected by a taste resembling *ghee*, and oiliness and stickiness in the mouth. An astringent taste indicates dyspepsia (weak digestive fire).

- ***Nakh parīkṣā*** **(Nail examination)**

A physician can also determine the nature of disease by observing the patient's nails. Aggravated *Vāta* is the cause of blue nails. Excess *Pitta doṣa* gives red or yellow color to the nails.White color indicates the predominance of *Kapha doṣa*. If the nails are yellow or red with a bluish haze, it indicates vitiation of both *Vata* and *Pitta doṣas*. If the nails become yellow or white it indicates vitiation of *Kapha* and *Pitta doṣas*. If the symptoms of all three *doṣas* are visible, it indicates *sannipātika roga* and the nails are blue, yellow, green or white with a reddish haze. Such a condition reflects incurability of a disease. Symptoms of abdominal disorders are reflected by white spots visible on the nails and fragile skin near the nails. Hence, by means of nail examination a physician can also diagnose and identify the disease.

Chapter 9

Therapeutic Methods

Due to inappropriate diet and lifestyle, the tissues in the body get vitiated. Also due to some external factors, trauma, injuries, bacterial and viral infections, the body may acquire a disorder (disease). In these cases, a clear four legged treatment procedure (as described in the previous chapter) brings the vitiated *dhātus* back to equilibrium, normalizes malfunctioning, and restores the body to order and health. The process that restores the normalcy is 'Treatment[(1), (2)].' Therefore treatment denotes the 'alleviation of disorders.' Treatments are of three types: (i) *Yuktivyapāśraya* (Rational), (ii) *Satvāvajaya* (*Psychic*), and (iii) *Daivavyapāśraya* (Godly).

(i) ***Yuktivyapāśraya*** (**Rational**): Treatment involving a proper food regimen and medicinal substances in a planned manner is *yuktivyapāśraya.*

(ii) ***Satvāvajaya*** (***Psychic***): Controlling the negative focus and emotions of the mind is *satvāvajaya* (*psychic*) treatment[(3)].

(iii) ***Daivavyapāśraya*** (**Godly**): Treatment with the help of hymns, herbs, precious stones, ritual sacrifices, fasting and so on is *daivavyapāśraya.*

Of these, these, the first and the second pertain to psycho-somatic disorders, while the third one is resorted when the two fail altogether. Among all, rational treatment prevails as it is based on reasoning. Some recommend simultaneous use of all the three on the levels of the body, mind and soul to bring perfect recovery. [PLATE 23]

1. *Yābhiḥ kriyābhirjāyante śarīre dhāta vaḥ samāḥ.*
Sā cikitsā vikārāṇāṁ karma tad bhiṣajāṁ smṛtam. (*Ca. sū.* 16:34)
Kathaṁ śarīre dhātūnāṁ vaiṣamyaṁ na bhavedi.
Samānāṁ cānubandhḥ syādityarthaṁ kriyate kriyā. (*Ca. sū.* 16:3)
2. *Caturṇāṁ bhiṣagādīnāṁ śastānāṁ dhātuvaikṛte.*
Pravṛttirdhātusāmyārthā cikitsetyabhidhīyate. (*Ca. sū.* 9.5)
3. *Punarapi ca trividhamauṣadham-Daivavyapāsrayaṁ yuktivyāpāśrayaṁ*
Satvāvajayaścetitatra daivavyapāśrayaṁ mantrauṣadhimaṇimaṅgalabalyupahāra-
homaniyamaprāyaścittopavāsasvastyayanapraṇipātagamanādi.
yuktivyapāśrayamāhārauṣadhayojanādi.sattvāajayaḥ punarahitānmanonigrah. (*A.saṅ.sū.* 12.5)

1. Different Methods of Treatment in *Āyurveda*

Āyurvedic treatments are completely different from the modern Medicine. These methods do not just confront a disease; rather, they aim for overall body purification. These methods facilitate such conditions inside the body which can easily eradicate the provoked *doṣas*, diseases and other root causes of the disease. Hence, a physician uses such a treatment procedure for strong, well-built and obese people, which can easily eliminate the accumulated *doṣas*, vitiated *dhātus* and *malas* from the body and bring back lightness to the body. Patients who are very lean, weak and emaciated with undernourished *doṣas* and *dhātus*, for them such treatment procedures are adopted which provide strength and nourishment to the *doṣas* and *dhātus*. *Āyurvedic* treatments vary from one condition to other. In the case of excessive oiliness or provoked *Kapha doṣa*, the treatment administered should be one that causes dryness (drying therapy). Whereas in excessive dryness or aggravated *Vāta*, oleation therapy is advisable. For these therapies, medicinal herbs with multiple properties are prescribed by a physician. All the above-said treatment modalities are basically divided in two parts[4].

1. ***Santarpaṇa cikitsā***[5] **(Stoutening therapy)**

This therapy includes those medicinal herbs and applications which bring heaviness to the body. They are meant to increase the body weight. This treatment facilitates nourishment and strengthening of the body and help in body building. Such medicinal herbs, food material and other applications are predominant in earth and water elements.

2. ***Apatarpaṇa cikitsā*** **(Lightning therapy)**

This category includes therapies involving such medicinal herbs and resources which are meant to bring lightness to the body and reduce the body weight. The medicinal herbs, food substances and other applications used in this therapy are predominant in fire, air and space (ether) elements.

Since the five elements possess both *santarpaṇa* and *apatarpaṇa* properties, the material substances formed by the combination of these elements, when used in the body, produce both types of effects.

Many procedures are used in *Āyurveda* for the above-said two types of treatments. All these therapies have been categorized into the following six types:

4. *Upakramyasya hi dvitvād dvidhaivopakramo mataḥekaḥ santarpaṇastatra dvitīyaścāpatarpaṇaḥ Bṛṁhaṇo laṅhanaśceti tatparyāyāvudāhṛtau.* (*A. saṅ. sū.* 24.2-4)

5. *Bṛṁhaṇaṁyad bṛhatvāya laṅghanaṁ lāghavāya tat.*
Dehasya bhavataḥ prāyo bhaumāpyamitaracca te. (*A. saṅ. sū.* 24.4-5)

1. *Laṅghana cikitsā* (Fasting therapy)
2. *Bṛṁhaṇa cikitsā* (Nourishing or Restorative therapy)
3. *Rūkṣaṇa cikitsā* (Drying therapy)
4. *Snehana cikitsā* (Oleation therapy)
5. *Svedana cikitsā* (Fomentation or Sudation therapy)
6. *Stambhana cikitsā* (Astringent or Binding therapy)

1. *Laṅghana cikitsā* (Fasting therapy)

The treatment procedure which brings lightness to the body is called as *laṅghana* therapy. It is of two types:

(A) *Saṁśodhana* or *śodhana cikitsā* (Purification or Detoxification therapy): The treatment in which vitiated *doṣas* and *malas* are eliminated through the excretory passages (anus, urinary tract, skin, nose and mouth) is called purification or detoxification therapy. There are five purification or detox therapies: *Vamana* (emesis) meaning expulsion of morbidity (*mala* or *doṣa*) through the oral route via vomiting; *Virecana* (purgation) meaning expulsion of morbidity through the anal route via loose motions; *Anuvāsana basti* (enema with medicated oil or *ghee* or other fatty substances); *Nirūha basti* (decoction enema); and *Nasya* (errhine or inhalation therapy) meaning pouring medicines into nostrils and thus expelling morbidity through them. Purification therapy is a part of *pañcakarma* therapy in *Āyurveda*, where oleation and sudation therapies are the *pūrvakarmas* (premonitoring procedures) of *pañcakarma*.

(B) *Śamana cikitsā* (Palliation or Alleviation therapy): In this treatment, without eliminating the vitiated *doṣas* and *malas* from the body, procedures are used that mitigate the *doṣas* and *malas* and bring them back into equilibrium. This is palliation or alleviation treatment. It includes:

(i) ***Dīpana* and *pācana* (stomachic and digestive):** These drugs are used to improve the digestive power, increase the appetite and improve the digestion of food. This quickly alleviates *doṣas* and *malas*.

(ii) ***Kṣutnigraha* or *upavāsa* (fasting)**: This includes starving or fasting or the intake of very light food. It quickly facilitates the expulsion of toxins.

(iii) ***Pipāsā nigraha* (thirst)**: To remain thirsty or to keep control over thirst is beneficial in water retaining and kidney disorders.

(iv) ***Śārīrika vyāyāma* (physical exercise)**: Physical fitness, *yogāsanas* and so on reduces obesity and bring the aggravated *doṣas* back to equilibrium, strengthens the body and develops immunity.

(v) ***Ātapa* and *māruta* (sun and air)**: Exposure to sun and inhalation of fresh air is beneficial in obesity and skin-related disorders.

If this therapy is used for weight reduction, it should be practiced on people who are stout, obese and capable of withstanding the therapy, and it can also be used on patients suffering from diseases generated by *Vāta* vitiation along with excess of *Kapha, Pitta*, blood and morbidity in the body.

If vomiting, diarrhea, cholera, fever, constipation, heaviness in the body, belching, nausea, anorexia and so on are caused by provocation of *Kapha* and *Pitta* and if these diseases are in their moderate form (neither very acute nor very low), they are initially treated with medicines capable of increasing the digestive power. If these diseases are in their mild form, then treatment includes fasting and control over thirst.

If a strong person is suffering from these diseases in a mild and moderate form, then the treatment adopted should be physical exercises and exposure to sun and air.

In *laṅghana* therapy, medicines used are light, hot, penetrating, non-slimy, dry, rough, minute, liquid and hard in quality.

2. *Bṛṁhaṇa cikitsā* (Nourishing or Restorative therapy)

One suffering from vitiated *Vāta* or *Vāta-Pitta* provocation, tuberculosis, debility, emaciation, senility and old-age, those who are addicted to excessive coitus and intoxication, those who get tired by frequent and long journeys and excessive physical work require nourishing therapy. The treatment that is strength-promoting and nourishing is *Bṛṁhaṇa cikitsā*. This treatment is very useful and much needed in the summer.

The treatment includes a healthy regime and intake of milk, *ghee*, cottage cheese, butter, honey and other nutritive and beneficial substances that provide nourishment and strength. In this therapy heavy, cool, emollient, slow, oily, stout, thick and dense substances are considered useful. A healthy regime involves baths, *ubaṭana*, good deep sleep; *basti* (enema) with sweet and oily medicines, to keep away grief and anxiety and related conditions.

3. *Rūkṣaṇa cikitsā* (Drying therapy)

This is useful in diseases which cause blockage in the body channels, excessive provocation of *Vāta* and other *doṣas* and when diseases affect the vital organs of the body such as stiffness of the legs, gout and obstinate urinary disorders.

Substances with pungent, bitter and astringent tastes, oil cakes prepared from sesame and mustard seeds and honey are used in this therapy. For this treatment rough, dry, light, penetrating, hot in potency, non-sticky and strong medicines are used.

4. *Snehana cikitsā* (Oleation therapy)

Treatment which increases smoothness of the body, fluidity, softness and moistness is oleation therapy. *Ghee*, oil, fat and other oily substances are used for oleation therapy. *Ghee* is considered the best among them. According to *Āyurveda*, when medicines are processed with ghee it absorbs various beneficial properties itself, it alleviates vitiated *Pitta* and *Vāta doṣas*, and it also nourishes *rasa* and *śukra dhātus*. Other than that, *ghee* clears the voice and enhances the complexion. It is useful for the skin. Its intake helps to treat diseases of the male and female genital tract. It strengthens the body and enhances sexual vigor and is also useful in trauma, fractures, prolapse of the uterus, otalgia (ear pain) and headache.

Bone marrow is also used as an emollient in oleation therapy. It enhances physical strength, especially of the bones. It nourishes *śukra dhātu* (semen), *rasa dhātu* (plasma), *meda dhātu* (adipose tissue), *majjā dhātu* (bone marrow) and increases *Kapha doṣa*.

For alleviation of *Pitta, ghee* is the best among all, followed by bone marrow, fats and oils respectively. To the contrary, in *Vāta* alleviation, oil is the best emollient whereas bone marrow and *ghee* are less effective, respectively.

5. *Svedana cikitsā* (Fomentation or Sudation therapy)

A treatment which cures stiffness, heaviness and coolness and produces sweat is called fomentation therapy. There are thirteen types of fomentation therapies described in *Āyurveda*. Their procedure, compatibility and contra-indications are different. They are useful for cold, cough, hiccoughs, bronchial asthma; heaviness in the body, bodyache, otalgia (ear pain), neck pain, headache and migraine; for hoarseness of the voice, sore throat and spasmodic obstruction in the throat; for hemorrhagic strokes or paralysis in a particular organ, of the full body or half the body; for excess yawning, body bending, contraction, chills, tremors, numbness, neuralgia of upper and lower extremities, and edema; for distention or flatulence, constipation, and abdominal cramps; for urinary obstruction, dysuria and testicular hypertrophy; for pain in the flanks, lumbago, sciatica, pain and cramps in legs, calf muscles and knee joints; for diseases produced due to abnormal digestive and metabolic activities; and for *Vāta* deformities in ankle joints and other *Vāta* disorders affecting the entire body. Hot, penetrating, smooth, dry, minute, stable, mobile, liquid and heavy substances are used in sudation therapy.

6. *Stambhana cikitsā* (Astringent or Binding therapy)

A procedure which can hamper the movement of any kind of flowing substances is an astringent or binding therapy. This procedure is useful in *Pitta* aggravation, burns caused by chemicals and fire, for those suffering from diarrhea, vomiting and for one who is a victim of poisoning and excessive sudation.

After *stambhana* treatment, if a patient gets relief and regains strength, it indicates that the therapy is succesfully accomplished. The substances which are liquid, less viscid with cool potency, stable, sweet, bitter and astringent in taste are used in astringent or binding therapy.

In all the above-mentioned therapies, drying therapy, fasting therapy and sudation therapy comes under *apatarpaṇa cikitsā*; and oleation therapy, nourishing therapy and astringent therapy comes under *santarpaṇa cikitsā*.

2. An Introduction to *Pañcakarma* Treatment

Pañcakarma, as the name specifies, includes five types of actions or processes which eliminate vitiated *doṣas* and *malas* from the body. *Pañcakarma* is an important part of *Āyurvedic* treatment, because disease aggravation recurs many a times, in spite of using different types of medicines.The methods of purification and detoxification for the prevention as well as eradication of a disease by the elimination of aggravated *doṣas* and *malas* from the body is *Pañcakarma* treatment. Several processes before the initiation of *Pañcakarma* treatment are pre-monitoring procedures, carried out with the help of palliation and purification therapies, especially include oleation and fomentation. These five basic processes are as follows:

1. *Vamana* (Emetic therapy)
2. *Virecana* (Purgative therapy)
3. *Nasya* (Inhalation therapy or Errhine)
4. *Anuvāsana basti* (A type of enema)
5. *Nirūha basti* (Another type of enema)

Ācharya Suśruta and other scholars described *rakta mokṣaṇa* (blood-letting therapy) in place of *nasya* (errhine) as a part of *pañcakarma*. Before administering all such treatments, it is necessary to find out whether the patient is capable; physically and mentally to bear such treatments. Otherwise it may inflict harm instead of benefitting a patient. The procedures carried before *pañcakarma* treatment are 'pre-monitoring procedures,' and some precautions and compatible diet must be followed along with and after the treatment which are 'post-treatment measures.' Special types of medicines and procedures are selected according to the patient and diseases. These *pañcakarma* procedures are described here in brief. [PLATE 24]

- For elimination of *Kapha* – Emesis is the best.
- For elimination of *Pitta* – Purgation is the best.
- For elimination of *Vāta* – Enema or *basti* (both *anuvāsana* and *āsthāpana basti*) is the best.
- For tenderness in the body – Fomentation is the best.

1) *Vamana*: Emetic therapy[6]

The treatment where emetic drugs are used to induce vomiting for detoxification of the abdomen is emetic therapy or therapeutic vomiting. This treatment can be followed throughout the year except in severe winter and extreme summer. Emetic medicines are used to expel toxic substances or wastes from the body.

6. *Doṣaharaṇamūrdhabhāgaṁ vamanākhyamadhobhāgaṁ virecanākhyamu bhayaṁ vā malavirecanādvirecanamityucyate.* (*A. saṅ. sū.* 27.3)

- **Use**

Emesis is beneficial for all those suffering from *Kapha* and *Pitta* disorders. Therapeutic vomiting is also useful when there is congestion in the lungs, causing cough, bronchial asthma, fever due to *Kapha*, tonsillitis, cold, inflammation of the nose, sinus and suppuration in the nose, palate and lips[(7)], and otorrhea (suppuration from the ears). It is also indicated in nausea, loss of appetite, indigestion, sprue syndrome, diarrhea, fat accumulation or diseases due to obesity, anemia, poisoning, intrinsic hemorrhage from lower channels of the body, dermatitis and other skin diseases (itching, erysipelas, etc.), boils, glandular swelling, edema, urinary disorders, excessive sleeping, drowsiness, hydrocele, epilepsy and insanity.

- **Indications**

Therapeutic vomiting is useful for those who are suffering from the above-mentioned diseases, who have strong vision, who have no problem while vomiting and have patience.

- **Contra-Indications**

Therapeutic vomiting is contra-indicated[(8)] in childhood, old age, debility, emaciation and hunger. Apart from this, people like heart patients, those having cavities in the lungs, bleeding from the upper body channels, during menstruation, during pregnancy, while in grief, afflicted by obesity or in any sort of disorder, intoxicated people, those having fear of vomiting, those who face difficulty in vomiting, those with eye diseases (cataract, blindness, pain in the eyes and so on), and those with a dry body constitution, jaundice, worm infestation and *Vāta* disorders.

Even in contra-indications if a person suffers from *Kapha* aggravation, indigestion or poisoning, emetic therapy can be administered in a mild form, using a decoction of liquorice root. But in childhood, debility and with fragile and fearful persons this therapy is not feasible.

- **Pre-emesis measures**

Before emesis, measures should be taken to aggravate *Kapha* in the patient's body. For this 1-3 days prior to emesis, a person is provided with medicated oils to drink 2-3 times a day until the feces become oily and he feels nauseated. A day before initiation of the treatment, oleation therapy (oil massage) followed by fomentation on the chest and back is administered to liquefy *Kapha*. To vitiate *Kapha*, a *Kapha* facilitating diet such as thin gruel, Basmati rice, milk, buttermilk and yogurt should be eaten with adequate salt in it. Emesis should be conducted in the morning (the time when *Kapha* is active).

7. *Navajvarātisārādhaḥ pittāsṛgrājayakṣmiṇaḥ. Kuṣṭhamehāpacīgranthiślīpadonmād akāsīnaḥ. Śvāsahṛllāsavīsarpastanyadoṣordharogiṇaḥ.* (*A. hṛ. sū.* 18.1-2)
8. *Avāmyā garbhiṇī rūkṣaḥ kṣudhito nityaduḥkhitaḥ. Bālavṛddhakṛśasthū lahṛdrogikṣatadurbalāḥ. Prasaktavamathuplīhatimirakrimikoṣṭhinaḥ. Urdhvapravṛttavāyvasradattabastihatasvarāḥ. Mūtrāghātyudarī gulmī durvamo, tyagnirarśasaḥ. Udāvartabhramāṣṭhīlāpārśvarugvātarogiṇaḥ. Rte viṣagarājīrṇaviruddhābhyavahārataḥ.* (*A. hṛ. sū.* 18.3-6)

- **Emetic substances**

Rock salt and honey are importantly used. Besides emetic nut, liquorice root, margosa, bitter sponge gourd, bitter bottle gourd, long pepper, bitter oleander and cardamom are the main emetic substances. In *Kapha* provocation pungent, penetrating and hot potency substances; and in *Pitta* provocation sweet and cool potency substances are used as emetics. In case of *Vāta* and *Kapha* aggravation sweet, salty, sour and hot potency substances are useful. All these medicines are used as decoctions, boiled and reduced to half the amount (in the ratio 170g in 3 liters of water).

- **Method**

During emesis a person should sit at ease on his legs with folded knees or on a chair of knee-height and drink the decoction in high, moderate or low doses of 7, 4.5 or 1.5 liter(s) respectively. After the intake, the person will feel nauseated. At this time the person should use his middle and index finger or use a tender and smooth castor twig to rub the tongue up to the throat to induce vomiting, continuing the process until it causes elimination of *Pitta* and *Kapha* followed by medicine taken, and finally *Pitta* is expelled in vomiting. If a person feels detoxified with lightness in the heart, throat, head and in the whole body, then emesis is successfully performed. The degree of success is determined by the number of vomits. Eight, six and four vomits are maximum, moderate and minimum, respectively.

- **Post-emesis measures**

When hungry, give vegetable soup, boiled rice and green gram to eat. For at least one day avoid cold drinks and cool substances, physical exercise, coitus, anger, *ghee* or oil massage. Be careful of getting indigestion.

- **Result of the therapy**

The symptoms observed after every treatment help to analyze the degree of success, whether it is successfully perfomed, less than required or more than required. The aim of the treatment is to pacify the disease. If the disease gets pacified, the body feels light, fresh and energetic, and the *doṣas* get expelled from the body. If all the medicine taken is vomited and this results in the carmination of *Vāta*, it can be considered that the procedure has been satisfactorily performed.

- **Minimal effect**

If more vitiation of *doṣas* is seen as compared to earlier and there is heaviness in the body, lethargy, oiliness, smoothness, nausea and itching, then the *doṣas* have not been eliminated properly. The effect of the therapy is then below normal.

- **Over-effect**

On the contrary, excessive dryness in the body, syncope, pain, excessive weakness, anorexia, stiffness, excessive thirst and excessive elimination of *doṣas* indicates the over-effect of the procedure.

- **Counter treatment**

According to the Scriptures, treatment should be given on the basis of the visible symptoms. If the effect of the procedure is low, then the therapy can be repeated, but if the effect is more, then cold or hot, restorative or fasting therapy can be provided accordingly.

2) *Virecana*: Purgative therapy[9]

Purgation is when medication is used to eliminate waste matter from the intestines through the anal passage. *Virecana* is the cleansing of *Pitta* and the purification of blood toxins. It is an important process of purification. It is normally given in the autumn, but if a disease is serious, then it can be administered in any season.

- **Use**

This therapy is normally used for the purification of the body. It also counters the effect of *Pitta* aggravation. Its parallel use also provides strength to the sensory and motor organs, refreshes the brain, increases the digestive fire, stabilizes the tissues and correspondingly increases body strength[10].

- **Indications**

Purgative therapy can be used for diseases due to *āma* (undigested or semidigested food), hemorrhoids, worms, flatulence and several skin diseases like dermatitis.

- **Contra-Indications**

Purgation is contra-indicated in children, people of old-age, debility, emaciation, a soft-natured person, pregnancy, a stout person, intoxication, the first stage of fever, post-delivery, diarrhea, persons with low digestive fire, wounds caused by weapons, a dry body constitution, immediately after *vamana*, ulcerative colitis and prolapsed rectum.

- **Nature of bowel movements**

The nature of bowel movements varies from person to person. These bowel movements are considered to be of three types according to the nature of peristaltic movements:

a) **Soft bowel movement**[11]: In some people, due to increased *Pitta*, purgation takes place very soon. Such persons have a 'soft bowel.' For them, mild laxatives in low doses are used for purgation. Mild medicines like milk, water, oil or grapes are beneficial for such people.

9. ----*Adhobhāgaṁ virecanākhyamubhayaṁ vā malavirecanādvirecanamityucyate.* (A. hṛ. sū. 27.3)
10. *Virekasādhyā gulmārśovisphaṭavyaṅgakāmalāḥ. Jīrṇajvarodaragaracchardiplīhahalīmakāḥ. Vidradhistimiraṁ kācaḥ syandaḥ paqvāśayavyathā. Yoniśukrāśrayā rogāḥ koṣṭhagāḥ kṛmayo vraṇāḥ. Vātāsramūrdhvagaṁ raktaṁ mūtrāghātaḥ śakṛdgrahaḥ. Vāmyāś ca kuṣṭhamehādyāḥ.* (A. hṛ. sū. 18.8.9)
11. *Bahupitto mṛdukoṣṭhaḥ kṣīreṇāpi viricyate.* (A. hṛ. sū. 18)

b) **Moderate bowel movement**: If the *Kapha doṣa* is predominant in the bowel, then one may require medicines with moderate strength (neither very strong nor very mild). For such people, peristaltic movements are of moderate intensity. For them, the laxatives used are Indian jalap, gentian and pods of Indian laburnum.

c) **Hard bowel movement**[(12), (13)]: If *Vāta* is prominent, then it results in hard stool. Purgation is very difficult for such persons and they are considered to have hard peristaltic movements. Strong purgative medicines like latex of the common milk hedge and purging nut are used.

Hence, before purgation therapy, the nature of bowel movements is an important factor to determine the type of medicine to be used.

3) *Nasya*: Inhalation therapy or Errhine

Therapy involving nasal administration to heal disorders of the head, eyes, ears, nose and throat is *'nasya'* or *'sirovirecāna.'* It is also known as '*nāvana.*' It is of two types[(14)]:

I) *Recana* or *karṣaṇa nasya* (purgative errhine)

II) *Snehana* or *bṛṁhaṇa nasya* (oleative or nutritive errthine)

I) ***Recana* or *karṣaṇa nasya* (purgative errhine)**[(15)]: This *nasya* therapy eliminates *Kapha* and other *doṣas* from the head. It involves the use of pungent oils and oils processed with extracts or decoctions of pungent drugs. The extracts or powders of pungent drugs are also used. This treatment is used in *Kapha* aggravated diseases (nose, ear, throat or head disorders), headache, hoarseness, chronic rhinitis, cold, edema, anorexia, epilepsy and skin disorders such as dermatitis.

II) ***Snehana* or *bṛṁhaṇa nasya* (oleative or nourishing errhine)**[(16)]: This therapy brings smoothness to the upper parts of the body like the head, nose and so on. It involves the use of oil or *ghee* or oil processed with extracts, decoctions, pastes or powders of medicines that are sweet in taste. This therapy is used in disorders of the head, nose, eyes, trigeminal neuralgia, migraine, headache, dry sinuses, premature graying of hair and hair fall, tinnitus, disorders of teeth, dryness in the mouth; stiffness in the neck, shoulders and steno-mastoid region, cervical spondylosis; lack of strength, *Vāta* and genetic disorders.

12. *Na tu recyo navajvarī. Alpāgnyadhogapittāsrakṣatapāyvatisāriṇaḥ.*
Saśalyāsthapitakrūrakoṣṭhātisnigdhaśoṣiṇaḥ. (A. hṛ. sū. 10.1-2)
13. *Prabhūtamārutaḥ krūraḥ kṛcchrācchayāmādikairapi* (A. hṛ. sū. 18)
14. *Virecanaṁ bṛṁhaṇaṁ caśamanaṁ ca tridhā, pi tat.* (A. hṛ. sū. 21.2)
15. *Virecanaṁ śiraḥśūlajāḍyasyandagalāmaye.*
Śophagaṇḍakṛmigranthikuṣṭhāpasmārapīnase. (A. hṛ. sū. 21.3)
16. *Bṛṁhaṇaṁ vātaje śūle sūryāvarte svarakṣaye.*
Nāsāsyaśoṣe vāksaṅge kṛcchrabodhe, vabāhuke. (A. hṛ. sū. 21.4)

- **Contra-Indications**

This therapy is not prescribed during pregnancy, menstruation, after sex, during eating and drinking alcohol.

- **Substances used in *nasya***

These include decoction, extract, paste or powder of sweet flag (calamus) root, onion, garlic, ginger and black pepper processed in *ghee* or oil.

4) *Anuvāsana basti*: A type of enema

Āyurvedic enema treatment involves elimination of waste and medications through the anal pathway. It includes introduction of medicines into the rectum in the form of oil or oily decoctions in a liquid form to eliminate *Vāta* disorders.

It includes oleation enema using *ghee*, oil and other oily substances and also the intake of such substances. It is known as *'anuvāsana'* or *'snehana basti'* (oleation enema). It is also known as '*mātrā basti*' because this basti is given in a specific dose of 100 ml or 50 ml.

- **Use**

This enema detoxifies the abdomen and brings back smoothness and tenderness. It increases the body mass and strength, improves health and longevity, and also enhances the complexion.

- **Indications**

Dryness in the body, acute digestive fire, chronic constipation and *Vāta* disorders are treated with *anuvāsana basti.*

- **Contra-Indications**

It is contra-indicated for children below seven years of age, people of old age, in dermatitis, obesity, diabetes, abdominal diseases, indigestion, anorexia, severe anemia, bronchial asthma, cough, tuberculosis, urinary diseases, excessive thirst, insanity and grief.

5) *Nirūha basti*: Another type of enema

The enema that includes herbal decoctions and milk for the purification of the bowels is *'nirūha basti.'* Since this *basti* supports *Vāta* and other *doṣas* and *dhātus* in the body, it is also known as *'āsthāpana basti.'* On the basis of its properties it is of many types like *dīpana basti*, *lekhana basti*, *bṛṁhaṇa basti*, *picchā basti*, *siddha basti*, *yuktarasa basti* and so on. All of these are used according to the disease and its nature. A general introduction of *nirūha basti* is given here.

- **Indications**

Nirūha basti is advisable in *Vāta* diseases, upward movement of *Vāta*, gout, malaria, abdominal disorders, flatulence, hyperacidity, low digestive fire, constipation, heart disease, calculi in the urinary bladder, pain, obstruction of urine, prameha (urinary abnormality) and metrorrhagia.

- **Contra-Indications**

It should not be administered if the *doṣas* are provoked, in debility, in pregnancy, vomiting, hiccoughs, cough, bronchial asthma, swelling of the rectum, hemorrhoids, diarrhea, dysentry, diabetes and skin diseases such as dermatitis.

- ***Rakta mokṣaṇa*** **(Blood-letting): Therapeutic blood cleansing**

'*Rakta'* means blood and '*mokṣaṇa*' is derived from '*mokṣa,*' which means to 'relieve' or 'let out.' Hence, letting out blood is known as '*rakta mokṣaṇa.*' Therapeutic blood cleansing is a localized action. The main focus of *pañcakarma* therapies like emesis and purgation is the purification of the vitiated *doṣa*, but the main aim of blood-letting procedures is extraction of blood. Blood is a very important tissue. On being vitiated, it leads to many diseases. A vast number of diseases originate due to vitiation of blood. Hence for the protection of health and prevention of the diseases, vitiated blood withdrawal is important. *Pitta* and blood are closely related. An increase in *Pitta* is manifested in the waste products of blood. Hence in many *Pitta* disorders, toxins circulate in the bloodstream. Therefore, withdrawal of vitiated blood also helps in the elimination of *Pitta* from the blood - the manifested site of *Pitta*. Hence for *Pitta* disorders blood-letting is formulated with precedence. Blood-letting gives an immediate result, but its improper application leads to many diseases. Blood-letting is of two types[17]:

1. *Śastra Visrāvaṇa*: Blood-letting with the aid of instruments.
2. *Anuśastra Visrāvaṇa*: Blood-letting without instrumental aids.

1. Blood-letting with the aid of instruments: It is again divided into two types:

(a) ***Pracchāna*** (Invasive procedure): To drain the accumulated blood from a particular point through incision.

(b) ***Sirā vedhana*** (Vene-section): Vene-puncture is devised whenever vitiated blood circulates in the body.

2. Blood-letting without instrumental aids: It is of four types[18]:

(a) ***Jalaukā*** (leech application): Deep-seated blood can be extracted by this method. It is advisable to extract blood vitiated by *Pitta* by the application of leech.

(b) ***Ghaṭī yantra*** (pot-cupping): This is used to drain vitiated blood which has settled in different layers of the skin.

(c) ***Alābu*** (vacuum extraction using bottle gourd): Blood vitiated by *Kapha* can be extracted by *alābu* as it contains penetrating and hot properties.

(d) ***Śṛṅga*** (cow's horn application) **:** This is used to extract blood vitiated by *Vāta*.

17. *Tatra śastravisrāvaṇaṁ dvividham. Pracchānaṁ sirāvyadhanaṁ ca.*(*Su. sū.* 14.26)
18. *Jalaukaḥ kṣāradahanakācopalanakhādayaḥ.*
Alauhānyanuśastrāṇi tānyevaṁ ca vikalpayet. (*A. hṛ. sū.* 26:27)

Different Types of Procedures Used in Blood-Letting

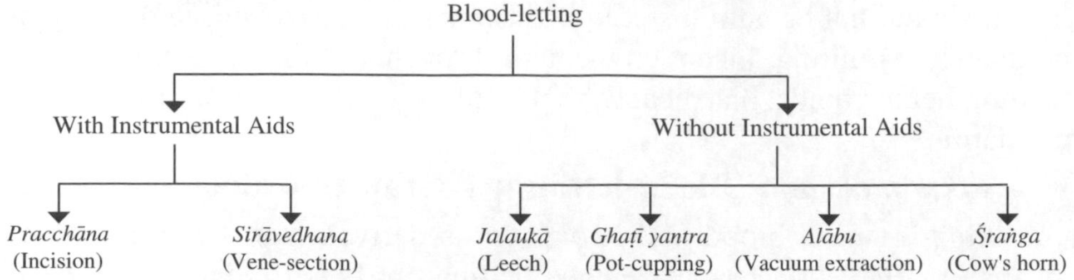

Different procedures are used according to the condition of *doṣa* at the time of blood-letting, the condition of vitiated blood and based on suffering.

- **According to *doṣa* vitiation**[(19), (20), (21)]: In the case of blood vitiated with *Vāta, Pitta* and *Kapha doṣa,* methods like *Śṛṅga*, *jalaukā* and *alābu* are used respectively.
- **According to the condition of blood**[(22), (23)]: Besides the condition of the *doṣas,* the method used in blood-letting also depends on the condition of blood (deep-seated or superficial). In glandular conditions leech therapy is used. In case of suppuration at one spot, invasion is followed. If vitiated blood spreads all over the body then vene-section is carried out for the flow of blood.
- **According to the suffering of a patient**[(24), (25), (26)]: Methods also differ on the basis of the body strength of the patient. Application of *alābu* and *śṛṅga* are used in delicate persons and leech therapy in very delicate and emaciated persons.

19. *Bhiṣag vātāvitaṁ raktaṁ viṣāṇena vinirharet.Pittānvitaṁ jalukābhiḥ.* (*Ca.ci.* 21.69-70)
20. *Tatra vāta-pittakaphaduṣṭaśoṇitaṁ yathāsaṅkhya śṛṅgajalaukālābubhiḥ avasecayetsarvāṇi sarvairvā. Viśeṣastu visrāvyaṁ śṛṅgajalaukālābubhiḥ gṛhaṇīyāt.* (*Su. sū.* 13.4)
21. *Uṣṇaṁ samadhuraṁ snigdhaṁ gavāṁ śṛṅgaṁ prakīrtitam. Tasmādvātopasṛṣṭe tu hitaṁ tadavasecane. Madhurā jalaukā vārisaṁbhavā. Tasmātpittopasṛṣṭe tu hitā sā tvavasecane. Alābukaṭukaṁ rūkṣaṁ tīkṣṇaṁ ca parikītitam. Tasmāt śleṣmopasṛṣṭe tu hitaṁ tadavasecane.* (*Su. sū.* 13.3-7)
22. *Pracchānenaikadeśasthaṁ grathitaṁ jalajanmabhiḥ. Haret śṝṅgādibhiḥ suptamasṛgvyāpi sirāvyadhaiḥ. Pracchānaṁ piṇḍite vā syād avagāḍhe jalaucasaḥ. Tvaksthe, lābughaṭī śṛṅgasiraiva vyāpake, sṛji.* (*A. hṛ. sū.* 26:50-51)
23. *Sirāviṣāṇatuṁ vastu jalaukābhiḥ padaistathā. Avagāḍhaṁ yathāpūrva nirhared duṣṭaśoṇitam. Avagāḍhe jalaukā syād pracchānaṁ piṇḍite hitam. Sirāgavyāpake rakte śṛṅgālābū tvaci sthite.* (*Su. śā.* 8:25-26)
24. *Ḍalhaṇaḥ:- śṛṅgālābū sukumāropāyau, jalaukasaḥ tu paramasukumāropāyaḥ. Asukumāropāyaś ca pracchānaṁ sirāvyadhanaṁ ca.* (*Su. sū.* 13:2)
25. *Jalaukasastu sukināṁ raktasrāvāya yojayet.* (*A. hṛ. sū.* 26:35)
26. *Nṛpāḍhyabalasthavira-bhīrū-durbalanārī-sukumārāṇāmanu-grahārthaṁ paramasukumāro, yaṁ śoṇitāvasecanopāyo, bhihito jalaukasaḥ.* (*Su. sū.* 13-2)

- **Uses**

Just as the body and other material substances have a combination of five elements, so does the blood. Blood is obviously very important. It is the blood which builds the body of a conscious person and also helps to sustain life. Hence it is important to save the blood in the body and prevent its excessive discharge.

In spite of being important, in certain circumstances blood has to be eliminated from the body. In skin diseases and carbuncles, blood-letting is an important procedure used for the treatment. Since such conditions develop due to increased toxins in the blood or due to an increase in the quantity of blood, blood-letting is vital to suck polluted blood from the body by means of leech therapy and through vene-section or vein puncturing.

- **Indications**

Blood-letting is indicated for tumors and glandular enlargement; burning; intrinsic hemorrhages; elephantiasis; alcoholism; drug addiction; toxicity of the blood; varicose veins; abscesses; breast diseases; heaviness or laxity in the body; drowsiness; hepato-splenic disorders; skin diseases such as erysipelas, eczema, herpes, acne, leucoderma, urticaria, scabies, ringworm, itching, redness of the skin, allergies, carbuncles, ulcers and so on; headache; gonorrhoea, suppuration in the eyes, ears, lips, nose and mouth; lymphadenitis, axillary and inguinal lymphadenitis; jaundice; gout and piles.

- **Contra-Indications**

Blood-letting is contra-indicated in anemia, debility, in babies and young children, people of old age, pregnancy, menstruation, leukemia, edema and cirrhosis.

- **Result**

If blood-letting is followed by relief, reduced intensity of pain and the disease, feeling of lightness in the body and decreased inflammation, then it is an indication that the therapy has been administered properly.

3. *Rasāyana Cikitsā*: Rejuvenation Therapy

The main aim of advanced medical treatments and of every action and all the latest discoveries in this world is the welfare of human beings by promoting happiness and amenities in life. In this link, scientists and doctors all over the world are engaged in the discovery of such medicines and other resources which may protect human beings from different types of diseases and also the complete eradication of the diseases they are suffering from. As a result of all these efforts and advancements in modern medical science and by achieving many other health promoting activities, the average life-span of human beings has increased tremendously. With an increase in average life-expectancy, various psychological and social problems have also originated.

A major problem has developed regarding the placement and negligence of aged persons in the society and family. Within this long span of life, several types of changes occur in social and environmental conditions, and often aged people no longer fit in and are unable to adjust accordingly. This generation gap results in a mutual dilemma on psychological grounds. Beside these mental disturbances, there is deterioration in the functioning of sensory and motor organs. Therefore, an older person can become physically incapable and dependent on others. He experiences monotony and loses enthusiasm in life and becomes a burden on society and the family. Along with an increased age-span, it is required to find out the solution for these problems too. In *Āyurveda*, such problems are treated with 'rejuvenation therapy.' Rejuvenation therapy is a medicine or treatment system which keeps away old age and its related infirmities and diseases, as well as other diseases, and results in anti-aging[(27), (28), (29), (30)].

- **The aim of rejuvenation therapy**

The main aim of rejuvenation therapy is to prevent or postpone the diseases and disabilities of old age. *Caraka Saṁhitā* describes the benefits of rejuvenation therapy as follows. One who undergoes rejuvenation therapy has a long life-span along with enhanced power of retention, increased intellect and improved health. Such persons maintain youthfulness, that is, the ill-effects of old age are not seen in their body. Their complexion becomes better. This helps to maintain the strength of sensory and motor organs. Their vocal strength and facial glow also increases. In brief, it can be said that its main aim is to maintain youthfulness in the body.

It aims to revive the society or to lay down the foundation of such a society where, instead of old, one who is physically and mentally strong (even in old age) may reside.

27. *Svasthasyorjaskaraṁ yattu tad vṛṣyaṁ tadrasāyanam.* (*Ca. ci.* 1:1:5)
Prāyaḥ prāyeṇa rogāṇāṁ dvitīyaṁ praśame matam.
Prāyaḥ śabdo viśeṣārtho hyubhayaṁ hyubhayārthakṛt. (*Ca. ci.* 1:1:6)
28. *Dīrghamāyuḥmṛtiṁ medhārogyaṁ taruṇaṁ vayaḥ. Prabhāvarṇasvaraudāryadehendriyabalaṁ param.*
Vāksiddhiṁ praṇatiṁ kāntiṁ labhate nā rasāyanāt.
Labhopāyo hi śastānāṁ rasādīnāṁ rasāyanam. (*Ca. ci.* 1:1:7)
29. *Svasthasyorjaskaraṁ tvetad dvividhaṁ proktamauṣadham. Yad vyādhinirghātakaraṁ vakṣyate taccikitsite.*
Cikitsārthaṁ etāvān vikārāṇāṁ yadauṣadham.Rasāyanavidhiśvāgre vājīkaraṇameva ca.(*Ca. ci.* 1:1:14)
30. *Dīrghamāyuḥ smṛtiṁ medhārogyaṁ taruṇaṁ vayaḥ.prabhāvarṇasvaraudāryaṁ dehendriyabalodayam-vāksiddhiṁ vṛṣatāṁ kāntimavāpnoti rasāyanam labhopāyo hi sastānāṁ rasādīnāṁ rasāyanam.* (*A. hṛ. utt.* 24:1-2)

- **Three levels at different stages of life**

According to *Āyurveda*, normal life-expectency of a human being is one hundred years. This life-span is divided into three stages, childhood, middle age and old age[31].

(1) **Childhood**: From birth up to 16 years, an individual is a child and this stage is called the childhood stage.

(2) **Middle age**: From age 16 to 65 years is a middle age and this stage is further divided into four phases:

(a) **Growth and developmental phase**: From 16-20 years is the period of rapid growth and development, corresponding to an increase in *dhātus* and body organs.

(b) **Youth phase**: From 21-30 years of age is considered the 'youth' or 'young adult' phase. It is the phase of achievement, characterized by energy, vitality and full potency of all *dhātus*, sense and motor organs.

(c) **Maturity (maintenance phase)**: From age 31-40 years is the phase of maintenance and maturity. During this phase growth and development of *dhātus* and other body organs decline, but stability in energy and strength is maintained.

(d) **Reduction phase**: After the above stages, the age up to 65 years is the reduction phase. This stage faces slow and steady reduction in the strength of *dhātus*, sensory and motor organs.

(3) **Old age**: After 65 to 70 years and up to100 years is the stage of old age or the geriatric stage. It is the phase of decay and degeneration. A gradual degeneration of all tissue elements sets in, and sensory and motor organs become lax, resulting in development of several diseases, leading towards eventual death.

According to the ancient saints the following ten attributes have been considered essential for an exhilarated and healthy life:

1) **Childhood (innocence)** is the early age characterized by tenderness, happiness, innocence and unstrained mind and stoicism.
2) **Growth** means growth and development of the body parts.
3) **Image** means splendor, brightness and glow of the face. Age affects the body but freshness, energy and vitality are maintained on the face.

31. *Vayastu trividhaṁ-bālyaṁ, madhyaṁ, vṛddhamiti.Tatronaṣoḍaśavarṣīyā bālāḥ. Te trividhāḥ:-kṣīrapāḥ, Kṣīrānnādāḥ, annādā iti. Teṣu saṁvatsaraparāḥ kṣīrapāḥ, dvisaṁ vatsaraparāḥ kṣīrānnādāḥ, parato, nnadā iti. Ṣoḍaśasaptatyorantare madhyaṁ vayaḥ. Tasya vikalpo vṛddhiḥ, yaunaṁ, sampūrṇatā, parihāṇiriti. Tatra āviṁśatervṛddhiḥ, ātriṁśato yauvanam, ācatvāriṁśataḥ sarvadhātvindriyabala-Vīryasampūrṇatā, ata ūrdhvamīṣatpari hāṇiryāvatsaptatiriti. Saptaterūrdhva kṣīyamāṇadhātvindriyabalavīryotsāhamahanyahani valitapalitakhālityajuṣṭaṁ kāsaśvāsapraphṛtibhirupadravairabhibhūyamānaṁsarvakriyā-svasamarthaṁ jīrṇāgāramivābhivṛṣṭamavasīdantaṁ vṛddhamācakṣate.* (*Su. sū.* 35:29)

4) **Intellect** means wisdom, power of judgment, patience, memory, retention and generation of ideas.
5) **Skin** means tenderness, luster, glow and healthy soft skin, the absence of wrinkles, freckles or dryness of the skin.
6) **Vision** means the power of watching, the power of vision, eyesight and good working capacity.
7) **Semen** means strength of life or life power. None of the body organs should be deformed, impotent or powerless.
8) **Valor or courage** means the power to perform brave deeds and the capacity to work accordingly.
9) **Brain or senses** means knowledge, visualizing, ability for thinking and planning.
10) **Motor organs (mobility)** means the power to move the motor organs, the hands, feet and other motor organs, and their strength to work.

Deficiency or absence of these factors makes the body vulnerable to diseases. Then the body cannot even perform normal life activities. Hence *Āyurveda* instructs us to keep the body healthy in all stages of life until there is life (Consciousness) in the body, and it emphasizes the above ten attributes to know whether the body is fit or not.

On the aggravation of disease, one has to take the support of medication. An expert practitioner has to keep in mind the age of the patient before selecting the treatment procedure. When treating a child or an aged person, a physician must focus on not practicing strong medicinal procedures like cauterization, alkali treatment or emesis and purgation therapy. In these stages, mild and light therapies are used. If strong treatment is required, then it must always be used in a mild form, then increase the potency and dose, slowly and carefully.

The physical strength and health of a person never remains constant. At a certain stage, growth rate and development of the body is very fast while in other stages it becomes slow or even arrested. Sometimes a condition arises when, instead of development, the body starts decaying. At various levels of age, strength of the body also changes. On this basis, human life is divided into four stages:

1. There is continuous development of the body up to the age of 20 years. In this phase body tissues grow and generate very fast. The *agnī* or enzymes present in the cells of these tissues provide quick nutrition to the tissues. They contain sufficient nutritive substances and favorable environment within them, which then facilitates quick development of *dhātus* and this also hastens their formation. This way, growth and development of the body is very quick.

2. From 20 to 40 years the number of cells in the tissues and their properties increases, but their multiplication and growth intensity is not as fast as it had been up to 20 years. In this phase there is an increase in the wisdom and experience of a person, the area of work expands a lot. In the initial phase, the life is not bound by any responsibility; it is restricted only in oneself. The only work is to gather knowledge. After 20-24 years, on the completion of education, a person is inspired to move ahead in life and earn. This is the phase of life where a person has to sensibly decide about her/his career pathway. There is enthusiasm and excitement, but simultaneously ego and ambition start dominating. A person becomes more constructive, more anxious for the accumulation of new objects, as a result of which life becomes more stressful and burdensome. Another important event at this stage of life is marriage that results in responsibility towards a person's life partner and children, which becomes a necessary duty that should be handled carefully. This is also the age to fulfill sexual desires. This is the age to gain strength, health, energy and *ojas*. It is also the time for one to fulfill all responsibilities properly, whether on emotional grounds, mutual relationship between a male and a female, responsibility towards society, the family or the nation. This is the time to sustain health by preserving the semen or *śukra dhātu*, which is a strength-promoting factor. At this stage of life one must keep a check over sexual indulgence and a balanced physical, mental and intellectual development to maintain complete health and good working ability.

3. Life between 41 to 65 years of age is the stage of stability. Growth and development become constant at this age, which means health remains constant during this period. This is possible only with a nutritious and balanced diet, by keeping away mental stress and anxiety, and by following a daily and seasonal routine, diet and lifestyle as recommended in *Āyurveda*, taking into consideration the compatibility of food and other requirements of the body. Otherwise, one is not likely to maintain even normal health. The slightest carelessness in habits can take a serious toll on health.

Generally, in this phase of life, one is occupied with ideology and thoughts, and deeds in diverse fields. The wisdom to make an appropriate decision is at its peak. Deviation from the ideal path, instability in mental thoughts and activities may disturb sleep, destroy peace and one loses the physical, mental and spiritual power to work. It is necessary to be logical, careful and patient while undergoing physical and sexual activities in this phase of life. Otherwise, body strength starts declining from this age onwards. The signs of old age such as wrinkles on the face, gray hair and baldness start appearing. Comparatively, there is reduction in the appetite, digestive power and productivity. Diet during this age should be decided keeping the above concerns in mind. At this age, avoid exposure to severe winter, summer, rain and other weather changes as vulnerability to seasonal illnesses increases. Another feature of this age is excessive deposition of fat on different parts of the body, particularly the stomach or waist, neck, face, thighs, buttocks and limbs, resulting in obesity. This indicates a slowing of the metabolism in the body. There is reduction in the metabolic activity of the body. The energy generated in the body due to diet and other sources declines as compared to previous stages, where tissues were properly nourished due to complete digestion and metabolism. This clearly indicates that regulating diet and lifestyle is crucial to maintain good health until 65 years of age.

4. After reaching the age of 65, the aging phase of the human body begins. Despite all efforts, the body begins to show the signs of decay and degeneration. Symptoms and ill-effects of old age predominate. Digestive and metabolic power gets eroded. Formation of waste products increases and they start accumulating in the body. In spite of nutritive and balanced food and even a regulated life with all cautions and precautions, it may not help in preventing weakness or providing strength and energy. Several changes occur in the bone tissues. Calcium accumulation (calcification) in the bones increases. Synovial fluid in the joints starts drying causing rigidity and loss of elasticity, and a person becomes unable to move the joints freely and work independently. Therefore, in this age, rheumatism, arthritis, osteo-arthritis, cervical spondylitis and other bone diseases occur. The nervous system slackens and weakens and does not work properly. Memory loss occurs. The eyesight starts deteriorating and hearing is also impaired. The nerves and arteries lose their elasticity and tenderness. The heart, kidneys, liver, lungs and other vital organs of the body lose their original strength and efficiency. These changes result in high blood pressure, insomnia, enlargement of the prostate gland and many other problems. The pancreas become less capable of secreting enough insulin which may lead to diabetes. Fractures during this age take a longer time to heal as regeneration of bones becomes difficult. The eyesight is affected by cataract (opacity of lens). The gums become weak, resulting in looseness and falling of teeth. In brief, an individual at this age becomes progressively helpless, both physically and mentally. He requires care from the family and society.

So as to prevent from being a burden to oneself and the family, and to prevent apathy towards life, follow a regulated routine and try to stay exhilarated and delightful even in the old age.

- **Importance of rejuvenation therapy**

To prevent or postpone diseases and disabilities related to old age and degeneration of *dhātus*, rejuvenation therapy as documented in *Āyurveda* can prove to be very effective and beneficial for life. The objective of this therapy is to maintain proper digestion and metabolism which provides strength to the tissues and promote the growth of new cells and tissues that give energy to the body. Rejuvenation therapy provides strength to the nerves and overall to the nervous system. It provides lubrication, tenderness and elasticity to the joints, nervous system and body organs. It maintains mental equilibrium and balance of the body. Physical and mental faculties remain strong and coordinate properly. Rejuvenation therapy helps to protect against diseases and disorders of old age and keeps the strength of sensory organs, which helps to maintain perfect vision and auditory activities. The glow of the face is restored and complexion is maintained. The skin remains smooth and maintains the youthful luster. This is the reason, why this therapy is very beneficial and is a must for every person. One should necessarily adopt rejuvenation therapy as a part of the lifestyle.

- **An appropriate time for rejuvenation therapy**

The main aim of rejuvenation therapy is to prevent diseases and disabilities of old age. If this therapy is followed after inevitable old age, it is not proven to be very beneficial. One should adopt rejuvenation therapy as a preventive measure to old age problems before reaching old age, during the youth or the adult phase. Rejuvenation therapy would be completely effective if adopted prior to old age, because of the normal functioning of the digestive system and metabolic activities during the youth and adult stages.

The following two conditions should be strictly followed prior to undergoing rejuvenation therapy:

1. **Purification of the body**: The very first thing to do is to purify the body, particularly the digestive system by the expulsion of unwanted and toxic substances from the body. This purification or detoxification therapy is to be adopted by induced vomiting and purgation. One cannot get full advantage of rejuvenation therapy without detoxifying the body. Hence, removing wastes from the body before practicing this therapy is necessary.
2. **Positive thinking and conduct**: A person practicing rejuvenation therapy should be taught to think positively, talk and perform in a way which helps to develop a good and healthy society. Such conduct and deeds itself rejuvenate the mind and body. A person remain young and

energetic even without the use of medicines and rejuvenating treatments. Such an optimistic attitude keeps an individual exhilarated, lively, enthusiastic and young. This is the reason why good conduct holds an important place in *Āyurveda.*

- **Indications**

An individual can be considered suitable for rejuvenation therapy, only if he/ she has a good moral character. In *Āyurveda*, character plays an important role while selecting a specific line of treatment. While selecting a person suitable for rejuvenation therapy, various characteristics of a person are considered.

- **Methods of use[32]**

According to *Āyurveda* scriptures, rejuvenation therapy can be used in the following two ways:

1. **Indoors or confinement to a cottage**: This method involves withdrawal from daily routine activities by being confined to a special type of cottage. It is identical to having indoor patient treatment.
2. **Outdoors or non-confinement**: In this method one can undergo rejuvenation therapy with their normal routine activities. It is similar to having out patient treatment. For most people this method is more appropriate as it is easier to do.

- **Incompatible food and habits in rejuvenation therapy**

A person undertaking rejuvenation therapy should avoid foods containing salty, sour and pungent tastes; oily foods, contaminated and left-over foods, sour *kāñji* (a fermented appetizer), alcohol, kodo millet (gingelli), wild rice (*nīvāra*), cottage cheese, yogurt, fatty foods, meat, wine, and dishes prepared from them; and habits such as coitus, wakening up late in the night, anxiety, fear, worry and anger.

- **Rejuvenating Medicines**

There are many herbs suitable for rejuvenation therapy in *Āyurveda* scriptures. The most important are Indian gooseberry (*āṁvalā*), myrobalan (*hara̱ra*), belleric myrobalan (*bahe̱rā*), tinospora (*giloya*), water hyssop (*brāhmī*), liquorice root (*muleṭhī*), bindweed (*śaṅkhapuṣpī*), hogweed (*punarnavā*), false pepper (*viḍaṅga*), Indian pennywort (*maṇḍūkaparṇī*) and vitality promoting *Āṣṭavarga* herbs. Along with herbal medicines, there are some other medicines which act as good rejuvenators. Besides plant medicines, some mineral and metal based medicines like the ones prepared

32. *Rasāyanānā dvividhaṁ prayogamṛṣayo viduḥ.*
Kuṭīprāveśikaṁ caiva vātātapikameva ca. (*Ca. ci.* 1:1:16)

from pure bitumen (*śilājīta*) and gold are also used as rejuvenators. Before using these minerals and metals in medicinal preparations, they are processed so that they become purified and are made compatible with the blood and other body fluids.

Āyurveda explains the processing, quantity, method and time of use of each rejuvenating substance and the compatibility and contra-indications while using rejuvenation therapy, which are different for different medicines. Hence, rejuvenation therapy should be undertaken in the supervision of a skilled physician and according to the scientific procedures mentioned in *Āyurveda* .

Besides using the above-mentioned medicines independently, there are certain preparations made by combining a mixture of several herbs and medicines having strong rejuvenating properties which are thus popularly used in rejuvenation therapy. Among them the common ones are *Cyavanaprāśa*, *Āmalakī Rasāyana*, *Brāhmī Rasāyana* and *Trifalā Rasāyana*. Out of these, *Cyavanaprāśa* is the most popular and commonly used. [PLATE 25]

4. *Vājīkarana*: Treatment for Infertility and Virility- The Science of Healthy Procreation

In *Āyurveda* classics, *dharma* (duty or ethical virtues), *artha* (wealth or material benefits and goals), *kāma* (desire or lust) and *mokṣa* (salvation or liberation) when compiled together form '*purusārtha catuṣṭaya,*' which means the above four factors are the main goals of human life. Following these principles of life, one can attain salvation. To achieve this *puruṣārtha catuṣṭaya*, it is important for a person to remain healthy. This is the reason why in *Āyurveda* health is accepted as the root of *dharma*, *artha, kāma* and *mokṣa*. Therefore, the first emphasis in *Āyurveda* is always on health protection.

Among the three goals, *dharma, artha* and *kāma*, the importance of *kāma* (lust or desire) is above all. This world is said to be '*agnisomātmaka,*' where '*agni'* means 'a female' and '*soma*' means 'a *male,*' and this whole world has originated from the union or fusion of both male (*soma*) and female (*agni*) energies, and an unabated tradition of life is based on this philosophy. This is the reason why some learned sages have accepted the importance of lust and described virilization or the science of aphrodisiacs as an independent branch among the eight branches of *Āyurveda.*

The following purposes of virilization are described in the classical texts by the learned sages:

1. Conception of the best progeny.
2. To enhance sexual vigor and support sexual vitality.

3. To eradicate disorders of semen, and for better strength, energy and improved complexion.
4. For the purpose of duty as it enhances the capacity to work due to the satisfaction of sexual desire, affection and attachment, and enhances pleasure and energy in the body.
5. To sustain long-term youth as one remains free from mental anxiety, distress and tribulation.
6. The treatment of semen and diseases associated with the male genital organs.

At present, due to revolutionary changes in lifestyle, dietary habits and transformed life parameters, various complications related to intercourse and conception are commonly diagnosed in day to day life. In this hard time, this specific *Āyurvedic* treatment system can turn out to be very useful. The need of the day is to rehabilitate virilization therapy based on modern scientific parameters.

- **Definitions**

1. Virilization includes the medicines, diet and lifestyle which enhance sexual vigor (like the horse), so that a person can undergo sexual indulgence repeatedly and satisfactorily or strengthen the frequency of intercourse.

   In *Āyurveda,* '*vājī*' means 'horse,' the symbol of sexual potency and performance. '*Vājī*' also means 'strength.' Those methods and therapies which enhance the strength and nourish the semen, increase libido and procreation power is '*vājīkaraṇa*.'

2. Lifestyle, diet and medicines including aphrodisiacs used in a proper way, so as to enhance the energy, sexual vigor, complexion, *ojas* and strong reproductive power that facilitates the origin of fit, healthy, intelligent and brilliant progeny is known as virilization.Virilization and the use of aphrodisiacs is mainly prescribed for males[33].

- **Aphrodisiac substances**

Aphrodisiacs include medicines, diet and lifestyle. Aphrodisiac substances are divided into three types on the basis of their use.

1. ***Śukrajanana* (spermopoietic)**: These ssubstances enhance the production of sperm, but do not affect the discharge of semen.

i. **Spermopoietic diet**: This diet calls for the addition of clarified butter (*ghee*), milk, almond and other substances.

ii. **Spermopoietic lifestyle**: One should engage in cheerfulness and good sleep.

33. *Vājīvātibalo yena yātyapratihato, ṅganāḥ. Bhavatyatipriyaḥ strīṇāṁ yena yenopacīyate. Tadvājīkararaṃaṁ taddhi dehasyorjaskaraṁ param.*(*A. hṛ. utt.* 40:2-3)

iii. **Spermopoietic medicines**: These include asparagus *(satāvarī), mūsalī,* country mallow *(balā), Āṣṭavarga* medicines (vitality promoting medicines) and so on.

2. ***Śukrapravartana* (Discharge of semen)**: These substances affect the discharge of semen, but produce no effect on sperm generation. They only provoke seminal discharge resulting in excitation for coitus. Generally, these substances have specific properties such that they are quickly absorbable or diffusible, produces looseness in the joints, hot in potency, penetrating and increases mobility. Do not use them for a longer duration.

i. ***Śukrapravartana* diet**: Black gram and so on.

ii. ***Śukrapravartana* lifestyle**: The touch and memory of a female, to watch seductive movies and photographs for excitement.

iii. ***Śukrapravartana* medicines**: Herbs which promote discharge of semen like pellitory *(akarakarā)*, cowhage (*kauṅca*), alcohol and so on.

Types of Aphrodisiac Substances

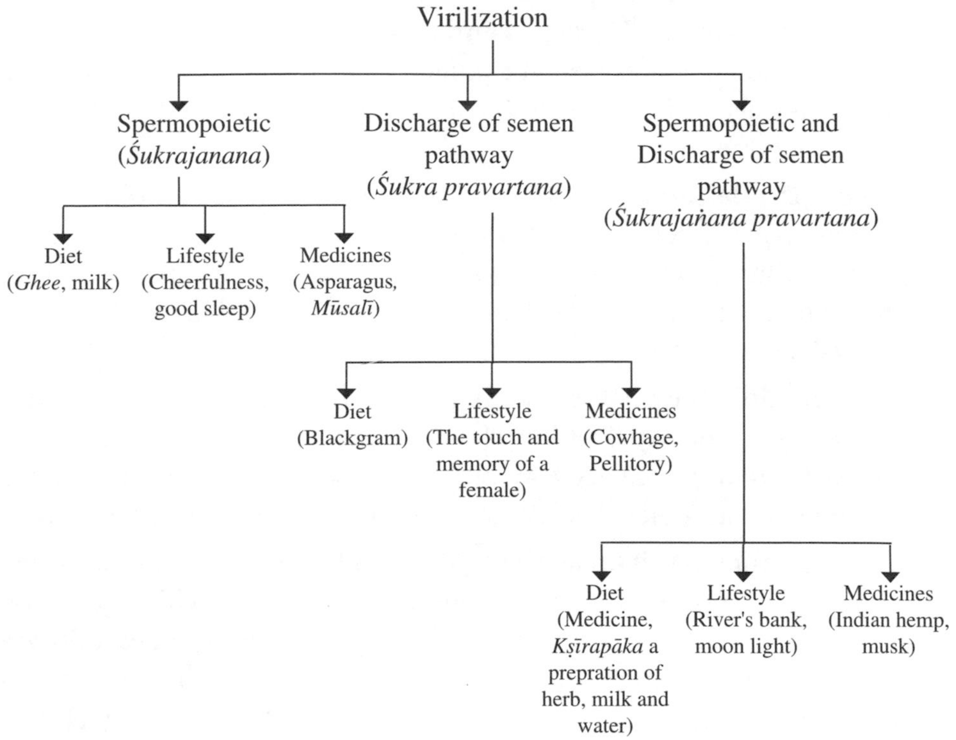

3. ***Śukrajanana pravartana* (that facilitates both spermopoiesis and discharge)**: These substances facilitate both spermopoiesis as well as discharge of semen; means it also contains property of excitation. These

substances are mostly hot in potency, light, minute, viscous, slack, quickly absorbable or diffusible and having mobility.

i. ***Śukrajanana pravartaka* diet**: Milk processed with medicated herbs like wintercherry *(aśvagaṇdha)*, *kṣīrapāka*, rice and rice pudding cooked with aromatic substances.

ii. ***Śukrajanana pravartana* lifestyle**: That which promotes spermopoiesis and discharge like walks in the moonlight, near river banks and beautiful flower valleys or other such romantic places or listening to melodious music.

iii. ***Śukrajanana pravartana* medicines**: Medicines which promotes spermatopoiesis and discharge like musk (*kastūrī*), Indian hemp (*bhāṅga*), snakewood *(kucalā)*, wild orchid *(sālamamiśrī)*, Himalayan marsh orchid (*sālamapañjā*) and so on.

- ## Incompatibility for virilization

1. **Incompatible for virilization as per the age**: According to *Ācārya Caraka*, aphrodisiacs should not be used without any specific disease and before marriage. The age of virilization is after 16 years and up to 70 years. It should not be used in childhood and youth. Sexual indulgence at a young age causes emaciation of the body, just as a pond containing less water dries up quickly.

2. **Incompatible for virilization according to marital status**: Coitus among married couples is also permitted within limits in a balanced manner. Our societal norms do not permit coitus for an unmarried male. Therefore, according to *Āyurveda* they are not suitable for the use of aphrodisiacs.

3. **Incompatible for virilization as per the principles of balance and harmony**: A person lacking physical and mental coordination, an unsteady brain and mind, over indulgence in sexual thoughts, with strong lust for sex and addicted people should not undergo virilization therapy.

4. **Incompatible for virilization as per the ailments**: A person suffering from venereal diseases such as gonorrhoea, syphilis, AIDS and so on should not indulge in sex. Therefore, they must not use aphrodisiacs until completely cured, because these diseases are contagious and can be transmitted from one person to another through sexual contact.

Chapter 10

Yoga Therapy and *Āyurveda*

Yoga and *Āyurveda* the basics of treatment in *Vedas*. In Indian culture, *Vedās* are known as '*apauruṣeya*,' which means that the knowledge of *Vedās* is revealed by God almighty, for the benefit of human beings. It is not created by man. Hence, *yoga* and *Āyurveda* are considered ancient sciences, as old as human civilization. Through long-lasting penance, constant research, studies and investigations our ancestral sages adviced that *yoga* and *Āyurveda* are useful for good health and benefit of lives. Besides, being great *yogis,* saints of *Vedic* period were great therapists. Being self aware, conscious, intellectual and wise, sages gained a deep insight of medicinal properties by getting into basic virtues of nature and universe which is described in *Yogaśāstra*. By the collective wisdom they established communication with herbs and medicinal plants. Its detail description is provided in *Āyurvedic* scriptures. Even in the practical laboratories, it is not possible to obtain complete knowledge about the qualities of each plant and herbal medicines. Similarly, *yogic* saints also had knowledge of *Āyurvedic* literature. Even in the present era, same saintly tradition is observed in India. Hence, *Āyurveda* and *yoga* are compatible treatment systems. *Āyurveda* includes a detail description of mutual association of body, sensory organs, mind and soul, making the existence of life possible through health conservation, by the knowledge of disease etiology and therapeutic suitability along with the philosophy of achieving eternal bliss and attaining liberation. Therefore, *yoga* and *Āyurveda* have the same principle and purpose; starting from the origin of life to ultimately the liberation of soul(1). Hence, it is clear that *Yogaśāstra* is a part of *Āyurvedic* literature. *Yoga* has been established as an independent branch with the development of psychological and spiritual aspects mentioned in *Āyurvedic* scriptures. The first authentic literature on *yoga* is known by the name '*Patañjali Yoga Darśana*.'

1. *Śarīrendriyasatvātmāsaṁyogodhārijīvitam.* (*Ca. sū.* 1:42)

1. Theoretical Similarities in the Principles of *Yogaśāstra* and *Āyurvedic* Treatises

According to the *Āyurveda* treatises, pleasure and pain is the result of mutual connection between mind, soul, sensory organs and their subjects. When mind becomes stable in the soul, psycho-somatic functions get suspended, as a result one gets free of the sense of pleasure and pain. At this stage, desires of mind are under the control of the soul. This stage is known as *yoga* by the scholars of *yoga*(2).

Similarly in *Yogasūtra,* prohibition of desires is called '*Yoga.*' When one is in the state of yoga, all misconceptions (*vṛttis*) that can exist in the mutable aspect of human beings (*citta*) disappears(3). It is because of these misconceptions associated with the mutable aspect, a person cannot understand the cosmic actions in their best or worst spiritual interest, as a result of which one has to bear the pleasure and pain in life, but these misconceptions can be controlled by *yoga*. As in *Āyurveda*, we find description of fourfold qualities of a physician such as friendship (friendly behavior with the patient), compassion, *śakyeprīti* (treating a patient with love and affection) and ignorance(4). Similarly, for eternal bliss *Yoga Darśana* describes about friendship, compassion, cheerfulness and ignorance(5). In the scripture of *Haṭhayoga,* the process of *ṣaṭkarma* is used for the purification of the body. These processes have many similarities with *pañcakarma* in *Āyurveda*. The introduction of *yamas* (moral restraints) and *niyamas* (observances) in *yoga* relates with good habits and conduct mentioned in *Āyurveda* for disciplined lifestyle in *sadvṛtta* (health horizons - an approach for healthy life). As the relaxing posture of the body is known as *āsana*, likewise many such physical positions are also described in *Āyurveda*. It is mentioned in *Caraka Saṁhitā* that to become a good physician, or while studying, sit in a relaxing posture on the plane surface(6). The same viewpoint is described in *Yogaśāstra* as ***'sthirasukhamāsanam.'*** Besides, the description of physical forms are found at many places in *Āyurveda*.

2. *Atmendriyamano, rthārnāṁ sannikarṣāt pravartate. Sukhadaḥ khamacārambhādātamasthe manasisthire. Nivṛttate tadubhayam vaśitvam copalāyate. Saśarīrasya yogaśāstrāṁ yogamṛṣayo viduḥ* (*Ca.Śā.*1/38-39)
3. *Yogacittavṛttinirodha* (*Yo.Da.*1.2)
4. *Maitrī kāruṇyamārteṣuśakye prītirupekṣaṇam. Prakṛtistheṣu bhūteśu vaidyavṛttiśraturvidhaḥ.* (*Ca.Sū.*9:26)
5. *Maitrīkaruṇāmuditopekṣāṇāṁ sukhadukhapuṇyāpuṇyaviṣayāṇāṁ bhāvanātaścittaprasādanam.* (*Yo.Da.*1/33)
6. *Tatrāyamadhyayanavidhiḥ-kalyaḥ kṛtakṣaṇaḥ prātarūkhśāyopavyūṣām vā. Kṛtva,,vaśyakamupaspṛśayodakaṁ devarṣi gobrāhamaṇaguruvṛddhācāryebhyo* (*Ca.Vi.*8/7)

Āsanas for Balancing *Vāta*, *Pitta* & *Kapha*

Doṣas and their location in the Body

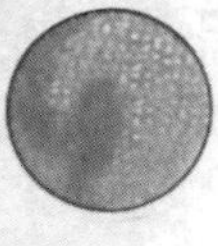

Vāta
(Movement Producing Humor)

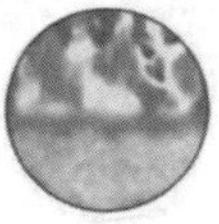

Pitta
(Heat Producing Humor)

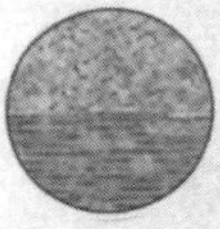

Kapha
(Structure Producing Humor)

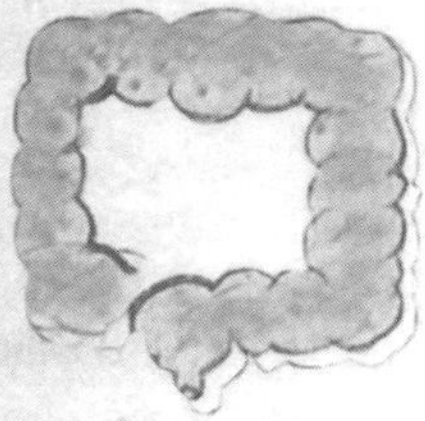

Seat of Vāta
Colon, Pelvic cavity, Large intestine, Stomach, Hypogastric region

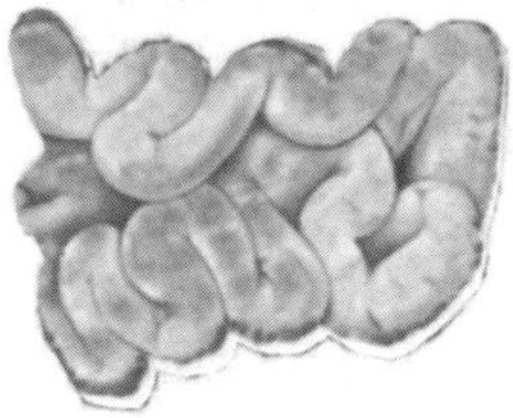

Seat of Pitta
Small intestine, Gastro-duodenal junction

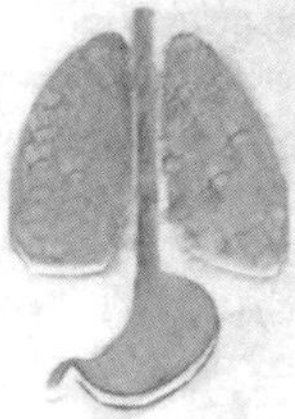

Seat of Kapha
Chest region, Stomach, Tongue, Head, Joints

Qualities

Vāta
Dry, Cold, Light, Subtle, Motile, Clear, Rough

Pitta
Oily, Hot, Sharp, Fluid, Sour, Tremulous, Pungent

Kapha
Heavy, Cold, Soft, Smooth, Sweet, Steady, Sticky

Yogāsanas and *Prāṇāyāmas* that Balance the *Doṣas*

Vāta

Āsanas that place pressure on the pelvic and colon areas. *Āsanas* done with slow, regular, silent breathing. Meditative *āsanas* that put pressure on lower abdomen & make body well grounded. Balancing *āsanas* that increase concentration making *Prāna* smoother and finer.

Padmāsana (Lotus), Backward Bend, *Paścimottānāsana* (Head knee), *Halāsana* (Plough), *Śalabhāsana* (Locust), *Bhujaṅgāsana* (Cobra), *Pavan Muktāsana* (Knee to Chest), *Śirsāsana* (Head stand), *Śavāsana* (Corpse), *Bhastrikā prāṇāyāma, Kapālabhāti prāṇāyāma, Anuloma-Viloma prāṇāyāma, Vāyu mudrā, Apāna mudrā, Apāna vāyu mudrā, Prāṇa mudrā, Varuṇa mudrā.*

Pitta

Āsanas that affect the navel area, increase gastric heat efficiency & stimulate digestion. *Āsanas* that stimulate liver, spleen & small intestines and strengthen gastric fire (*Agni*).

Padmāsana (Lotus), *Dhanurasāna* (Bow), *Matsyāsana* (Fish), *Sarvāṅgāsana* (Shoulder stand), *Ardhacakrāsana* (Half wheel), *Kapālabhāti prāṇāyāma, Anuloma-Viloma prāṇāyāma, Śītalī prāṇāyāma, Gyāna mudrā, Śūnya mudrā*

Kapha

Āsanas that work on the chest, stomach & head areas, bringing energy into the seat of *Kapha*. Strengthening *āsanas* that increase flexibility & reduce fat and *Kapha*.

Ardha Matsyendrāsana (Spinal Twist), *Naukāsana* (Boat), *Siṁhāsana* (Lion), *Paścimottānāsana* (Head knee), *Tāḍāsana* (Palm tree), *Ardhacakrāsana* (Half wheel), *Bhastrikā prāṇāyāma, Kapālabhāti prāṇāyāma, Anuloma-Viloma prāṇāyāma, Ujjāyī prāṇāyāma, Sūrya mudrā, Liṅga mudrā*

Regulated breathing in each exhalation and inhalation of *prāṇa vāyu* is known as *prāṇāyāma* in *yoga*. Even in *Āyurveda, vāyu* is considered as a vital source and is described as ***'vāyurstantrayantradhara.'*** The balance of *vāyu* is considered very important for the body and health.

Besides the above examples, the subjects related to psycho-interpretation, self-interpretation, *sātvikīvṛttī, puruṣa, karma* (deed), theory interpretation and other subjects have the same philosophical viewpoint in both the literatures on *yoga* and *Āyurveda*. Therefore, there is a close connection between both the subjects.

2. Importance of *Yoga* in the Treatment of *Āyurveda*

The main purpose of *Āyurveda* is to protect a healthy person and to alleviate disorders in a diseased. To fulfill this aim the tri-dimensional system of medicines, diet and lifestyle are described in *Āyurveda*.

Treatments are carried in two ways, with medicines (*dravauṣadhi*) and non-medicinal (*adravyauṣadhi*). When tablets, powders, decoctions and other medicinal pastes are used in the treatment, then the treatment is medicinal. When chants (*mantra*), prayers (*japa*), penance (*tapa*), fast (*upavāsa*), insight, science, patience, memory, *samādhi* (total equilibrium), *āsanas* and *prāṇāyāmas* are used in the treatment, then the treatment is non-medicinal (*adravyauṣadhi*).

Health can be protected by practicing *aṣṭāṅga yoga* as described in *Yogaśāstra*. In the form of non-medicinal treatments, *āsanas*, *prāṇāyāmas*, prayer, penance and fast help to provide psycho-somatic health resulting in complete fitness.

Compatibility and incompatibility of food, and dietary system are also the part of *yoga*. Whereas *yamas* (moral restraints) and *niyamas* (observances) are directly related to lifestyle. This emphasizes that *yoga* also support the importance of different *Āyurvedic* tacts.

Āyurveda defines health on physical, mental, social and spiritual aspects. Physical health is obtained through *yogāsanas, prāṇāyāmas* and *ṣaṭkarma*. Mental and spiritual health is achieved by *pratyāhāra* (sensory withdrawal), *īśvara prāṇidhāna* (surrender to God), *dhāraṇa* (concentration) and *dhyāna* (meditation). Social health is achieved by *yamas* (moral restraints) and *niyamas* (observances).

The use of yoga in *Āyurvedic* treatment could be understood by the following points:

1. By following good moral conduct and ethics (*yamas*) and observances (*niyamas*), one gets benefitted in leading a disciplined life which acts as a best rejuvenator. The disorders caused due to intellectual blasphemy (*prajñāparādha)* are not generated by the use of *yama-niyama* and *sadavṛtta* (good habits for healthy living).

2. With the practice of *āsanas*, body becomes healthy, well-shaped and strong. Different *āsanas* provide positive effects on endocrine gland, blood circulation, nervous system, bones, joints and metabolic activities.
3. *Prāṇāyāma* benefits in chest and respiratory disorders, cardiovascular and blood circulation system.
4. By means of *pratayāhāra* (sensory withdrawal), *dhāraṇa* (concentration) and *dhyāna* (meditation), psychological disorders such as sorrow and depression are relieved.
5. The practice of *ṣaṭkarma* defined in *yogaśāstra*, helps in the purification of the body by the elimination of toxic wastes from the body, resulting in good health.

Hence, it is a true and proven fact that *yoga* is used for the medical benefits in *Āyurvedic* treatment.

3. Relationship Between *Tridoṣa* and Alleviation of Diseases Through *Yoga*

Āyurveda consider physical exercise as a very important aspect to keep the body healthy. However, it does not describe anywhere how to keep the *doṣas* in balance by means of *yoga* therapies and physical exercise. Just as the aggravated *doṣas* can be balanced by means of medicines and other *Āyurvedic* practices; in a similar manner by means of physical exercise, various *yoga* practices such as *sūrya namaskāra, āsanas*, *prāṇāyāmas*, morning walk and other activities, not only the aggravated *doṣas* can come back to equilibrium, but it also helps to sustain the equilibrium of *doṣas* and prevent their aggravation. Therefore, an *Āyurvedic* scholar should be aware of the fact that *yogic* exercises have both preventive and curative value.

The correlation between alleviation of *tridoṣa* (*Vāta, Pitta* and *Kapha*) is hardly discussed when we talk to achieve health by means of *yoga* and related practices. A brief description of *āsanas*, *prāṇāyāmas*, exercises and other therapies to keep the body fit and healthy (by keeping the *doṣas* in equilibrium) is provided here for the general information of the readers, which is based on years of research carried out by *Yogarṣi* Swami Ramdev*. These breathing exercises clean and detoxify the body at all levels, increase immunity and balance all the three *doṣas*. It is an overall package for complete health and fitness.

* For detailed methods consult Swami Ramdev's '*Prāṇāyāma Rahasya*' and '*Yog Sādhanā* & '*Yog Cikitsā*' published by Divya Prakashana, Divya Yog Mandir (Trust), Patanjali Yogpeeth, Haridwar

4. Effective Solutions and Sources to Obtain Good Health

Yogaśāstra is also based on a multi-dimensional and vast literature like *Āyurveda*. Therefore, one who wants to acquire complete knowledge and expertise in the *yoga*, should deeply study *Yogaśāstra* and get expertise in *yoga* practice in the supervision of a *yoga gurū*. *Yogarṣi* Swami Ramdev has established a world-record in his contribution towards achievement of perfect health and fitness by eradicating several diseases through *āsanas* and *prāṇāyāmas*. For the general awareness of the reader, we are briefly describing the functional and practical aspects of *yoga* designed by Respected Swami Ramdev. Although from treatment point of view various *yogāsanas, mudrās* and *kṛyās* are also beneficial, but on the basis of our experience with millions of people, we have concluded that for the alleviation of majority of diseases main eight *prāṇāyāmas* and twelve *āsanas* are sufficient. By doing so one can get rid of number of diseases without using modern medicines (allopathy) and going through a surgery. Some specified *prāṇāyāmas* and *āsanas* can be practiced in certain special conditions. We are presenting here the main practice sequence which balances *tridoṣa,* regulate thirteen *agnīs*, nourishes seven *dhātus* and *ojas* along with the purification of *srotas*, complete purification of sensory organs and mind, and self-actualization. This stage is known as perfect health in *Āyurveda*. Those who suffer from chronic respiratory disorders, cancer, arthritis, psoriasis, diabetes, urinary abnormalities and other incurable diseases should perform *Kapālabhāti* and *Anulom-viloma prāṇāyāma* for atleast half an hour and practice meditation for a longer duration. [PLATE 26]

Regularly practice Swami Ramdev's one hour package of *yoga* therapy which has been scientifically designed to keep the body fit and promote good health, in general. It includes eight-step *prāṇāyāma* (breathing techniques) package along with light exercises and *āsana* postures. Sit straight while performing and start the program as follows:

1. Start with 'OMKAR.' Perform it loudly with full concentration, three times.
2. Perform 'chanting of *mantras*.' The healing vibrations of the *mantras* penetrate deeper and deeper into the heart and nourishes the individual soul. *Mantras* awakens the *cakras*.

Chant *Gāyatrī Mantra* (Prayer for energizing and for wisdom):

"Om bhūr bhuvaḥ svaḥ! Tatsavitur vareṇyaṁ bhargo devasya dhīmahi! Dhiyo yo naḥ pracodayāt !!"

means,

"O Omnipotent God! We meditate on your glory. Thou are our dearest life-breath. Keep us away from evil intentions and physical sufferings. May we ever have Thy pure vision in our mind. O Divine Enlightener! Lead us kindly to the light. May Thy splendor nature direct our minds towards the righteous path. May we attain not only physical progress, but also the ultimate emancipation."

Mahāmṛtuñjaya Mantra (Great Death-conquering *Mantra*):

"Om trayambakaṁ yajāmahe sugandhiṁ puṣṭivardhanam! urvārukamiva bandhanānmṛtyormukṣīya mā, mṛtāt!!"

means,

"Om! We Worship the Three-Eyed One (Lord Shiva), Who is Fragrant (Spiritual Essence) and Who Nourishes (increase in health, wealth and well-being) all beings, May He severe our Bondage of Worldly Life (Bondage by deadly and over-powering diseases) like a Cucumber (Severed from the bondage of its creeper), and thus Liberate us from the Fear of Death, by making us realize that we are never separated from our Immortal Nature."

Prārthanā Mantra (Hymn of peace):

"Om asato mā sadgamaya! Tamaso mā jyotirgamaya! mṛtyormā, mṛtaṁ gamaya!" Om śāntiḥ sāntiḥ sāntiḥ!

means,

"Lead me from ignorance to Truth, Lead me from darkness to light, Lead me from mortality (death) to realization of That which is immortality."

Om! peace, peace, peace.

- ## Main *Prāṇāyāmas* and *Āsanas*

1. ***Bhastrikā prāṇāyāma***: Take a deep breath. Fill in the breath till the diaphragm is full and exhale with full force. It can be performed according to an individual°s capacity in three ways: slow, medium and fast. This *prāṇāyāma* should be practiced minimum for three minutes and maximum upto five minutes. Practice it at a slow pace and for lesser duration in summer.
2. ***Kapālabhāti prāṇāyāma***: It emphasize on exhaling vigorously. Here inhalation is natural without any effort, but breath is thrown out forcefully. Perform three rounds of 5 minutes each (15 minutes).
3. ***Bāhya prāṇāyāma***: Sit in *padmāsana* or *sidhāsana* and exhale out all at once completely and forcefully. Now apply *mūlabandha*, *uddiyāna bandha* and *jālandhara bandha* and control the breath outside as long as possible. Relax the *bandhas* slowly and breath in normally. Repeat this three to five times. Follow *bāhya prāṇāyāma* with *agnisāra kṛyā*.

   ♦ ***Agnisāra kṛyā***: As in *bāhya prāṇāyāma,* exhale out all at once completely and forcefully and contract or flap your abdominal muscles in and out. When you feel like breathing inhale normally. Repeat the procedure three to five times.
4. ***Ujjāyī prāṇāyāma***: Contract the throat and inhale while doing this *prāṇāyāma*. Snoring sound is produced while contracting the throat.

Repeat this three to five times.

5. ***Anuloma-viloma prāṇāyāma***: Press the right nostril with right thumb and take a deep breath from left nostril. Now close the left nostril and perform *(vice-versa)* this rhythmic breathing repeatedly. Inhale with full strength and exhale in the same manner. Perform upto 15 minutes in three cycles of 5 minutes each.
6. ***Bhrāmarī prāṇāyāma***: Inhale completely and press lightly at the root of the nose with middle fingers of both the hands and concentrate on *ājñā cakra* in between the eye brows. Close both the ears with thumbs. Now perform humming like a bee and resonate "OM" chanting while breathing out. Repeat it three to seven times.
7. ***Udgītha prāṇāyāma***: Concentrate on breathing, inhale in a rhythmic flow, breathe out and chant "OM" with full concentration methodically. Repeat it three times.
8. ***Praṇava prāṇāyāma***: Meditate for one minute by sitting quietly with closed eyes and natural breathing, concentrate on the mind and think of God. You can increase the time of meditation as per your desire.

- ***Hāsyāsana*** (laughter) followed by ***siṁhāsana*** (lion's posture) three times each and ***Śītalī prāṇāyāma*** where hands are kept on the knees. Fold the tongue inward, open the mouth and inhale from the mouth and fill the air in the lungs. Control the breath for sometime and close the mouth. Exhale through both nostrils. Repeat it three times. Reduce the practice during winter. [PLATE 27]

• Some important *āsanas* to be followed by *prāṇāyāma*

After *prāṇāyāma*, perform *yogic jogging*, light exercises of hands, legs, wrists, elbows, shoulders and eyes. These light exercises can also be perfomed between the *prāṇāyāma* sequence. Besides, follow Indian exercises including types of *dandāsanas* (sit-ups) and "*Sūrya Namaskāra*" (3-5 rounds) [PLATE 28]

1. ***Āsanas* in sitting posture**: *Maṇḍūkāsana* Part 1 and 2 (Frog posture), *Śaśakāsana* (Rabbit posture), *Gomukhāsana* (Cow face posture) and *vakrāsana* (Spinal twist).
2. ***Āsanas* while lying down on the belly**: *Makrāsana* (Crocodile posture), *Bhujaṅgāsana* Part 1, 2 and 3 (Cobra posture) and *Salabhāsana* Part 1 and 2 (Locust posture).
3. ***Āsanas* while lying on the back**: They include *Markaṭāsana* part 1, 2 and 3 (Spinal twist), *Pavanamuktāsana* part 1 and 2 (Knee to Chest), *Ardhahalāsana* (Half plough posture), *Pādavṛttāsana* (Leg rotation), *Dvi-cakrikāsana* part 1 and 2 (Knees rotation) and *Śavāsana* or *Yoganidrā* (Corpse).
4. ***Śāntīpāṭha* (for peace, harmony and happiness)**: It infuses the body and mind with positive feelings and vibrations. It creates a feeling of well-being and peace in our environment, and ultimately in the whole

Universe:

"Om dyauḥ śāntirantarikṣaṁ śāntiḥ pṛthivī śāntirāpaḥ śāntiroṣadhayaḥ śāntiḥ! Vanaspatayaḥ śāntirviśvedevāḥ śāntirbrahma śāntiḥ sarvaṁ śāntiḥ śāntireva śāntiḥ sā mā śāntiredhi!" Om śāntiḥ, śāntiḥ, śāntiḥ!

means,

"Unto Heaven be Peace, Unto the Sky and the Earth be Peace,
Peace be unto the Water,
Unto the Herbs and Trees be Peace, Unto all the Gods be Peace,
Unto *Brahma* and unto All be Peace, And may We realize that Peace."
Om! Peace, Peace, Peace.

This module will take about an hour. But it can be adapted according to individual capacity and requirement. Also for the purification of the body *ṣaṭkarma* therapies such as *neti, dhouti, vamana* and *saṅkha prakṣālana* can also be practiced. All these therapies should be performed only under the guidance of an expert *gurū*. [PLATE 29]

- **Important to Note**

1. In this package of *yoga* practice, exercises and *āsanas* can be altered. In winter, exercises and *āsanas* can be performed in the beginning, followed by *prāṇāyāma*. In summer, it can be performed *vice-versa*, begin with *prāṇāyāma*, followed by exercises and *āsanas*.
2. All *prāṇāyāmas* should be performed moderately and according to individual capacity. Do not exert yourself.
3. *Yogāsanas* and *prāṇāyāmas* should be practised in a calm, peaceful, clean and properly ventilated place. During winter, maintain room temperature according to your adaptability.
4. The best time for all exercises and *āsanas* is empty stomach in the morning. Maintain a gap of almost 4 hours after meals if practicing *yogāsanas* in the evening.
5. Extreme forward bending is contra-indicated in backpain and disc-related problems.
6. Do not perform backward bending or *āsanas* that pressurize the abdomen in case of hernia, after thoraco-abdominal surgery/injury, heart problem, ulcer and complicated conditions.
7. The main cause for disease genesis in *Āyurveda* is the aggravation and vitiation of the three *doṣas* (*Vāta*, *Pitta, Kapha*). All three *doṣas* affect different systems of the body and their physiology on whose basis *yoga* therapies can be performed. *Yogic* activities and *prāṇāyāma* should be practiced according to individuals capacity and body constitution.

Appendix

Health Tips: Suggestions for Maintaining Good Health

1. To sleep early at night and to wake up early, at least one and half hour before sunrise (the ambrosial hour), is good for health.
2. Health is not merely the physical fitness, it also includes an exhilarated, calm and peaceful mind and brain.
3. To meditate and worship for 10-15 minutes in the morning after awakening, initiates mental peace and happiness.
4. To remain healthy and for the prevention of ailments, always take a compatible and beneficial diet. A person following compatible diet does not require any medication.
5. Spare some time for yourself during meals and be in a peaceful and cheerful state of mind.
6. Eat with a gap in between two meals as food consumed before the digestion of the previous meal is harmful to health. A golden rule in *Āyurveda* advises to eat only when one is hungry. Otherwise, one can fast for one meal of the day.
7. Yogurt at night and sleep during the day (except for summers) is harmful for health.
8. Exercise is beneficial for the body, but over exercising or taking it beyond the body's strength is very harmful.
9. Obesity and emaciation both are unwanted. One must be aware that obesity is the root cause of several ailments.
10. Any disease should not be taken lightly as ignorance may cause grave consequences.
11. A diet should be in accordance with the seasons, environment and physical needs. Also one must eat for less than their appetite for good health.
12. A glass or two of lukewarm water should be taken the first thing in the morning as this lukewarm water intake mixed with the juice of half a lemon and a teaspoon of honey is quite useful in hydrating the digestive system. Tea or Coffee should be avoided early in the morning on an empty stomach.
13. Locking jaws while defecation prevents loss of teeth even in old age.
14. In the morning, hold water in the mouth and sprinkle cold water in the eyes. Also clean the palate with the thumb to keep away diseases of eyes, ears, nose and throat.
15. Massaging feet with mustard oil before bathing helps in keeping a normal vision even in old age. Walking barefoot on green grass early in the morning also helps in improving vision. Full body massage including the soles and thumbs with mustard oil once a week proves beneficial in promoting blood circulation and relieves the body of excess Vata.
16. Gazing on Sun at dawn if possible for five minutes daily improves eyesight.
17. Brushing teeth after every meal and even before sleeping at night removes food particles otherwise stuck between the teeth thus preventing bad breath.
18. Add lemon juice to bathing water to keep away from the body odor and stay fresh.

19. Practice *yogāsanas* and *prāṇāyāmas* regularly after morning relieve and bath. Thi keeps away all kinds of diseases. It not only keeps the mind peaceful but also makes the body healthy and strong along with enhancing mental strength.
20. Breakfast should include easily digestible, light and fibrous foods, sprouts, fruits and porridge. While eating, chew the food properly to facilitate assimilation.
21. After a meal, sit in the position of Vajrāsana for at least10 minutes, and if possible, walk at night after dinner.
22. Take at least 8-12 glasses of water (3-4 liters) per day.
23. Always sit in a straight posture, and if sitting on the floor, avoid any support while getting up.
24. Always keep the nails trimmed and clean and never bite your nails.
25. Do not drink water while eating food. Take water half an hour before and after the meal. Always drink water in small sips.
26. Always thanks God for the food He has provided for and then consume it as a sacrament of God.
27. Include green vegetables and salad in your meal/food plate as much as possible. Excessive warm or cold food is harmful for digestion. Use of minimum spices is suggested in the food along with daily intake of seasonal fruits, which is very useful for health. It is strongly advised not to eat fruits with food but to eat them seperately before the meals.
28. Never suppress natural urges of the body such as defecation, urination, sneezing and so on, as it may result in various diseases.
29. To deal with faulty language, conduct and thoughts and also to move ahead in the journey of life, daily at night close your eyes and think patiently, peacefully and introspectively. Work accordingly to achieve and adopt *Aṣṭāṅga yoga* in life. Do not cover the mouth while sleeping. Maintain proper ventilation in the room while sleeping. Sleeping in the left lateral posture helps in proper breathing from right nostril which facilitates digestion of food.
30. Do not read or sleep on the belly.
31. Application of oil on the head calms the mind and induces sound sleep.
32. Drinking water and other edibles should be clean and fresh as unhygenic conditions invite various diseases.
33. Dry hair immediately after washing to prevent sinus problem.
34. Blowing the nose forcefully may be injurious to the ears, eyes and nose.
35. Continuous nose picking and scratching the anus may be the sign of worms in the body.
36. Cracking of joints may be injurious to the body, as it causes derangement of Vāta.
37. It is harmful to have sex during menstruation, which causes derangement of Vāta.
38. Avoid physical exertion such as yoga or running during menstruation.
39. After coitus, milk heated with raw cashews and sugar promotes strength and maintains sexual vigor.

Properties and Actions of Different Substances

In the below mentioned table, some variations may be found in context to *Rasa, Vīrya, Vipāka,* Properties and Actions of different substances in various treatises such as *Caraka Saṁhitā, Suśruta Saṁhitā, Aṣṭāṅga Hṛdaya, Bhāvprakāśa* and other *Āyurvedic nighanṭus.* Following mentioned Properties and Actions are based on various *Āyurvedic nighanṭus.*

Substances	*Rasa* (Taste)	*Vīrya* (Potency)	*Vipāka* (Post-Digestive Effect)	Properties and Action on *Tridoṣa*
Animal products				
Chicken	Sweet and Astringent	Heating	Pungent	Light, oily, strengthening. Moderately fit for *Vāta, Pitta* and *Kapha.*
Eggs	Sweet	Heating	Pungent	Heavy, oily, smooth. Increases *Pitta* and *Kapha*. Decreases *Vāta.*
Fish (general)	Sweet	Heating	Sweet	Heavy, oily, smooth. Promotes heat. Increases *Pitta* and *Kapha*. Reduces *Vāta.*
Pork	Sweet and Astringent	Heating	Sweet	Heavy, oily, smooth, appetizing. Promotes perspiration. Increases *Vāta, Pitta* and *Kapha*
Dairy				
Butter (unsalted)	Sweet and Astringent	Cooling	Sweet	Oily, smooth. Reduces hemorrhoids, promotes intestinal absorption. Increases *Kapha*. Reduces *Vāta* and *Pitta.*
Cheese (unsalted)	Sweet and Sour	Cooling	Sweet	Heavy, smooth. Increases *Pitta* and *Kapha.* Decreases *Vāta.*
Cow's milk	Sweet	Cooling	Sweet	Light, oily, smooth. Increases *Kapha*. Decreases *Vāta* and *Pitta* and alleviates all disorders
Ghee	Sweet	Cooling	Sweet	Light, oily, smooth, strengthening. Promotes digestion. If taken in excess, increases *Kapha.* If taken moderately, good for *Vāta, Pitta* and *Kapha.*
Goat's milk	Sweet and Astringent	Cooling	Sweet	Light. Relieves cough, fever, diarrhea. Increases *Vāta.* Decreases *Pitta* and *Kapha.*
Mother's milk	Sweet	Cooling	Sweet	Light, oily, smooth. Enhances *ojas*. Keeps balance of *Vāta Pitta* and *Kapha.*
Yogurt	Sour and Astringent	Heating	Sour	Smooth, oily, *grāhī*, aphrodisiac. Promotes strength. Good for digestion, diarrhea, painful urination.
Oils				
Castor oil	Sweet and Bitter	Heating	Sweet	Heavy, sharp, oily. Relieves rheumatic fever and constipation. Increases *Pitta, Kapha* and potency. Decreases *Vāta.*

Substances	*Rasa* (Taste)	*Vīrya* (Potency)	*Vipāka* (Post-Digestive Effect)	Properties and Action on *Tridoṣa*
Coconut oil	Sweet	Cooling	Sweet	Relatively light, oily, smooth. Increases *Kapha*. Relieves *Vāta* and *Pitta*.
Corn oil	Sweet	Heating	Sweet	Relatively light, oily, smooth. Increases *Pitta*. Moderate for *Vāta* and *Kapha*.
Oil (general)	Sweet	Heating	Sweet	Heavy, oily, smooth, strengthening. Increases *Pitta*. Relieves *Vāta*.
Safflower oil	Sour	Heating	Sweet	Heavy, sharp, oily, irritating in excess, harmful for eyes. Increases *Kapha*.
Sunflower oil	Sweet	Cooling	Sweet	Heavy and thick. Increases *Pitta* and *Kapha*. Reduces *Vāta*.
Mustard oil	Pungent	Heating	Pungent	Light, sharp, oily, digestive, stomachic. Increases *Pitta*. Decreases *Vāta* and *Kapha*.
Sesame oil	Sweet, Bitter and Astringent	Heating	Sweet	Heavy, oily, smooth. Good for memory, skin and hair, uterus purifier. Increases *Pitta*. Decreases *Vāta* and moderate for *Kapha*.
Sweetener				
Cane sugar	Sweet	Cooling	Sweet	Heavy, smooth, oily. Increases fat and *Kapha*. Relieves *Vāta* and *Pitta*.
Legumes				
African gram	Sweet	Cooling	Sweet	Light, *grāhī*, reduces fever. Increases *Vāta*. Decreases *Pitta* and *Kapha*.
Black gram	Sweet	Heating	Sweet	Strengthening, aphrodisiac. Increases *Vāta*, *Pitta* and *Kapha*.
Black lentil	Sweet	Heating	Sweet	*Grāhī*, strengthening. Increases *Vāta*. Decreases *Pitta* and *Kapha*.
Bengal gram	Astringent	Cooling	Sweet	Light, dry, reduces fever. Increases *Tridoṣa*.
Horse gram	Astringent	Heating	Pungent	Reduces fever, hiccough, burning, flatus. Increases *Pitta*. Decreases *Kapha*.
Kidney beans	Sweet and Astringent	Cooling	Sweet	Heavy, dry, rough, laxative. Increases *Vāta* and *Kapha*. Decreases *Pitta*.
Linseed	Sweet and Pungent	Heating	Pungent	Heavy. Alleviates *Tridoṣa*.
Mung beans	Sweet and Astringent	Cooling	Sweet	Light, rough, *grāhī*, good for eyes,reduces fever. Increases *Vāta*. Decreases *Pitta* and *Kapha*.

Substances	*Rasa* (Taste)	*Vīrya* (Potency)	*Vipāka* (Post-Digestive Effect)	Properties and Action on *Tridoṣa*
Pigeon Pea	Sweet and Astringent	Cooling	Sweet	Light, *grāhī,* Increases *Vāta.* Decreases *Pitta* and *Kapha.*
Red lentil	Sweet and Astringent	Cooling	Sweet	Easy to digest. Increases *Pitta.* Relieves *Vāta* and *Kapha.*
Soyabeans	Sweet and Astringent	Cooling	Sweet	Heavy, oily, smooth, laxative. Increases *Vāta* and *Kapha.* Decreases *Pitta.*
Vegetables				
Beet	Sweet	Heating	Sweet	Heavy, smooth. Relieves Anemia. May increase *Pitta* and *Kapha,* when taken in excess. Decreases *Vāta.*
Broccoli	Sweet and Astringent	Cooling	Pungent	Rough, dry. Increases *Vāta.* Decreases *Pitta* and *Kapha.*
Cabbage	Sweet and Astringent	Cooling	Pungent	Rough, dry. Increases *Vāta.* Decreases *Pitta* and *Kapha.*
Carrot	Sweet and Bitter	Cooling	Pungent	Heavy. Reduces hemorrhoids. Increases *Pitta,* if taken in excess. Reduces *Vāta* and *Kapha.*
Cauliflower	Astringent	Cooling	Pungent	Rough, dry, light. Promotes flatus. Increases *Vāta.* Relieves *Pitta* and *Kapha.*
Cucumber	Sweet and Astringent	Cooling	Pungent	Heavy, *grāhī,* tastant. Increases *Kapha.* Relieves *Vāta* and *Pitta.*
Flat beans	Sweet and Astringent	Heating	Sour	Heavy, causes constipation. Alleviates *Kapha.*
Lettuce	Astringent	Cooling	Sweet	Light, rough, watery. Easy to digest, creates lightness in the body, promotes flatus, if taken in excess. Increases *Vāta.* Relieves *Pitta* and *Kapha.*
Lady finger	Sweet and Astringent	Cooling	Pungent	Rough, slimy. Moderate for *Vāta, Pitta* and *Kapha*
Onion (raw)	Pungent	Heating	Pungent	Heavy, appetizing, strengthening. Stimulates libido. Relieves fever when applied externally. Increases *Vāta* and *Pitta.* Relieves *Kapha.*
Pea	Sweet	Cooling	Sweet	Light, dry. Alleviates *Tridoṣa.*
Potato	Sweet and Astringent	Cooling	Sweet	Light, dry, rough. Increases *Vāta.* Decreases *Pitta* and *Kapha.*
Radish leaves	Pungent	Heating	Pungent	Relieves flatus, promotes digestion. May increases *Pitta.* Decreases *Vata* and *Kapha.*
Spinach	Astringent	Cooling	Pungent	Rough, dry. Increases *Vāta* and *Pitta.* Decreases *Kapha.*

Substances	*Rasa* (Taste)	*Vīrya* (Potency)	*Vipāka* (Post-Digestive Effect)	Properties and Action on *Tridoṣa*
Sprouts (general)	Mildly Astringent	Cooling	Sweet	Light to digest. May aggravate *Vāta* if taken in excess, good for *Pitta* and *Kapha*.
Tomato	Sweet and Sour	Heating	Sour	Light, moist. Increases *Vāta, Pitta* and *Kapha*
Fruits				
Apple	Sweet and Astringent	Cooling	Sweet	Heavy, nourishing, tastant. Increases *Vāta* and semen. Decreases *Pitta*. Moderate for *Kapha* in small quantity.
Banana	Sweet and Astringent	Cooling	Sweet	Heavy, smooth. Laxative, if taken in excess. Increases *Pitta* and *Kapha*. Decreases *Vāta*.
Coconut	Sweet and Astringent	Cooling	Sweet	Oily, smooth, nourishing, strengthening. Increases *Kapha,* if taken in excess. Relieves *Vāta* and *Pitta*.
Figs (ripe)	Sweet and Astringent	Cooling	Sweet	Heavy, nourishing. Delays digestion. Increases *Kapha*. Relieves *Vāta* and *Pitta*.
Grapes (purple)	Sweet, Sour and Astringent	Cooling	Sweet	Smooth, watery, strengthening, laxative. Increases *Kapha*. Decreases *Vāta* and *Pitta*.
Melons (general)	Sweet	Cooling	Sweet	Heavy, watery. Increases *Kapha*. Relieves *Vāta* and *Pitta*. Watermelon increases *Vāta*.
Orange	Sweet and Sour	Heating	Sweet	Heavy. Promotes appetite. Increases *Pitta* and *Kapha*. Decreases *Vāta*.
Peaches	Sweet and Astringent	Heating	Sweet	Heavy, watery. Increases *Pitta* and *Kapha*. Decreases *Vāta*.
Pears	Sweet and Astringent	Cooling	Sweet	Light, aphrodisiac. Alleviates *Tridoṣa*.
Plums (Sweet)	Sweet and Astringent	Heating	Sweet	Heavy, watery. Increases *Pitta* and *Kapha*. Decreases *Vāta*.
Pomegranate	Sweet, Sour and Astringent	Cooling	Sweet	Smooth, oily. Stimulates digestion, helps to form red blood cells in anemia. Increases *Vāta*. Decreases *Pitta* and *Kapha*.
Spices and Condiments				
Bay leaves	Pungent and Bitter	Heating	Pungent	Dry. Increases *Pitta*. Decreases *Vāta*. and *Kapha*.
Black pepper	Pungent	Heating	Pungent	Light, dry, rough. Promotes digestion. Increases *Pitta*. Stimulates *Vāta*. Relieves *Kapha*.
Cardamom	Sweet and Pungent	Heating	Sweet	Promotes digestion, good for heart. May stimulate *Pitta,* if taken in excess. Relieves *Vāta* and *Kapha*.
Cinnamon	Sweet, Bitter and Pungent	Heating	Sweet	Relieves thirst and dryness of mouth, stimulates salivation. Stimulates *Kapha*. Decreases *Vāta* and *Pitta*.

Substances	*Rasa* (Taste)	*Vīrya* (Potency)	*Vipāka* (Post-Digestive Effect)	Properties and Action on *Tridoṣa*
Clove	Pungent	Heating	Pungent	Promotes digestion. Improves taste and flavor of food. Increases *Pitta.* Decreases *Vāta* and *Kapha.*
Coriander leaves	Sweet	Cooling	Sweet	Specially reduces *Pitta.*
Coriander seeds	Pungent and Astringent	Cooling	Sweet	Light, oily, dry. Reduces burning sensation in the urine. Helps absorption. Increases *Vāta* and *Kapha.* Relieves *Pitta.*
Cumin	Bitter, Pungent and Astringent	Heating	Pungent	Light, oily, smooth. Promotes digestion, relieves diarrhea. Stimulates *Pitta.* Decreases *Vāta* and *Kapha.*
Fenugreek seeds	Bitter and Astringent	Heating	Pungent	Dry. Helpful in fever and arthritis. Increases *Vāta* and *Pitta,* if taken in excess. Decreases *Kapha.*
Garlic	Pungent	Heating	Pungent	Heavy, oily, smooth. Anti-rheumatic. Good for cough and worms. Increases *Pitta.* Relieves *Vāta* and *Kapha.*
Ginger powder	Pungent	Heating	Sweet	Light, dry, rough. Promotes digestion. Detoxifying agent. Increases *Pitta,* if taken in excess. Relieves *Vāta* and *Kapha.*
Mustard seeds	Salty	Heating	Pungent	Light, oily, sharp. Relieves muscular pain. Increases *Pitta.* Decreases *Vāta* and *Kapha.*
Saffron	Sweet and Astringent	Cooling	Sweet	Smooth. Relieves hemorrhoids, reduces vomiting, helps stop hemoptysis. Increases *Vāta* and *Kapha.* Relieves *Pitta.*
Salt (general)	Salty	Heating	Sweet	Heavy, rough. Promotes digestion, causes retention of water and hypertension. Increases *Pitta* and *Kapha.* Relieves *Vāta.*
Sesame (seeds)	Sweet, Bitter and Astringent	Heating	Pungent	Heavy, oily, smooth, strengthening. Increases *Pitta* and *Kapha.* Decreases *Vāta.*
Thymol	Bitter and Pungent	Heating	Pungent	Light, antihelmintic. Increases *Pitta.* Relieves *Vāta* and *Kapha.*
Turmeric	Bitter, Pungent and Astringent	Heating	Pungent	Helps in diabetes, promotes digestion. Increases *Vāta* and *Pitta* if taken in excess. Relieves *Kapha.*

Substances	*Rasa* (Taste)	*Vīrya* (Potency)	*Vipāka* (Post-Digestive Effect)	Properties and Action on *Tridoṣa*
Grains				
Barley	Sweet and Astringent	Cooling	Sweet	Light, diuretic. Increases *Vāta*. Decreases *Pitta* and *Kapha*.
Basmati rice	Sweet	Cooling	Sweet	Light, soft, smooth, nourishing. Decreases *Vāta* and *Pitta*. Moderate for *Kapha* in small quantity.
White rice (polished)	Sweet	Cooling	Sweet	Light, soft, smooth. Little nutrient value. Moderate for *Kapha* in small quantity. Reduces *Vāta* and *Pitta*.
Brown rice	Sweet	Heating	Sweet	Heavy. Increases *Pitta* and *Kapha*. Decreases *Vāta*.
Corn	Sweet	Heating	Sweet	Light, dry. Increases *Vāta* and *Pitta*. Reduces *Kapha*.
Oats (dry)	Sweet	Heating	Sweet	Heavy. Dry oats increases *Vāta* and *Pitta,* reduces *Kapha*. Cooked oats increases *Kapha,* reduces *Vāta* and *Pitta*.
Wheat	Sweet	Cooling	Sweet	Heavy. Increases *Kapha*. Reduces *Vāta* and *Pitta*.
Nuts				
Almond	Sweet	Heating	Sweet	Heavy, oily, energizer, aphrodisiac, rejuvenator. Increases *Pitta* and *Kapha*. Decreases *Vāta*.
Cashew	Sweet	Heating	Sweet	Heavy, oily, aphrodisiac. Increases *Pitta* and *Kapha*. Decreases *Vāta*.
Peanut	Sweet and Astringent	Heating	Sweet	Heavy, oily. Increases *Pitta* and *Kapha*. Moderate for *Vāta* in limited quantity.
Walnut	Sweet and Astringent	Heating	Sweet	Heavy, dry. Increases *Pitta* and *Kapha*. Decreases *Vāta*.

Tastes and Their Actions

Tastes	Properties	Examples	Actions	Disorders
Sweet (Earth+Water)	Cooling	Wheat, Rice, Milk, Candy, Sugar, Dates, Licorice Root, Peppermint.	Anabolic. Decreases *Vāta* and *Pitta.* Increases Kapha. Adds wholesomeness to the body. Increases *rasa,* water and *ojas.* Promotes strength. Relieves thirst. Creates burning sensation. Nourishes and soothes the body. Cold, heavy.	Increases obesity, causes excess sleep. Heaviness, lethargy, loss of appetite, cough, diabetes and abnormal growth of muscles.
Sour (Earth+Fire)	Heating	Yogurt, Cheese, Green Grapes, Lemon, Tamarind.	Anabolic. Decreases *Vāta.* Increases *Pitta* and *Kapha.* Adds deliciousness to food. Stimulates appetite and sharpens the mind. Strengthens the sense organs. Causes secretions and salivation. Light, hot and unctuous.	Increases thirst, sensitivity of teeth, closure of eyes, liquefy *Kapha.* Toxification of blood, edema, ulceration, heart burn and acidity.
Saline (Salty) (Water+Fire)	Heating	Sea salt, Rock salt.	Anabolic. Decreases *Vāta.* Increases *Pitta* and *Kapha.* Helps digestion. Acts as an anti-spasmodic and laxative. Promotes salivation, nullifies the effect of all other tastes. Retains water. Heavy, unctuous and hot.	Affects blood. Causes fainting and heating of the body. Increases skin diseases, causes inflammation, blood disorders, peptic ulcers, rashes, pimples and hypertension.
Pungent (Fire+Air)	Heating	Onion, Radish, Chili, Ginger, Garlic, Asafoetida, Pepper.	Catabolic. Decreases *Kapha.* Increases *Vata* and *Pitta*. Keeps the mouth clean. Promotes digestion and absorption of food, purifies the blood, cures skin diseases, helps to eliminate blood clots, cleanses the body. Light, hot, unctuous.	Increases heat, sweating, fainting, causes burning sensation in throat, stomach and heart. Can cause peptic ulcers, dizziness and unconsciousness.
Bitter (Air+ Space/ Ether)	Cooling	Rhubarb, Fresh Turmeric Root, Fenugreek, Gentian Root, Tinospora.	Catabolic. Decreases *Pitta* and *Kapha*. Increases *Vāta*. Promote other tastes. Acts as an anti-toxic and germicidal. Is an antidote for fainting. Itching and burning sensations in the body. Light and cold.	Increases roughness, emaciation, dryness. Reduces bone marrow and semen. Can cause dizziness and eventual unconsciousness.
Astringent (Air+Earth)	Cooling	Unripe Banana, Myrobalan, Lebbeck, Alum, Pomegranate.	Catabolic. Decreases *Pitta* and *Kapha*. Increases *Vāta*. Has a sedative action, but is constipative. Causes constriction of blood vessels, coagulation of blood. Dry, rough and cold.	Increases dryness in the mouth, distension, constipation, obstruction of speech. Too much astringent taste can adversely affect the heart.

Glossary of *Āyurvedic* Vocabulary

Āyurvedic Terminology	Description
***Agni* (Digestive fire)**	• There are mainly three types of *agni- jaṭharāgni, pañcabhutāgni* and *saptadhātvāgni.*
***Āhāra* (Diet, Food)**	➤ ***Āhāryate galād adho nīyate iti āhāraḥ.*** That which is made to gallop or swallow is called *āhāra.* ➤ ***Āhāraḥ prīṇanaḥ sadyo balakṛddehadhārakaḥ. Āyustejaḥ samutsāhasmṛtyojognivivardhanaḥ.*** (*Su. ci.* 24.68-69) Food provides contentment, gratification, immediate strength and supports the body, increases life-span, radiance, enthusiasm, memory, valiance and digestive capacity.
◆ ***Sātmya* (Wholesome, Compatible)**	• ***Sātmyaṁ nāma yad yadātmanyupaśete.*** (*Ca. vi.*1.20) *Sātmya* means that which is favorable and suits the body.
◆ ***Asātmya* (Incompatible)**	• *Asātmya* means that which is unfavorable and does not suits the body.
◆ ***Pathya* (Wholesome, Compatible diet)**	• A compatible diet for the body.
◆ ***Apathya* (Incompatible diet)**	• An incompatible diet for the body.
***Āma* (Indigestion)**	➤ ***Jaṭharānaladaurbalyādavipaqvastu yo rasaḥ.*** (*Ca.ci.*15.44) Weak digestive fire that causes improper digestion of the ingested food which remains as it is, this undigested *rasa* of the ingested food is called *Āma.* ➤ ***Ūṣmaṇo, lpabalatvena dhātumādyamapācitam. Ṣṭamāmāśayagataṁ rasamāmaṁ pracakṣate.*** (*A.Hṛ.sū.* 13.25) The *rasā dhātu* that remains undigested because of feeble *āgni* (weak metabolism) and gets accumulated in stomach is known as *āma.*
◆ ***Sāmāvāsthā***	• ***Āmena tena sampṛktā doṣā dūṣyāśca dūṣitāḥ. Sāmā ityupadiśyante ye ca rogāstadudbhavāḥ.*** (*A.Hṛ.sū.* 13.27) The *doṣas* and *dhātus* (*rasa,* etc.) associated with this *āma* (toxins produced from undigested food) are known as *sāma*. The disorders arise by it are also termed as *āma.*
◆ ***Nirāmāvāsthā***	• *Doṣas* and *dhātus* devoid of *āma*. When *sāma doṣa*, *dhātu* and *mala* (excreta) becomes devoid of *āma* by means of purification methods is '*Nirāmā*' condition.
***Anupāna* (Adjuvant, Vehicle)**	➤ ***Annādanu paścāt pīyat ityanupānam.*** (*Su.sū.* 46.419) *Anupāna* is the liquid such as buttermilk, milk, juice, etc. consumed immediately after meals or other solid foods.

Āyurvedic Terminology	Description
	➤ ***Auṣadhabhakṣaṇopari yatpītaṁ tadan upānamityarthaḥ.*** (*Śā.saṁ.ma.kha.*6.4-5) The one which is consumed immediately after the administration of medicines is called '*Anupāna.*' ➤ ***Anu paścāt pīyata ityanupānam.*** (*A.Hṛ.sū.* 8.47) Consumption of medicinal recipes mixed along with fluids or the intake of fluids immediately after the consumption of medicines is called '*Anupāna.*' It facilitates easy movement, absorption and quick action of the medicine.
Āpta **(Authority)**	➤ ***Rajastamobhyāṁ nirmuktāstapojñānabalena ye.Yeṣāṁ trikālamamalaṁ jñānamavyāhataṁ sadā. Āptāḥ śiṣṭā vibuddhāste teṣāṁ vākyamasaṁśayam. Satyaṁ vakṣyanti te kasmādasatyaṁ nīrajastamāḥ.*** (*Ca.sū.* 11.19) Those who are free from *rajas* and *tamas* and endowed with strength of penance and knowledge. Whose knowledge is defectless, always non-contradictory and true universally about past, present and future are known as *āpta* (who have acquired all the knowledge), *śiṣṭa* (expert in the discipline) and *vibuddha* (enlightened), their words are free from doubts and is true because being devoid of *rajas* and *tamas*. ➤ ***Aptastu yathārthavaktā-*** (*Tarkasaṅgraha-śabdakhaṇḍa*) Those whose sayings or quotations are always true.
Āptopadeśa **(Scriptual Testimony)**	• ***Aptopadeśaḥ śabdaḥ.*** (*Sāṅkhyasū.* 1.101) Authoritative words of an authentic person is called *Āptopadeśa*. It is also known as *śabda pramāṇa* (true words).
Āsana	• *Yoga* postures or poses.
Ātmā **(The Soul, The True Self)**	➤ ***Atati satataṁ gacchati, śarīrāntaraṁ prāpnotīti ātmā.*** Who continuously obtains a new body after rebirth. It always withholds a new body or transmutate from one body to another after next birth is called *Ātmā*. ➤ ***Jñānādhikaraṇamātmā.*** That which is the tribunal (basis) of consciousness is *Ātmā*. ➤ ***Icchā dveṣaḥ sukhaṁ duḥkaṁ prayatnaścetanā dhṛtiḥ. Buddhismṛtirahaṅkāro liṅgāni paramātmanaḥ.*** (*Ca.śā.* 1.72) Aversion, happiness, misery, determination, desire, efforts, consciousness, control, intellect, memory and ego are the signs of the self. Self is identified with the presence of these attributes.

Āyurvedic Terminology	Description
Āyurveda	➤ ***Āyurvedayatītyāyurvedaḥ.*** (*Ca.sū.*30. 20) That which gives knowledge about life is called *Āyurveda.* ➤ ***Hitāhitaṁ sukhaṁ duḥkhamāyustasya hitāhitam. mānaṁ ca tacca yatroktamāyurvedaḥ sa ucyate.*** (*Ca.sū.* 1.41) *Āyurveda* is the science that teaches about the benefits or harm, the reason for joy and sorrow, compatibility and incompatibility of substances, their properties and actions, as well as the duration and characteristics of life. ➤ ***Āyurasmin vidyate, anena vā, yurvindanti, ityāyurvedaḥ.*** (*Su.sū.* 1.15) *Āyurveda* is that (science) in which 'life' (knowledge of life) is endowed or by which 'life' (long and healthy life) is achieved. ➤ ***Āyurhitāhitaṁ vyādhernidānaṁ śamaṁ tathā. Vidyate yatra vidvadbhirāyurvedaḥ sa ucyate. Anena puruṣo yasmādāyurvindanti vetti ca. Tasmānmunivaraireṣa āyurveda iti smṛtaḥ.*** *(Bhāvaprakāśa)* That scripture or science in which scholars had given their opinion about the compatibility, incompatibility for life, etiology of diseases and their treatment is called *Āyurveda.* By means of this scripture person attains a healthy life and knowledge about how to remain healthy for whole life. Hence it is called '*Āyurveda*' by the saints.
Bala **(Strength)**	• ***Prakṛtastu balaṁ śleṣmā vikṛto mala uccyate.***(*Ca. sū........*) *Kapha* or mucus in its natural condition forms the strength and vitiated *Kapha* forms the waste products.
Bheṣaja **(Medicine)**	• ***Bheṣajaṁ dvividhaṁ ca tatsvasthasyorjaskaraṁ kiñcit kiñcidārtasya roganut.*** (*Ca.ci.*1.4) Therapeutics are of two types: That which promotes strength (immunity) in a healthy person. That which alleviates disorders.
Brahmacarya **(Celibacy)**	➤ ***Indriyasaṁyamo vedādhyayanaṁ vā.***(*Su.ci.* 28.28) Control over sensory organs is celibacy or continuous study of *Vedas* by following controlled daily regimen is known as celibacy. ➤ ***Brahmaṇe mokṣāya caryaṁ brahmacaryam upasthanigrahādi*** (*Ca.sū.*1.6-7.*cakrapāṇi-ṭīkā*) The spiritual act and religious vow taken to get salvation is known as celibacy. It mainly deals with self-control over genital organs and other sensory organs.

Āyurvedic Terminology	Description
Buddhi **(Intellect)**	• ***Adhyavasāyo buddhiḥ.*** (*Sāṁkhyakārikā*-23) To decide or determine the particular subject is the function of intellect.
Cakra	• Energy centers in the body that are responsible for different levels of consciousness; they correspond physiologically to the nerve plexus centers in the body.
Caraka	• Great *Āyurvedic* physician who wrote one of the classic texts of *Āyurveda* : *Caraka Saṁhitā.*
Cikitsā **(Treatment)**	• ***Yā kriyā vyādhiharaṇī sā cikitsā.*** (*Bhāvaprakāśa*.......) That which helps in alleviation of diseases is called *Cikitsā.*
◆ ***Agadatantra*** **(Toxicology)**	• ***Agadatantraṁ nāma sarpakīṭalūtāmūṣakādidaṣṭav iṣavyañjanārthaṁ vividhaviṣasaṁyogopasamanārt hañca.*** (*Su.sū.*1.9) The branch of *Āyurveda* which describes the treatment of bites by poisonous animals like snakes, insects, spiders, rat etc., diseases due to different kinds of poisons and their treatment.
◆ ***Bhūta Vidyā*** **(Psychiatry & Exorcism)**	• ***Bhūtavidyā nāma devāsuragandharvayakṣara kṣaḥpitṛpiśācanāgagagagrahādyupaśṛṣṭacetāṁ śāntikarmabaliharaṇā digrahopaśamanārtham.*** (*Su.sū.*1.7) The branch of *Āyurveda* that deals to counter the bad effect of spirits, giants, demons, demigod, ghouls, evil, etc. and methods of propitiating them such as *śāntikarma* (pacificatory rites), offerings, oblations, exorcism, etc.
◆ ***Kaumārabhṛtya tantra*** **(Pediatrics)**	• ***Kaumārabhṛtyaṁ nāma kumārabharaṇadhātrīkṣīradoṣa saṁśodh anārthaduṣṭastanyagrahasamutthānāṁ ca vyādhīnāmupaśamanārtham.*** The branch of *Āyurveda* that describe about the methods of bringing up (looking after) children, purification of breast milk of the mother, diseases arising from drinking vitiated breast milk and their treatment.
◆ ***Kāyacikitsā*** **(Internal Medicine)**	• ***Kāyacikitsā nāma sarvāṅgasaṁśritānāṁ vyādhīnāṁ jvararaktapittaśoṣonmādā, pasmāra kuṣṭhamehā, tisārā- dīnāmupaśamanārtham.*** (*Su.sū.*1.6) The branch of *Āyurveda* which describes the diseases and treatment affecting all parts of the body such as fever, blood disorders, consumption, insanity, epilepsy, leprosy, diabetes, diarrhea, etc. It relates to the treatment of all diseases arising from disordered digestive activity.

Āyurvedic Terminology	Description
◆ *Rasāyana tantra* (Rejuvenation Therapy)	• *Rasāyanatantraṁ nāma vayaḥ sthāpanamāyurmedhābalakaraṁ rogāpaharaṇasamarthañca.* (*Su.sū.*1.10) The branch of *Āyurveda* that describes about the methods to restore youth, increasing life-span, intelligence, strength and capacity to get rid of diseases.
◆ *Śālākya tantra* (Otolaryngology & Ophthalmology)	• *Śālākyaṁ nāmordhvajatrugatānāṁ rogāṇāṁ śravaṇavadananayanaghrāṇādisaṁśritānāṁ vyādhīnāmupaśamanārtham.* (*Su.sū.*1.5) The branch of *Āyurveda* dealing with the diseases and treatment of parts above the shoulders such as ears, eyes, mouth, nose, etc.
◆ *Śalya tantra* (Surgery)	• *Tantra, śalyaṁ nāma vividhatṛṇakāṣṭhapāṣāṇapāṁ śulohaloṣṭhāsthibālanakhapūyāsrāduṣṭavraṇāntar garbhaśalyoddharvaaṇārthaṁ, yantraśastrakṣārāg nipraṇidhānavraṇaviniścayārthañca.* (*Su.sū.* 1.14) The branch of *Āyurveda* which describes the methods of removal of different kinds of foreign objects such as grass, wood, stone, sand, metal, bone, hair and nail; pus, exudation, vitiated ulcer, use of caustic alkalies and fire (cauterization) and diagnosis of ulcers and wounds.
◆ *Vājīkaraṇa tantra* (Infertility & Virility Treatment)	• *Vājīkaraṇatantraṁ nāmālpaduṣṭaksīṇaviśuṣkaretasā māpyāyanaprasādopacayajananānimittaṁ praharṣaṁjananā nārthaṁ ca.* (*Ca.si.*1.11) The branch of *Āyurveda* which deals with methods of increasing semen which is either less, vitiated, decreased or dried up of bestowing pleasure and growth of the body.
Dhātu	➤ Body's seven basic constituents, synonymous with "tissues" in Western medicine. ➤ *Ta ete śarīradhāraṇāt dhātavaḥ ityucyate.* (*Su. sū.*14.20) These (*rasa, rakta, māṁsa, medas, asthi, majjā* and *śukra*) are called *dhātus* because they nourish & support (maintain) the body.
Doṣa	➤ *Dūṣayantīti doṣāḥ* That which vitiate the *dhātus* is known as *doṣa.* ➤ The three biological energy pillars of the body- *Vata, Pitta & Kapha.*
◆ *Vāta*	• *Vātīti vātaḥ* (*Su.sū.*21.5, *Ḍalhaṇa ṭīkā*) The *doṣa* responsible for all movements in the body and for the flow of consciousness is *Vāta doṣa.* It controls all bodily activities and it is the vital power of the body.

Āyurvedic Terminology	Description
◆ *Apāna Vāyu*	• ***Vṛṣaṇau vastimeḍhraṁ ca nābhyūrū vaṁkṣaṇau gudam. Apānasthānamantrasthaḥ śukramūtraśakṛnti ca.*** (*Ca.ci.*28.10) ***Sṛjātyārtavagarbhau ca.*** (*Ca.ci.*28.11) Testicles, urinary bladder and penis, navel region, thighs, kidney and anus are the seats of *apāna vāyu*. It is seated in the colon and helps in the downward movement of *vāyu*. It control all processes of elimination of waste, ejaculation of semen, regulate all sexual functions, foetus expulsion and menstruation.
◆ *Prāṇa Vāyu*	• ***Vāyuryo vaktrasañcārī sa prāṇo nāma dehadhṛk. So, nnaṁ praveśayatyantaḥ prāṇāṁścāpyavalambate.*** (*Su. ni.*1.13) *Prāṇa vāyu* is located in the head, chest, throat, tongue, mouth and nose. Its functions are spitting, sneezing, belching, respiration, digestion, etc.
◆ *Samāna Vāyu*	• ***Svedadoṣāmbuvāhīni sratāṁsi samadhiṣṭhitaḥ. Antaragneśca pārasthaḥ samāno, gnibalapradaḥ.*** (*Ca.ci.*28.8) It is located in channels carrying sweat, *doṣas* and water, seated in the stomach and intestinal tract. Besides it provides strength to *agni* (digestive fire) and helps in the digestion of food.
◆ *Udāna Vāyu*	• ***Udānasya punaḥ sthānaṁ nābhyuraḥ kaṇtha eva ca. Vākpravṛttiḥ prayatnorjo balavarṇādi karma ca.*** (*Ca.ci.*28.7) *Udāna vāyu* is located in the navel, chest and throat; speech, effort, energy, strength, complexion are its functions.
◆ *Vyāna Vāyu*	• ***Dehaṁ vyāpnoti sarvaṁ tu vyānaḥ śīghragatirnṛṇām. Gatiprasāraṇākṣepanimeṣādikṛyaḥ sadā.*** (*Ca.ci.*28.9) It is being quick moving pervades the entire body and perform the functions of movements, extension, contraction, blinking, etc.
◆ *Pitta*	• ***Tapatīti pittam.*** (*Su.sū.*21.5-*ḍalhaṇaṭīkā*) The *doṣa* responsible for biotransformation and metabolism, by which heat is created, it is the form of *agni*. It helps to maintain heat in the body and digestive activities.
◆ *Alocaka Pitta*	• ***Yadṛṣṭyāṁ pittaṁ tasminnālocako, gniriti saṁjñā.*** (*Su.sū.*21.10) *Pitta* residing in the *dṛṣṭi* (eye) is *ālocakāgni* (*ālocaka pitta*), it is responsible for vision.
◆ *Bhrājaka Pitta*	• **Yattu tvaci pittaṁ tasmin bhrājako, gniriti saṁjñā.** (*Su.sū.* 21.10) *Pitta* that resides in the *tvak* (skin) and gives luster to the skin and maintain the body temperature.

Āyurvedic Terminology	Description
◆ ***Pācaka Pitta***	• ***Taccādṛṣṭahetukena viśeṣeṇa pakvāśayamadhyasyaṁ pittaṁ caturvidhamannapānaṁ pacati.*** (*Su.sū.*21.10) *Pitta* that is found localized between *pakvaśāya* (large intestine) and *āmāśaya* (stomach and small intestine) in *grahaṇī* and it promotes digestion of food.
◆ ***Rañjaka Pitta***	• ***Yattu yakṛtplīhnoḥ pittaṁ tasmin rañjako, gniriti saṁjñā.*** (*Su.sū.*21.10) *Pitta* located in the *yakṛit* (liver) and *plīhā* (spleen) is *rañjakāg*ni (*rañjaka pitta*); it bestows red color to *rasa dhātu.*
◆ ***Sādhaka Pitta***	• ***Yat pittaṁ hṛdayasthaṁ tasmin sādhako, gniriti saṁjñā.*** (*Su.sū.*21.10) *Pitta* residing in the *hṛdaya* (heart) is *sādhakāgni* (*sādhaka pitta*); it is responsible for fulfilling the desires of the mind like intellect, etc.
◆ ***Kapha***	➤ ***Śliṣyatīti śleṣmā.*** (*Su.sū.* 21.5, *Ḍalhaṇaṭīkā.*) That which is *śliṣyat* (adhering) is called *Kapha*. Its action is embracing (adhering), it lubricates the joints and makes the body firm. ➤ ***Kena jalena phalati iti kaphaḥ*** (*Halāyudhakoṣa vyākhyā* page.200) In *Sanskrit* term *'Jala'* is derived from *'Ka'* and ' *Pha*' means result or production, hence that which is produced from water is *Kapha.*
◆ ***Avalambaka Kapha***	• ***Urasthaḥ sa trikasya svavīryataḥ. Hṛdayasyānnavīryācca tatstha evāmbukarmaṇā. Kaphadhāmnāṁ ca śeṣāṇaṁ yat karotyavalambanam. Ato, valambakaḥ śleṣmā.*** (*A.Hṛ.sū.* 12.15) The *śleṣmā* (mucus or *Kapha*) located in the chest, by its impact holds '*tṛka*' (the junction of shoulder, neck and back) region and strengthens the heart by nourishing it and support other *Kapha* sites by controlling the lubrication and the fluids around the heart, lungs, upper back and other *śleṣmā* sites, therefore known as *avalambaka kapha* (the supporter).
◆ ***Bodhaka Kapha***	• ***Rasabodhanāt. (Bodhako rasanāsthāyī.)*** (*A.Hṛ.sū.*12.17) It controls the perception of taste and is located in the tongue.
◆ ***Kledaka Kapha***	• ***Yastvāmāśayasaṁsthitaḥ. Kledakaḥ son, nnasaṁghātakledonāt.*** (*A.Hṛ.sū.* 12.16) The mucus (*Kapha*) that lies in stomach and helps in moistening and softening of solid food material is known as *kledaka kapha* (moistness).
◆ ***Śleṣaka Kapha***	• ***Sandhisaṁśleṣācchleṣakaḥ sandhiṣu sthitaḥ.*** (*A.Hṛ. sū.* 12.18) The *Kapha* which is located in joints and lubricates and associates them is known as *śleṣaka kapha.*

Āyurvedic Terminology	Description
◆ *Tarpaka Kapha*	• ***Śiraḥ saṁstho, kṣatarpaṇāt. Tarpakaḥ.*** (*A.Hṛ.sū.* 12.17) The *Kapha* which is located in the head and nourishes organs of senses is known as *tarpaka kapha*.
Dravya (Substance, Matter)	➤ ***Dravati gacchati saṁyogavibhāgādiguṇāniti vā dravyam.*** That which has properties of conjunction and disjunction is *dravya.* ➤ ***Dravati gacchati pariṇāmamabhīkṣṇamiti dravyam.*** That which regularly gets transformed is *dravya.* ➤ ***Yatrāśritāḥ karmaguṇāḥ kāraṇaṁ samavāyiyat, taddravyam.***(*Ca.sū.*1:51) *Dravya* (substance including drugs) is a substratum of actions and properties and is the co-existent cause (of its effect). ➤ ***Dravyalakṣaṇaṁ tu kriyāguṇavatamavāyi kāraṇāmiti.*** (*Su.sū.* 40.3) That having functions and qualities as its inherent (inseperable) cause. Functions and qualities are considered as component of the substances.
◆ *Ākāśīya dravya*	• ***Nābhasaṁ sūkṣmaviśadalaghu śabdaguṇolbaṇam.*** (*A.Hṛ.sū.*9.9) Those substances that possess qualities like subtleness, non-sliminess, lightness and hearing sensation. They are derived from element of Space (ether).
◆ *Apya dravya*	• ***Dravaśītagurusnigdhamandasāndrarasolbaṇaṁ dravgaṁ snehanaviṣyandakledaprahṛdabandhakṛt.*** (*A.Hṛ.sū.* 9.6-7) Those substances that possess qualities like coldness, heaviness, smoothness, dullness, increases determination; it bestows lubrication, emission, wetness, fulfillment and consistency. They are derived from the element of Water.
◆ *Audbhida dravya*	• ***Udbhidya pṛthivīṁ jāyata iti audbhidaṁ vṛkṣādi*** (*Ca.sū.* 1.681-*Cakra*) The substances that emerges from the earth, e.g., plants.
◆ *Jāṅgama dravya*	• ***Gacchatīti jaṅgamam.***(*Ca.sū.*1.64 *cakra*) Living beings having locomotary functions are called as *jaṅgama*. Substances derived from animal products are *jaṅgama dravya.*
◆ *Pārthiva dravya*	• ***Tatra dravyaṁ gurusthūlasthi ragandhaguṇolbaṇam. Pārthivaṁ gauravasthairyasaṅgātopacayāvaham.*** (*A.Hṛ.sū.* 9.5-6) ***Pṛthivīvikāraḥ pārthivam.*** (*Ca.sū.*1.69-*cakra*) Those substances that possess qualities like heaviness, thickness, stability and have an odor; it imparts immensity, constancy, firmness and intensification. They are derived from element of Earth.

Āyurvedic Terminology	Description
• *Taijasa dravya*	• ***Rūkṣṇatīkṣṇoṣṇaviśadasūkṣmarūpaguṇolvaṇam. Āgneyaṁ dāhabhāvarṇaprakāśacayanātmakam.*** (*A.Hṛ.sū.* 9.7-8) Those substances that possess qualities like dryness, sharpness, warmness, non sliminess, minuteness and are attractive in form. It produces burning sensation, glow, gleam, appearance of color and digestion. They are derived from the element of Fire.
• *Vāyavya dravya*	• ***Vāyavyaṁ rūkṣaviśadalaghusparśaguṇolbaṇam.Raukṣyalāghavavaiśadyavicāraglānikārakam.*** (*A.Hṛ.sū.* 9.8-9) Those substances that possess qualities like dryness, non-sliminess, lightness and touching sensation. It causes dryness, lightness, clarity, activities and tiredness. They are derived from the element of Air.
***Gaṇḍūṣa* (Gargle)**	• ***Sukhaṁ saṁcāryate yā tu gaṇḍūṣe sā prakīrtitā.*** (*Su.utt.* 53.8) Gargle with medicated fluids by withholding the fluid in the mouth without any movement is called *gaṇḍūṣa.*
***Guṇa* (Property)**	➤ ***Samavāyi tu niśceṣṭaḥ kāraṇaṁ guṇa.***(*Ca.sū.*1.57) *Guṇa* (property) is related with inherence (to *dravya*), is devoid of action and is *asamavāya* (non-inherent) cause (of its effect). ➤ ***Viśvalakṣaṇā guṇāḥ*** (*Ra.vai.*1.168) Properties of the substance (*dravya*) is called *Guṇa*. ➤ It is any fundamental natural quality of a substance. Also applied to *sattva, rajas* and *tamas* - the three mental attributes (*gunas*).
Haṁsodaka	• ***Divā sūryāṁśusaṁtaptaṁ niśi candrāṁśītalam.Śu Kālena paqvaṁ nirdoṣamagastyenāvīṣīkṛtam. Haṁsodakamiti khyātaṁ śāradaṁ vimalaṁ śuci.*** (*Ca.sū.*6.46-47) The water treated with sun rays during the daytime and cooled with moon light at night becomes free from defects and detoxified by the effect of star Canopus (*Agastya*) is known as *haṁsodaka.*
Kāla	➤ ***Kālo hi nityagaścāvasthikaśca, tatrāvasthiko vikāramapekṣate, nityagastu ṛtusātmyāpekṣaḥ.*** (*Ca.vi.*1.21.6) *Kāla* is eternally moving (time) as well as condition. The one conditionally related to disorder while the eternally moving one to seasonal suitability. ➤ ***Yena mūrtīnāmupacayāścāpacayāśca lakṣyante taṁ kālamāhuḥ.*** (*Mahābhāṣyam.* 2.2.5) That which denotes the wear and tear of the worldly matters. ➤ ***Kālayati sarvāṇi bhūtā iti kālaḥ.*** That which causes death is *kāla.*

Āyurvedic Terminology	Description
◆ *Ādāna kāla* (Summer Solstice)	• ***Ādadāti kṣapayati pṛthivyāḥ saumyāṁśaṁ prāṇināṁ ca balamityādānam.*** (*Ca.sū.* 6.4. *Cakrapāni-ṭīkā)* It is the period where the sun absorbs the calmness (*saumya)* of nature and wind due to the predominance of *agney* (heat) is called *ādāna kāla.* It is also known as *Uttarāyaṇa* (summer).
◆ *Visarga kāla* (Winter Solstice)	• ***Visṛjati janayati āpyamāṁśaṁ prāṇināṁ ca balamiti visargaḥ.*** (*Ca.sū.* 6.4, *Cakrapāṇī-ṭīkā*) During this period moon having unobstructed strength replenishes the world continuously with its cold rays, thus *visarga* is *saumya*. It is also known as *Dakṣiṇayāna* (winter).
◆ *Ṛtu* (Season)	• ***Iyartti iti ṛtuḥ- kālaviśeṣaḥ. 'at kātyaḥ-ādāya mārgaśīrṣācca dvau dvau māsavṛturmataḥ.*** (*Abhidhānacintāmaṇi-svopajñavyākhyā*-155) That which has movement is *ṛtu*. Each *ṛtu* has 2-2 months, as told by the *kātyaḥ*. According to him, year starts from *Hemant ṛtu.*
Karma	➤ ***Kriyate iti karma.*** Any action is *karma.* ➤ ***Prayatnādi karma ceṣṭitamucyate.*** (*Ca.sū.*1.49) The movement initiated by effort is called *karma.* ➤ ***Pravṛttistu ceṣṭā kāryārthā, saiva kriyā prayatnaḥ kāryasamārambhaśca.*** (*Ca.vi.*8) ***Saṁyoge ca vibhāge ca kāraṇaṁ dravyamāśritam.*** (*Ca.sū.* 1.52) The causative factor in conjunction and disjunction, located in *dravya* and its performance is *karma.*
Kavala (Gargle, Rinsing Therapy)	• ***Asaṁcāryā tu yā mātrā kavale sā prakīrtitā.*** (*Su. utt.* 53.8) Withholding of fluid in mouth so that it can easily move within the oral cavity to alleviate the *kapha* is called *kavala.*
Koṣṭha (Abdominal cavity, Gastro-intestinal tract)	In *Āyurveda* whole abdomen is considered as *koṣṭha.*
Mala (Excretory Products, Waste Matter)	➤ ***Śarīramalinīkaraṇāt.*** (*Ca.sū.*17.115-118, *cakrapāṇi. ṭīkā*) Urine, fecal matter and sweat are known as *malās* due to their befouling property. ➤ ***Malanīkaraṇādāhāramalatvānmalāḥ.*** (*A.saṁ.sū.*20) ***Malā mūtraśakṛtsvedādayo, pi ca.*** (*A.Hṛ.sū.* 1.13) That toxifies and tarnishes the body are known as *mala.*
◆ *Mūtra* (Urine)	• ***Annādyaḥ kiṭṭāṁśastato mūtrapurīṣebhavato vāyuśca.*** (*Ca.sū.*28.14) The liquid waste product produced after digestion is urine.

Āyurvedic Terminology	Description
• *Purīṣa* (Feces)	• ***Annādyaḥ kiṭṭāṁśastato mūtrapurīṣe bhavati vāyuśca.*** (*Ca.sū.*28.14) The excretory waste semi-solid product which is produced after digestion of food is *purīṣa* (fecal matter).
• *Sveda* (Sweat)	• ***Malaḥ svedastu medasaḥ.*** (*Ca.ci.*15.18) The waste product of *medā* is sweat. It produces moistness in the body.
Mana (Mind)	➤ ***Manyate budayate anena iti manaḥ.*** Mean by which a subject can be understood is known as *mana* or mean of understanding any subject is known as *mana* (mind) ➤ ***Ātmendriyārthasannikarṣe jñānasya bhāvo, bhāvaśca manaso liṅgam.*** (*Vai. sū.* 3.2.1) ***Manaḥ purassarāṇīndriyāṇi arthagrahaṇasamarthāni bhavanti.*** (*Ca.sū.* 8.7) Conjunction between self, sense organs and their subjects resulting in perception of knowledge or absence of knowledge is one of the specific feature of *mana*.
Muni (A Sage, A *Vedic* Seer)	• ***Mananātjñānaprakarṣaśālitvānmuniḥ.*** (*Ca.sū.*1.25-26, *cakrapāṇi ṭīkā*) Those who are always involved in practice of attaining self-knowledge are sages. According to *Āyurvedic Saṁhitās, Bhāradvāja, Ātreya, Punarvasu, Kāśyap, Caraka, Suśuta* are all *Āyurvedic* seers.
Nidāna (Etiology)	➤ ***Tatra nidānaṁ kāraṇamityuktamagre.*** (*Ca.ci.*1.7) The cause of the disease is called *nidāna* (etiology). It is the cause in both genesis and knowledge of disease. ➤ ***Nidānaṁ heturucyate*** (--------) The cause of the disease is called etiology. ➤ ***Nitarāmasādhāraṇatayā dayate kāryam, roga nirṇaye, roga hetau.*** (*Vācaspatyam* page. 4065) Which maintain the disease in a specific form is known as etiology. In general the cause of disease is known as etiology.
Nidrā (Sleep)	➤ ***Śleṣmāvṛteṣu srotaḥsu śramāduparateṣu ca. Indriyeṣu svakarmabhyo nidrā viśati dehinam.*** (*A.saṁ.sū.*9:39) When the body channels are enveloped with *Kapha* and sensory organs become relaxed, it produces sleep. ➤ A natural periodic state of rest for the mind and body where responsiveness (consciousness) to external stimuli is partially suspended and decreased, to restore the power of the body.

Āyurvedic Terminology	Description
Ojas	• The purest expression of metabolism; the final end product of correct digestion and assimilation of food.
Pañcakarma	• The purification therapies; literally the five actions.
Pañcamahābhūta	• The five basic elements - *Ākāśa, Vāyu, Agnī, Jala* and *Pṛthvī* which governs the universe.
Poultice	• A soft, moist substance applied hot to the surface of the body for the purpose of supplying heat and moisture.
Prabhāva	➤ ***Prabhavati sāmarthyaviśiṣṭaṁ bhavati dravyamaneneti prabhāvaḥ*** By which *drava* obtains specific potency is known as *prabhāva*. ➤ ***Viśeṣaḥ karmaṇāṁ caiva prabhāvastasya sa smṛtaḥ.*** (*Ca.sū.* 26.27) There is difference in action, this (difference) is said to be due to *prabhāva* (specific potency).
Prakṛti	➤ ***Tatra prakṛtirucyate svabhāvo yaḥ, sa punarāhārauṣadha dravyāṇāṁ svābhāviko gurvādiguṇayogaḥ tadyathā māṣamudgayoḥ*** (*Ca. vi.*1.21.1) *Prakṛti* is *svabhāva* (nature) which is the natural property of a substance used as food and drug; such as black gram (heavy) and green gram (light) are their nature. ➤ The body constitution or the natural makeup of the body governed by the *dosas*.
Prajñā aparādha	• The mistakes of the intellect.
Prāṇa	• It is the vital energy (life-force) which activates the body and mind. *Prāṇa* is responsible for higher cerebral functions, and the motor and sensory activities. The *prāṇa* located in the head is the vital *prāṇa*, while the one which is present in the cosmic air is the nutrient *prāṇa*. There is a constant exchange of energy between the vital *prāṇa* and the nutrient *prāṇa* through respiration.
Prāṇāyāma	• A series of respiratory exercises involving regulated breathing.
Rajas	• The innate impulse to act.
Rakta Mokṣaṇa	• Blood-letting; expulsion of impure blood vitiated by *Pitta* associated diseases is known as blood-letting.
Rasa (Dhātu)	• ***Tatra rasa gatau dhātuḥ, ahararhagacchatīti rasaḥ.*** (*Su.sū.*14.13) That which is moving in the entire body (Plasma) is known as *rasa* and it is the first *dhātu* of the body.
Rasa (Pārada)	• ***Rasati bhakṣati sarvān lohān iti rasaḥ.*** (*Dr.gu.vi...*) The one which absorbs all metals is known as *rasa* (*pārada*).
Rasa (Svarasa)	• ***Vastraniṣpīḍito yaḥ sa rasaḥ svarasa ucyate.*** (*Śā. saṁ.ma.kha.*1.2) The juice extracted from fresh drugs or medicinal substances is known as *rasa* (*svarasa*).

Āyurvedic Terminology	Description
Rasa **(Taste)**	• ***Rasyate āsvādyate rasanena iti rasaḥ*** (*Cakradatta.....*) The one which is detected by tongue is known as *rasa* (taste).
◆ ***Ṣaḍrasa***	• ***Madhura-amla-lavaṇa-kaṭu-tikta-kaṣāyāḥ*** (*Ca sū.* 26.9) Sweet, Sour, Salty, Bitter, Pungent and Astringent are the six *rasas*.
Samādhi	• A state of equilibrium, supreme joy and bliss.
Ṣaṭkarma	• Six *yogic* practices involving purification of the body
Sattva	• Purity; the innate impulse to evolve.
Srota **(Channels)**	➤ ***Sravaṇāt srotāṁsi.*** (*Ca.sū.* 30.12) The path by which the plasma and other substances transport from one place to another in the body is called *srota* (channel). ➤ ***Srotāṁsi khalu pariṇāmamāpadyamānānāṁ dhātūnāmabhivāhīni bhavantyayanārthena.*** (*Ca.vi.* 5.3) ***Ākāśīyāvakāsānāṁ dehe nāmāni dehinām. Sirāḥ sratāṁsi mārgāḥ khaṁ dhamanyo nāḍya āśayāḥ.*** In which the plasma, waste products and water flow from one place to another or from one *dhātu* to another within the *ākāśa mahābhūta* predominant body is called *srota* (channel).
Sūtra	• ***Sūcanāt sūtraṇāccārthasantateḥ sūtram.*** (*Ca. sū.*1.24.*Cakrapāṇi-ṭīkā*) That which indicates specific meaning is known as *sūtra.*
Svapna **(Dream)**	➤ ***Sarvendriya Vyuparatau mano, nuparataṁ yadā. Viṣayebhyastadā svapnaṁ nānārūpaṁ prapaśyati.*** (*A.saṁ.sū.*9.40) When the sense organs lose contact with their subjects, but the mind is still in conjunction with the subject, this stage is known as *svapna* (dream). ➤ ***Nidropalutena tandrāyuktena manasāviṣayagra haṇam svapnaḥ*** (*Ḍalhaṇa*) The conjunction of subject by the mind with sleep is called as *svapna.* ➤ A state of mind involving a series of thoughts, actions, images, ideas, emotions and sensation that occur involuntarily in the mind, during certain stages of sleep.
Svasthavṛtta	➤ ***Utthāyotthāya satataṁ svasthenārogyamicchatā. Dhīmatā yadanuṣṭheyaṁ svasthavṛttaṁ taducyate.*** The regular activities carried out to maintain the health is known as *svasthavṛtta.* ➤ The science telling about the disciplined behavior of a person leading to long and healthy life. It is a code for healthy conduct or an *Āyurvedic* approach to a healthy life.

Āyurvedic Terminology	Description
• ***Dinacaryā***	• The *Āyurvedic* daily routine.
• ***Ṛtucaryā***	• The *Āyurvedic* seasonal routine.
Tamas	• Inertia; the innate impulse to remain the same.
***Tarpaṇa* (Nourishment)**	• ***Tarpayatīti tarpaṇaṁ.*** (*Ca.sū.*7.5-25-*Cakrapāṇiṭīkā*) Those substances which provides nourishment and gratification, for example: water, juice, etc.
Tridoṣa	➤ It relates to the functional (psycho-somatic) aspect of the body governed by the three biological energy pillars of the body - *Vāta, Pitta* and *Kapha.* ➤ ***Vāyuḥ pittaṁ kaphaśceti trayo doṣāḥ samāsataḥ.*** (*A.Hṛ.sū.* 1.6) In brief, the three *doṣas* in *Āyurveda* - *Vāta, Pitta* and *Kapha* are *tridoṣa.*
Upadhātu	• *Upadhātu* is that which nourishes and witholds the body but it does not play any role in the nourishment of tissues (*rasa rakta,* etc.)
Vipāka	➤ ***Pariṇāmalakṣaṇo vipākaḥ***(.......) Transformation is called *vipāka,* such as food transformed into different *rasas* is called *vipāka*. For example, the taste of sugar is sweet and it's *vipāka* is sour. ➤ ***Avasthāpākāpekṣayā viśiṣṭaḥ pākaḥ vipākaḥ*** (*Su. sū.*40.10) The taste after digestion of food is *vipāka.* ➤ ***Jaṭhareṇāgninā yogādyadudeti rasāntaram.*** ➤ ***Jaṭhareṇāgninā yogādyadudeti rasāntaram. Rasānāṁ pariṇāmante sa vipāka iti smṛtaḥ.*** (*A.Hṛ. sū.*9.20) The *rasa* (taste) produced in the end of digestion of food by the impact of *jātharāgni* (digestive fire) is *vipāka.*
Vīrya	• ***Dravyāṇi hi dravyaprabhāvād guṇaprabhāvā ddravyaguṇaprabhāvācca tasmistasmin kāle tattadhikaraṇamāsādya tāṁ tāṁ ca yuktimarthaṁ ca taṁamabhipretya yat kurvanti tat karma, yena kurvanti tad vīryaṁ.*** (*Ca.sū.*26.13) ***Viryamutsāḥ*** (*Yogasūtra-uyāsabhāsya* 1.13) Potency of the drug. *Vīrya* is characterized by the factor, which is responsible for drug action.
• ***Śīta vīrya***	• ***Śītapicchilāvambuguṇabhūyiṣṭhau.*** (*Su.sū.*41.11) *Jalamahābhūta* is predominant in drugs/ substances which are having cold potency.
• ***Uṣṇa vīrya***	• ***Tīkṣṇoṣṇāvagneyau.*** (*Su.sū.*41.11) *Agnimahābhūta* is predominant in substances which are having hot potency.

Āyurvedic Terminology	Description
***Vyādhi* (Disease)**	➤ Vitiation of physical, psychological and spiritual action of the body is called as *vyādhi* (disease). ➤ ***Vyādhīyate kupathyairvyādhiḥ puṁ liṅgaḥ, vividhā ādhayo, treti vā; yad vācaspatiḥ. vividhān yaḥ karotyādhīn vyādhiḥ sa hi nirucyate.*** (*Abhidhānacintāmaṇi-svopajñavyākhyā*.462) The one which is produced due to incompatibility is known as *vyādhi* (disease). According to *Vācaspatiḥ,* which causes different types of pains and miseries is termed as disease. ➤ ***Tadduḥkhasaṁyogā vyādhaya ucyante.*** (*Su.sū.* 1.23) The conjunction of miseries with *purusa* (body) is known as disease. ➤ ***Vividhaṁ duḥkhamādadhatīti vyādhayaḥ*** (*Ḍalhaṇa*) That which introduces different types of pains in the body is known as *vyādhi*.
Yoga	➤ ***Yagaścittavṛttiniradhaḥ, yogaḥ samādhiḥ.*** (*Yo.sū. vyāsabhāsya*.1.2) Mental concentration is known as *yoga*. According to *Caraka Saṁhitā,* the deeds of people in this world and in the other world depends upon the concentration of the mind i.e. ***Manaḥ saṁādhau tatsarvamāyattaṁ sarvadehinām.*** (*Madātyaya Cikitsā Prakaraṇa Chi.* 24.52). ➤ *Vedic* knowledge for attaining union with the domain of pure consciousness.
Yogavāhī	• ***Yogādyogino guṇaṁ vahatīti yogavāhaḥ.*** (*Ca. ci.*3.38-*Cakrapāṇī.ṭīkā*) The substances that absorbs the property of other substances. In *Āyurveda*, honey is popularly used as *yogavāhī*.

Glossary of *Āyurvedic* Pharmacodynamics: Properties and Actions

Ayurvedic Terminology	Description
Abhiṣyāndī	• ***Paicchilyāt gauravāt dravyam rūdhvā rasa sirāḥ. Dhatte yad gauravaṁ tat syādabhiṣyandi yathā dadhi.*** (*Śā.pra.* 4.25) Substances which obstruct the passage of *rasa* in blood vessels and veins and causes heaviness in the body.
Aṅgamardapraśamana	• Substances which alleviates body ache (mild muscle cramps and pains are called *aṅgamardapraśamana* (relieves body pain).
Anuloma **(Carminative)**	• ***Kṛtvā pākaṅ malānāṁ yadbhitvā bandhamadho nayet taccānulomanaṁ jñeyaṁ yathā proktā harītakī.*** (*Śā.pra.*4.4) A substance that relieves flatus and expel out waste in downward direction, after breaking their dense and compact structure is known as carminative.
Āśukārī	• ***Aśukārī tathā,, śulvāddhāvatyambhasi tailavat.*** (*Su.sū.* 46) Substances which quickly spreads in body *srota* within no time like oil drops spreading on water.
Āyuṣya **(Longevity)**	• ***Āyuṣyastu āyuḥprakarṣakāritvena.*** (*Ca.sū.*26.430 *Cakrapani*) Substances which promote long life, e.g., Indian gooseberry (*Āṁvalā*), milk.
Balya **(Tonic)**	• Substances which strengthens the body is known as *balya* (tonic).
Bhedana **(Emmolient Laxative)**	• ***Malādikamabaddhaṁ ca baddhaṁ vā piṇḍitaṁ malaiḥ. Bhittvā, dhah pātayati yad bhedanaṁ kaṭukī yathā.*** (*Śā.pra.*4.6) Those substances which helps to expel condensed, hard, loose or bolus feces through the anus, e.g., gentian (*kuṭakī*).
Bṛṁhaṇa **(Restorative Substances)**	• ***Bṛhatvaṁ yaccharīrasya janayettacca bṛṁhaṇam.***(*Ca. sū.*22.10) ***Bṛhaṇaṁ padhivyambuguṇabhūyiṣṭhām.*** (*Su.sū.*41.6) Substances that causes *bṛṁhaṇa* (stoutening, heaviness or obesity), especially increase *māṁsa dhātu* in the body. These substances have excess of two *mahābhūta, pṛthvī* (earth) and *jala* (water), which means these substance have an excess of earth and water content.
Chardinigrahaṇa **(Anti-emetic)**	• Substances which stops emesis (vomit) are known as *chardinigrahaṇa*.
Chedana **(Expectorant)**	• ***Śliṣṭān kaphādikān doṣānunmūlayati yad balāt. Chedanaṁ tadyathā kṣārā maricāṅi śīlājatu.*** (*Śā.pr.kha.*4.10) Substances which forcefully detaches *Kapha* and *doṣās* sticking in the stomach and expels it out from the body, e.g., black pepper and black bitumen *(śilājīta)*.
Dīpana **(Stomachic)**	• ***Pacennāmaṁ vahnikṛcca dīpanaṁ tadyathā miśiḥ.*** (*Śā.pra.*4.1) Substances which does not digest *āma* (undigested food material) but enhance digestive power, e.g., fennel seeds.

Ayurvedic Terminology	Description
Dīpana-pācana **(Stomachic and Digestive)**	• ***Pacatyāmaṁ na vahniṁ ca kuryādyattaddhi pācanam Nāgakeśaravadvidyāccitro dīpana-pacanaḥ.*** (*Śā.pra.* 4.12) Substances which cause digestion of undigested food material are known as *pācana* (digestive), e.g., *nāgakesara* while substances which are digestive as well as stomachic is known as *dīpana-pācana*, e.g., white leadwort (*citraka*).
Gaṇḍūṣa **(Gargle)**	• ***Asaṁcārī mukhe pūrṇe gaṇḍūṣaḥ.*** (*Śā.sa.utt.kha.*10.4) Withholding of water, oil and other oily substances like ghee, milk, honey in the oral cavity without allowing the movement of substances in the oral cavity.
Grāhī	• ***Dipanaṁ pācanaṁ yatsyāduṣṇātvaḍ dravaśoṣakam. Grāhi tacca yathā śuṇṭhi jīrakaṁ gajapippilī.*** (*Śā.pra.*4.12) Substances which digest *Āma* (undigested food material). Act as stomachic and absorb fluids due to heat generated after pācana (digestion) are called *Grāhī* e.g., cumin, dry ginger and scindapsus (*gaja pīppali*).
Jīvanīya **(Vitality Promoting)**	• ***Jīvanam āyuḥ tasmai hitaṁ jīvanīyam.*** (*Cakra. Dra.gu. vi.* I.page 359) Substances which enhance vitality power are *jīvanīya* or vital substance. According of *Ācārya Caraka*, milk is the best *jīvanīya dravya* (vital substance).
Kavala **(Gargle, Rinsing Therapy)**	• ***Kavalaścaraḥ*** (*Śā.sa.utt.kha.* 10.4) Withholding of water, oil and other substances so that they can easily move inside the oral cavity.
Lekhana **(Scraping Substances)**	• ***Dhātūnmalānvā dehasya viśoṣyollekhayecca yat. Lekhanaṁ tadyathā kṣaudraṁ nīramuṣṇaṁ vacā yavāḥ.*** (*Śā.pra.*4.11) Medicinal substances which initially causes drying of *rasa, rakta* and other *dhātus* and *malas* and then decrease them are known as scraping or curative substances, e.g., honey, warm water, sweet flag (*vaca*) and barley.
Madakārī **(Intoxicating Substances)**	• ***Buddhiṁ lumpati yad dravyaṁ madakāri taducyate.*** (*Śā. pra.*4.21-22) Substances which destroy intellect are known as intoxicating or alcoholic substances.
Medhya **(Brain Tonic)**	• ***Medhāyai hitaṁ medhyam.*** Substance which promote intellect are known as *medhya*.
Nāvana nasya **(Errhine)**	• Method of putting oil and other oily substances in the nostrils (nasal inhalation).
Pramāthī **(Expelling Substances)**	• ***Nijavīryeṇa yad dravjaṁ srotobhyo doṣa sañcayam. Nirasyati pramāthi syāttadyathā maricaṁ vacā.*** (*Śā.pra.*4.24) Medicinal substances which expel vitiated or pathological matter present in *srota* or body channels through ear, mouth or other body passages, e.g., black pepper and sweet flag (*vaca*).

Ayurvedic Terminology	Description
***Rakṣoghna* (Anti-bacterial)**	• Substances that destroy or kills bacteria, e.g., fumigation with white and yellow mustard.
***Rasāyana* (Rejuvenating Substances)**	• ***Rasānāṁ raktadīnāmayamāpyāyanam.*** (*Su.sū.* 1.7) ***Rasāyanaṁ ca tajjñeyaṁ yajjarāvyādhināśanam.*** ***Yathā, mṛtā rudantī ca gugguluśca harītakī.*** (*Śa.pra.*4.23) Medicinal substances which keep away aging and related diseases and specifically enhances *rasa,* blood and other tissues are known as rejuvenating substance, e.g., *amṛtā* (*giloya*), gum guggula, Indian gooseberry (*āṁvalā*) and myrobalan (*harar̲a).*
Recana	• ***Vipaavaṁ yadapaqvaṁ vā malādi dravatāṁ nayet.*** ***Recayatyapi tajjñeyaṁ recanaṁ trivṛtā yathā.*** (*Śa.pra.*4.6-7) Substances which excrete digested (*pakva*) and undigested (*apakva*) food material in liquid form from the body.
***Saṁśamana (*Alleviation, Balanced Dosa)**	• ***Na śodhayati na dveṣṭi samān doṣāṁstathoddhatān.*** ***Samīkaroti viṣamān śamanaṁ tadyathāmṛtā.*** (*Śā.pra.*4.3) Substances which bring the vitiated *doṣas* in a balanced state internally without eliminating it by means of purification therapy are known as *saṁśamana*, e.g., *amṛtā (giloya)*
***Saṁśodhana* (Purification)**	• ***Sthānād bahirnayedūrdhvamadho vā malasañcayam.*** ***Dehasaṁśodhanaṁ tatsyād devadālīphalaṁ yathā.*** (*Śā.pra.* 4.8-9) Substances that relieves the vitiated *doṣa* accumulated in stomach through upward passage (oral cavity) and *malas* accumulated in intestine through lower passage (anal region), e.g., fruit of bitter sponge gourd (*devadālī phala*).
***Śleṣmapūtihara* (Purulent Mucus)**	• Substances which cures the purulent smell of *śleṣmā or Kapha* (mucus).
***Snehana* (Oleation)**	• ***Stanyaradhaka, snehana, svedana.*** Substances which causes smoothness, moisture and softness.
***Sraṁśana* (Bulk Laxative)**	• ***Paktauyaṁ yadapaktvaiva śliṣṭaṁ koṣṭhe malādikam.*** ***Nayatyadhaḥ saṁsanaṁ tadyathā syāt kṛtamālakaḥ.*** (*Śā.pra.*4.5) Substances which help to eliminate the hard excreta that is either *pakva* or *apakva* from the large intestine by smooth action without causing irritation in the process, e.g., Indian laburnum (*amalatāsa).*
***Staṁbhana* (Styptic Substances)**	• ***Raukṣyācchaityāt kaṣāyatvāllaghupākācca yad bhavet.*** ***Vātakṛt stambhanaṁ tatsyādyathā vatsakaṭuṇṭukau.*** (*Śā.pra.*4.13) Substances having *rūkṣa, kaṣāya guṇa*, (dry and astringent property), easy to digest and increases *Vāta doṣa*, it also causes the stoppage of flow in downward direction are styptic substances, e.g., chenopodium (*vatsaka*), bitter oleander (*kuṭaja)* and Indian trumphet plant (*śyonāka* or *sonāpāṭhā*).
***Stanyarodhaka* (Anti-galactagogue)**	• Substances which obstruct or stop lactation are anti-galactagogues.
***Śukrala* (Spermatic)**	• ***Yasmācchukrasya vṛddhiḥ syācchukralaṁ ca taduccyate.*** ***Yathāśvagandhā musalī śarkarā ca śatāvarī.*** (*Śā.pra.*1.15-16) Substances which increase the *śukra* (semen) or seminal production are spermatic substances, e.g., wintercherry (*aśvagandhā*), muscle (*mūsalī*), sugar and asparagus (*śatāvarī*).

Ayurvedic Terminology	Description
Sūkṣma **(Subtle)**	• ***Dehasya sūkṣmacchidreṣu viśedyat sūkṣmamucyate. Tadyathā saindhavaṁ kṣaudraṁ nimbatailaṁ rabūdbhavam.*** Medicinal substances which enter into fine pores of the body are called as subtle substances, e.g., rock salt, margosa oil.
Svarya **(Voice enhancer)**	• ***Kaṇṭhasya svarāya hitaṁ svaryam.*** Substances that improve the voice quality are known as voice enhancer.
Svedana **(Sudation, Diaphoretic)**	• Substances which cause sweating in the body are diaphoretic.
Tvakprasādana **(Complexion enhancer)**	• Substances which enhances the complexion are known as *tvakprasādana* (complexion enhancer).
Upanāhasveda **(Poultice Sudation)**	• It is a type of *āgni śveda* (Thermal sudation). Perspiration caused by a kind of poultice.
Vājikaraṇa **(Aphrodisiac)**	• ***Yasmād dravyādbhavetstrīṣu harṣa vājīkaraṁ ca tat. Yathā nāgabalādyāḥ syurvījam ca kapikacchukam.*** (*Śa.pra.* 4.15) Substances which increases *śukra* (semen) and heighten the sexual desire are known as aphrodisiac substances, e.g., veronicalolia (*nāgabalā),* cowhage seed (*kevāṁca bīja*).
Vamana **(Emetic Substances)**	• ***Apaqvapittaśleṣmāṇau balādūrdhvaṁ nayettuyatā vamanaṁ tattu vijñeyaṁ madanasya phalaṁ yathā.*** (*Śā.pra*.4.6-8) Medicinal substances which expel undigested food material, *Pitta* and *Kapha* present in the stomach via upward passage (oral cavity) are known as emetic substances, e.g., emetic nut (*madana phala*).
Varṇya **(Complexion)**	• Substances which enhances the complexion, natural color, appearance and texture of the skin, especially of the face.
Vikāsī **(Slackening Substances)**	• ***Sandhibandhāstaṁ śithilānyatkaroti viśi tat. Viṣleṣyaujaśca dhātubhyo yathā kramukakodravāḥ.*** (*Śā.pra.* 4.21) Substances which separates *ojas* from the body tissues and causes looseness or slackness of joints are known as *vikāsī dravya,* e.g., betelnut, gingelli (*kodo*).
Virecaka **(Purgative)**	• Substances which expel *malas* (toxins) and *doṣas* from the lower channels of the body are known as purgative.
Vraṇaropaṇa **(Vulnerary Substances)**	• ***Śuddhaṁ vraṇaṁ yāni dravyāṇi ropayanti, tāni ropaṇāni ityucyante.*** (*Dr.gu.vi.*) Substances which causes healing of fresh wound.
Vyavāyī **(Quickly Absorbing Substances)**	• ***Pūrvaṁ vyāpyākhilaṁ kāyaṁ tataḥ pākaṁ ca gacchati. Vyavāyi tadyathā bhaṅgā phenaṁ cāhisamudbhavam.*** (*Śā.pra*.4.20) Substances which get absorbed immediately all over the body and then undergo digestion during circulation in the body, e.g., cannabis and poppy (opium).

Glossary of *Ayurvedic* Attributes

Attributes	Description
Drava (Liquid)	• ***Dravyasya viloḍane karmaṇi śaktiḥ dravaḥ.*** (*A.Hṛ.sū.*1.18, *Hemādri-ṭīkā*) Power of a substance to dissolve or liquify. Promotes salivation, cohesiveness and agitation.
Guru (Heavy)	• ***Dravyasya bṛṁhaṇe karmaṇi śakti guruḥ.*** (*A.Hṛ.sū.*1.18 *Hemādri-ṭīkiā*) When there is gravity in a substance then it possesses *guru guṇa*, it causes heaviness or stouten the body.
Kaṭhina (Hard)	• ***Dravyasya dṛḍhīkaraṇe śaktiḥ kaṭhinaḥ.*** (*A.Hṛ.sū.*1.18 *Hemādri-ṭīkā*) Ability of a substance to promote sturdiness and strengthening are said to be hard in property.
Khara (Rough)	• ***Dravyasya lekhane karmaṇi śaktiḥ kharaḥ.*** (*A.Hṛ.sū.*1.18 *Hemādri-ṭīkā*) Substance which has the ability to scrap, thus helps to scrap fat and causes weight reduction or bring about emaciation.
Laghu (Light)	• ***Dravyasya laṅghane karmaṇi śaktiḥ laghuḥ.*** (*A.Hṛ.sū.*1.18, *Hemādri-ṭīkā*) Power of a substance to bring lightness in the body.
Manda (Slow, Dull)	• ***Dravyasya śamane karmaṇi śaktiḥ mandaḥ.*** (*A.Hṛ.sū.*1.18. *Hemādri ṭīkā*) Power of a substance to pacify imbalanced *doṣa.*
Mṛdu (Soft)	• ***Dravyasya ślathane karmaṇi śaktiḥ mṛduḥ.*** (*A.Hṛ.sū.*1.18, *Hemādri-ṭīkā*) Power of a substance to bring looseness in the body.
Picchila (Slimy, Mucilaginous, Cloudy)	• ***Dravyasya lepane karmaṇi śaktiḥ picchilaḥ.*** (*A.Hṛ.sū.*1.18, *Hemadri-ṭīkā*) Binding property of a substance that causes cohesion.
Rūkṣa (Dry)	• ***Dravyasya śoṣaṇe karmaṇi śaktiḥ rūkṣaḥ.*** (*A.Hṛ.sū.*1.18, *Hemādri-ṭīkā*) Power of a substance to cause dryness and roughness.
Sāndra (Solid, Dense)	• ***Dravyasya prasādane karmaṇiśaktiḥ sāndraḥ.*** (*A.Hṛ.sū.*1.18, *Hemādri-ṭīkā*) It is thick and dense and has the property of nourishing and strengthening.
Sara or *Cala* (Mobility)	• ***Dravyasya prasaraṇe karmaṇi śaktiḥ saraḥ.*** (*A.Hṛ.sū.*1.18, *Hemādri-ṭīkā*) Substances that causes mobility and are not stable.
Śīta (Cold)	• ***Dravyasya stambhane karmaṇi śaktiḥ śītaḥ.*** (*A.Hṛ.sū.*1.18, *Hemādri-ṭīkā*) Power of a substance that causes stiffness are said to be cold in attribute.
Slakṣaṇa (Smooth)	• ***Dravyasya ropaṇe karmaṇi śaktiḥ ślakṣṇaḥ.*** (*A.Hṛ.sū.*1.18, *Hemādri-ṭīkā*) Power of a substance to heal the wounds.
Snigdha (Oily, Greasy)	• ***Dravyasya kledane karmaṇi śaktiḥ snigdhaḥ.*** (*A.Hṛ.sū.*1.18, *Hemādri-ṭīkā*) Power of a substance to provide lubrication and softness.
Sthūla (Gross, Bulky)	• ***Dravyasya saṁvaraṇe karmaṇi śaktiḥ sthūlaḥ.*** (*A.Hṛ.sū.*1.18, *Hemādri-ṭīkā*) Channel obstructing power of a substance is said to be due to grossness or bulkiness.
Sthira (Stable, Static)	• ***Dravyasya dhāraṇe karmaṇi śaktiḥ sthiraḥ.*** (*A.Hṛ.sū.*1.18, *Hemādri-ṭīkā*) Power of a substance to withhold the tissues.
Sūkṣma (Subtle)	• ***Dravyasya visaraṇe karmaṇi śaktiḥ s1ukṣmaḥ.*** (*A.Hṛ.sū.*1.18, *Hemādri-ṭīkā*) Substances which have the property to penetrate the minute body channels and subtle capillaries.
Tīkṣṇa (Sharp or Pungent)	• ***Dravyasya śodhane karmaṇi śoktiḥ tīkṣṇaḥ.*** (*A.Hṛ.sū.*1.18 *Hemādri-ṭīkā*) Power of a substance to penetrate and purify the *doṣa.*
Uṣṇa (Hot)	• ***Dravyasya svedane karmaṇi śaktiḥ uṣṇaḥ.*** (*A.Hṛ.sū* 1.18.*Hemādri-ṭīkā*) Substances that induce sweating are said to be hot in attribute.
Viśada (Non-slimy, Non-mucilaginous, Clear)	• ***Dravyasya kṣālane karmani śaktiḥ viśadaḥ.*** (*A.Hṛ.sū.*1.18.*Hemādri-ṭīkā*) Power of a substance to destroy sliminess or stickiness.

List of Diseases in *Āyurveda*

Diseases	Description
Acne	An inflammatory eruption occurring usually on face, neck and shoulders.
Allergy	A hypersensitive reaction to substances in the individual's environment.
Anemia	A below-normal level in the number of red blood cells.
Arthritis	An inflammatory condition of the joints, characterized by pain and swelling.
Ascites	An excessive accumulation of fluid in the abdominal cavity.
Bile	A bitter fluid secreted by the liver which flows into the small intestine; stored in the gall bladder, it helps to metabolize fat.
Bronchial Asthma	A respiratory disorder in which there is breathlessness, wheezing and cough (dry or with expectoration).
Bronchitis	Inflammation of the bronchi in the lungs.
Cholesterol	A fatty substance in a crystallized form found in all animal fats, oil, milk, egg yolk, bile, blood, brain tissue, liver, kidney and adrenal glands.
Cirrhosis	A chronic liver disease marked by degeneration of cells, inflammation and fibrous thickening of tissue.
Colitis, Sprue	A chronic disease characterized by excessive secretion of mucus in the large intestine and the passage of mucus and membranous shreds in the feces.
Conjunctivitis	An inflammation of the membrane that lines the eyelids.
Dermatitis	An inflammatory condition of the skin, characterized by redness, pain and itching.
Diabetes	A clinical pathological condition characterized by the excessive excretion of urine and increased blood-sugar level.
Diarrhea	Excessive frequency of stool.
Depigmentation	The loss of color of the skin.
Distention	Bloating in the abdomen from internal pressure.
Dysurea	Painful urination.
Eczema	Acute or chronic skin inflammation.
Edema	A condition in which the body tissues retain an excessive amount of fluid resulting in swelling.
Elephantiasis	A syndrome describing the gross enlargement of the cutaneous and sub-cutaneous tissues of the limbs or other parts of the body resulting from lymphatic obstruction with a filarial worm.
Epilepsy	A group of neurological disorders characterized by recurrent episodes of convulsive seizures, sensory disturbances, abnormal behavior, loss of consciousness, or all of these.
Erysepelas	Disease which spreads in upward, downward, right and left directions or spreads like an abscess or edema.
Fatigue	Feeling of tiredness without exercise or any physical activity.
Goiter	Swelling of the thyroid gland, that can lead to the swelling of the neck or larynx.
Gonorrhea	A common venereal disease affecting the genito-urinary tract.
Gout	Metabolic disease marked by acute arthritis and inflammation of the joints.
Hemorrhoids	Enlarged veins in the lower rectum or anus causing oozing of blood in the feces.
Hiccough (hiccups)	An involuntary contraction of the diaphragm and respiratory organs, with a sudden closure of the glottis and a sound like a cough that may repeat several times per minute.
Hives	Eruption of very itchy skin caused by an allergic substance or food.

Diseases	Description
Hydrocele	Accumulation of fluid in a sac surrounding the testicles characterized by swelling of the scrotum underneath the penis.
Jaundice	A condition of liver malfunctioning characterized by yellowness of the skin.
Leprosy	A chronic skin disease; primarily a granulomatous disease of the peripheral nerves and mucosa of the upper respiratory tract, characterized by skin lesions as the primary external sign. It causes skin sores, nerve damage and muscle weakness that gets worse over time.
Leucoderma	Localized loss of skin pigment.
Leucorrhea	A condition that causes a whitish, viscid discharge from the vagina and uterine cavity.
Leukemia	A malignant progressive disease; a type of cancer of the blood or bone marrow.
Lockjaw	An early sign of tetanus involving muscular stiffness in the jaws; an acute and serious infection of the central nervous system caused by bacterial infection, where the jaw is tightly locked closed because of tonic spasm of the muscles of mastication.
Lymphadenitis	Inflammation of lymph node, a complication of bacterial (microbial) infection of a wound.
Metrorrhagia	Uterine hemorrhage; non-menstrual discharge of blood from the uterus.
Migraine	Pricking or splitting pain in half of the head.
Naevi	A skin disease characterized by chronic lesions on the skin.
Osteopenia	A condition where bone mineral density (BMD) is lower than the normal peak but not low enough to be classified as osteoporosis.
Osteoporosis	Porous bones; when bones lose an excessive amount of their protein and mineral contents, particularly calcium. Overtime bone mass and strength gets decreased as a result bone become fragile and break easily.
Prameha	A urinary abnormality. It is a *Sanskrit* word formed from the verb root '*Mih Secane*' or '*Migh*' which means watering, involving excess of urine in both frequency and volume. It is of 20 types.
Psoriasis	A common genetically-determined skin inflammation.
Psycho-somatic	Pertaining to the mind-body relationship; having bodily symptoms of a psychic, emotional or mental origin and diseases originated as a consequence of both.
Rheumatism	Any of a large number of inflammatory conditions of the joints, ligaments or muscles, characterized by pain or limitation of movement.
Rhinitis	Inflammation of the mucus membrane of the nose.
Scabies	A contagious skin disease characterized by itching and peeling of skin.
Sciatica	Inflammation of the sciatic nerve characterized by lower back pain which radiates down the leg.
Scrophula	Glandular swelling; a form of tuberculosis affecting the lymph nodes, especially of the neck.
Sinus	A cavity within the bone.
Spondylosis	A condition of the spine characterized by stiffness of the vertebral joint.
Syphilis	A venereal infection transmitted through sexual contact.
Tinnitus	Perception of sound (ringing, swishing or other types of noise) originating within the human ear.
Torticollis (*Manyāstambha*)	Stiffness of muscles on dorsal surface of the neck.
Urticaria	A blood reaction of the skin, marked by the transient appearance of smooth, slightly elevated patches which are red or pale than the surrounding skin, accompanied by severe itching.
Varicose vein	Superficial veins that have become enlarged, tortous, stretched and swollen with blood, usually seen in the legs.

List of Botanical Names of Medicinal Plants Used in the Text

S.No.	Common Names	*Hindi / Sanskrit* Names	Botanical Names
1.	Aconite	*Ativiṣā*	*Aconitum heterophyllum* Wall. ex Royle Syn. *A. petiolare* Royle ex Stapf
2.	African gram, Wildgram	*Mudgaparṇī* (*Mūgavana*)	*Vigna trilobata* (Linn.) Verdcour Syn. *Phaseolus trilobus* Ait.
3.	Almond	*Bādāma*	*Prunus dulcis* (Mill.) D.A. Webb Syn. *P. amygdalus* Batsch
4.	Aloe vera	*Gvārapāṭhā* (*Ghṛtakumārī*)	*Aloe vera* (Linn.) Burm. f. Syn. *A. barbadensis* Mill.
5.	Angled loofah	*Toraī*	*Luffa acutangula* (Linn.) Roxb. Syn. *Cucumis acutangulah* Linn.
6.	Apple	*Seba* (*Mahābadara*)	*Malus sylvestris* (Linn.) Mill. Syn. *Pyrus malus* Linn.
7.	Apricot	*Khūbānī*	*Prunus armeniaca* Linn.
8.	Asafoetida	*Hiṅga, Hiṅgū*	*Ferula narthex* Boiss.
9.	Ash coloured fleabane	*Sahadevī*	*Vernonia cineria* (Linn.) Less. Syn. *Conyza cinerea* Linn.
10.	Ash gourd	*Kūṣmāṇḍa* (*Peṭhā*)	*Benincasa hispida* (Thunb.) Cogn. Syn. *B. cerifera* Savi
11.	Asparugus	*Śatāvarī*	*Asparagus racemosus* Willd. Syn. *A. petitianus* A.Rich.
12.	Avocado, Butterfruit	*Makhanphal*	*Persea americana* Mill.
13.	Bamboo	*Bāṁsa* (*Vaṁśa*)	*Bambusa bambos* (Linn.) Voss Syn. *B. arundinacea* Willd.
14.	Banana	*Kelā* (*Kadalī*)	*Musa paradisiaca* Linn. Syn. *M. sapientum* Kuntze
15.	Barley	*Jau* (*Yava*)	*Hordeum vulgare* Linn. Syn. *H. sativum* Pers.
16.	Beet root	*Cukandara*	*Beta vulgaris* Linn.
17.	Belleric myrobalan	*Baheṟā* (*Vibhītaka*)	*Terminalia bellirica* (Gaertn.) Roxb. Syn. *Myrobalanus bellirica* Gaertn.
18.	Bengal gram	*Canā* (*Caṇaka*)	*Cicer arietinum* Linn. Syn. *C. grossum* Salisb.
19.	Bengal quince	*Bela* (*Bilva*)	*Aegle marmelos* (Linn.) Correa Syn. *Crateva marmelos* Linn.
20.	Betel leaf	*Pāna* (*Tāmbūla*)	*Piper betel* Linn. Syn. *Chavica betle* (Linn.) Miq.
21.	Betel nut	*Supāṟī* (*Pūga*)	*Areca catechu* Linn. Syn. *A. hortensis* Lour.
22.	Bindweed	*Saṅkhapuṣpī*	*Convolvulus pluricaulis* Choisy Syn. *C. microphyllus* Sieb.
23.	Bitter gourd	*Karelā*	*Momordica charantia* Linn. Syn. *M. indica* Linn.

S.No.	Common Names	*Hindi / Sanskrit* Names	Botanical Names
24.	Bitter oleander, Telicherry bark	*Kuṭaja*	*Holarrhena antidysenterica* (Roth) DC. Syn. *Wrightia antidysenterica* J. Grah.
25.	Blackberry	*Jāmuna* (*Jambū*)	*Syzygium cumini* (Linn.) Skeels Syn. *Eugenia jambolana* Lam.
26.	Black gram	*Uṟada* (*Māṣa*)	*Phaseolus mungo* Linn. Syn. *Vigna mungo* (Linn.) Hepper
27.	Black henbane	*Khurāsānī ajavāyaṇa*	*Hyoscyamus niger* Linn.
28.	Black nightshade	*Makoya*	*Solanum nigrum* Linn. Syn. *S. americanum* Mill.
29.	Black pepper	*Marica* (*Kālī marica*)	*Piper nigrum* Linn.
30.	Blue water lily	*Kamala-Nīlophara* (*Utpala*)	*Nymphaea stellata* Willd. Syn. *N. nouchali* Burm. f.
31.	Blue wiss	*Māṣaparṇī*	*Teramnus labialis* (Linn.) Spreng. Syn. *Glycine labialis* Linn.f.
32.	Bottle gourd	*Laukī*	*Lageaneria siceraria* (Molina) Standl. Syn. *L. vulgaris* Seringe
33.	Box myrtle	*Kokilākṣa* (*Tālamakhanā*)	*Hygrophila auriculata* (Schumach.) Heine Syn. *Hygrophila spinosa* T. Anders.
34.	Brinjal	*Baiṁgana*	*Solanum melongena* Linn. Syn. *S. esculentum* Dunal
35.	Broccoli	*Harī phūlagobhī*	*Brassica oleracea* var. *italica* Plenck
36.	Cabbage	*Gobhī patra* (*Bandagobhī*)	*Brassica oleracea* (Linn.) var. *capitata* Linn.
37.	Caltrope, Puncture vine	*Gokharū*	*Tribulus terrestris* Linn. Syn. *T. lanuginosus* Linn.
38.	Calumpang tree	*Ciraunjī* (*Priyāla*)	*Buchanania lanzan* Spreng. Syn. *B. latifolia* Roxb.
39.	Camphor	*Karpūra*	*Cinnamomum camphora* (Linn.) Sieb. Syn.*C. officinarum* Nees
40.	Carambola, Star fruit	*Kamarakha* (*Karmaraṅga*)	*Averrhoa carambola* Linn. Syn. *A. acutangula* Stokes
41.	Cardamom	*Idlāyacī Choṭī* (*Elā*)	*Elettaria cardamomum* (Linn.) Maton Syn. *Alpinia cardamomum* (Linn.) Roxb.
42.	Carrot	*Gājara* (*Gṛñjana*)	*Daucus carota* Linn. var. *sativa* DC.
43.	Cashewnut	*Kājū*	*Anacardium occidentale* Linn.
44.	Castor plant	*Eraṇḍa*	*Ricinus communis* Linn. Syn. *R. africanus* Mill.
45.	Cauliflower	(*Phūla gobhī*)	*Brassica oleracea* (Linn.) var. *botrytis* Linn. sub var. *cauliflora* DC.
46.	Catechu	*Khaira* (*Khadira*)	*Acacia catechu* (Linn. f.) Willd. Syn. *A. wallichiana* DC
47.	Celery	*Ajamodā*	*Apium graveolens* Linn.
48.	Chenopodium, Lambs quarters	*Bathuā* (*Vāstūka*)	*Chenopodium album* Linn. Syn. *C. agreste* E.H.L.Krause

S.No.	Common Names	*Hindi / Sanskrit* Names	Botanical Names
49.	Cherry	*Elavāluka*	*Prunus cerasus* Linn.
50.	Chili, Cayenne	*Marica lāla*	*Capsicum frutescens* Linn. Syn. *C. minimum* Roxb.
51.	Chiretta	*Cirāyata* (*Kirātatikta*)	*Swertia chirayita* Roxb. Syn. *Gentiana chirayita* Roxb.
52.	Cinnamon, Bayleaf	*Dālacīnī, Tejapattā*	*Cinnamomum zeylanicum* Breine
53.	Clove	*Lavaṅga* (*Lauṅga*)	*Syzygium aromaticum* (Linn.) Merr. & L.M. Perry. Syn. *Eugenia aromatica* Kuntze
54.	Cobras saffron	*Nāgakeśara*	*Mesua ferrea* Linn. Syn. *M. roxburghii* Wight.
55.	Coconut	*Nāriyala* (*Nārikela*)	*Cocos nucifera* Linn. Syn. *C. indica* Royle
56.	Coffea	*Kām̐phī*	*Coffea arabica* Linn. Syn. *C. corymbulosa* Bertol.
57.	Colocynth	*Indrāyaṇa* (*Indravāruṇī*)	*Citrullus colocynthis* (Linn.) Schrad. Syn. *Cucumis colocynthis* Linn.
58.	Coomb teak	*Gambhārī*	*Gmelina arborea* Roxb. Syn. *G. sinuata* Link
59.	Coriander	*Dhaniyām̐* (*Dhānyaka*)	*Coriandrum sativum* Linn. Syn. *C. globosum* Salisb.
60.	Corn, Maize	*Makkā*	*Zea mays* Linn. Syn. *Z. curagua* Molina
61.	Couch grass, Devil's grass	*Dūba* (*Dūrvā*)	*Cynodon dactylon* (Linn.) Pers. Syn. *Panicum dactylon* Linn.
62.	Country mallow	*Balā*	*Sida cordifolia* Linn. Syn. *S. herbacea* Cav.
63.	Cranberry, Black cherry	*Karaudā* (*Karamarda*)	*Carissa congesta* Wight, Syn. *C. carandas* Linn.
64.	Croton oil seed	*Dravantī*, *Jamālagoṭā*	*Croton tiglium* Linn. Syn. *C. acutus* Thunb.
65.	Cucumber	*Khīrā* (*Trapuṣa*)	*Cucumis sativus* Linn. Syn. *C. rumphii* Hassk.
66.	Cumin	*Jīrā Śveta-Śveta Jīraka*	*Cuminum cyminum* Linn. Syn. *C. odorum* Salisb.
67.	Dabra	*Pṛśniparṇī*	*Uraria picta* (Jacq.) Desv. ex DC. Syn. *Hedysarum pictum* Jacq.
68.	Date	*Kharjūra*	*Phoenix sylvestris* (Linn.) Roxb. Syn. *Elate sylvestris* Linn.
69.	Drumstick tree	*Sahijana* (*Śigru*)	*Moringa oleifera* Lam. Syn. *M. pterygosperma* Gaertn.
70.	Eagle wood	*Agaru*	*Aquilaria malaccensis* Lam. Syn. *A. agallocha* Roxb.
71.	Edible pinenut	*Cilagojā*	*Pinus gerardiana* Wall. ex Lamb.
72.	Elephant creeper	*Vidhārā*	*Argyreia speciosa* Sweet Syn. *A. nervosa* (Burm. f.) Bojer
73.	Eucalyptus	*Nīlagirī*	*Eucalyptus globulus* Labill.
74.	False pepper	*Vāyaviḍaṅga*	*Embelia ribes* Burm. f. Syn. *Antidesma grossularia* Raeusch.
75.	Fenugreek	*Methī* (*Methikā*)	*Trigonella foenum-graecum* Linn.

S.No.	Common Names	*Hindi / Sanskrit* Names	Botanical Names
76.	Fennel	*Sauṁpha*	*Foeniculum vulgare* Mill. Syn. *F. officinale* All.
77.	Fig	*Añjīra (Phalgū)*	*Ficus carica* Linn. Syn. *F. caprificus* Risso
78.	Fine leaved fumitary	*Pittāpāpaṟā Parpaṭa*	*Fumaria indica* (Hassk.) Pugsley Syn. *F. parviflora* Lam.
79.	Flat bean	*Sema (Niṣpāva)*	*Dolichos lablab* Linn. Syn- *Lablab purpureus* (Linn.) Sweet
80.	Fragrant swamp mallow	*Sugondhabāla* (*Bālaka*)	*Pavonia odorata* Willd. *Udicya* Syn. *Diplopenta odorata* Alef.
81.	Garcinia	*Amlavetasa*	*Garcinia pedunculata* Roxb.
82.	Garlic	*Lasuna* (*Rasona*)	*Allium sativum* Linn. Syn. *A.pekinense* Prokh.
83.	Gentian	*Kuṭakī*	*Picrorhiza kurrooa* Royle ex Benth.
84.	Gingelli, Kodo millet	*Kodo* (*Kodrava*)	*Paspalum scrobiculatum* Linn. Syn. *P. adelogaeum* Steud.
85.	Ginger	*Soṁṭha, Śuṇṭhī* (*Ārdraka*)	*Zingiber officinale* Rosc. Syn. *Z. majus* Rumph.
86.	Glue cherry, Indian cherry	*Lisoṟa*	*Cordia dichotoma* Forst. f. Syn. *C.indica* Lam.
87.	Grapes	*Aṅgūra* (*Ḍrākṣā*)	*Vitis vinifera* Linn. Syn. *Cissus vinifera* (Linn.) Kuntze
88.	Green gram, Munga bean	*Mūṁga (Mudga)*	*Vigna radiata* (Linn.) Wilczek var. *radiata* Verdcourt. Syn. *Phaseolus radiatus* Linn.
89.	Guava tree	*Amarūda* (*Amṛtaphala*)	*Psidium guajava* Linn. Syn. *Guajava pumila* (Vahl) Kuntze
90.	Gum arabica tree	*Babūla* (*Kīkara*)	*Acacia arabica* Willd. Syn. *A. nilotica* ssp. *indica* (Benth.) Brenan
91.	Gum guggula	*Guggulu*	*Commiphora mukul* (Hook. ex Stocks) Engl. Syn. *C. wightii* (Arnott) Bhandari *Balsamodendron mukul* Hook. ex Stocks
92.	Hedge mustard	*Kūṁbakalā*	*Sisymbrium irio* Linn. Syn. *S. pinnatifidum* Forssk.
93.	Himalayan marsh orchid	*Śālamapañjā*	*Orchis latifolia* Linn. Syn. *Dactylorhiza hatagirea* (D.Don) Soo
94.	Himalayan silver fir	*Tāliśapatra*	*Abies webbiana* Lindl. Syn. *A. spectabilis* (D.Don) Spach.
95.	Hog weed	*Punarnavā*	*Boerhaavia diffusa* Linn. Syn. *B. repens* Linn.
96.	Holy basil	*Tulasī*	*Ocimum sanctum* Linn. Syn. *O. tenuiflorum* Linn.
97.	Honey tree, Butter tree	*Mahuwā*	*Madhuca longifolia* Linn. Syn. *Bassia longifolia* Linn.
98.	Horse gram	*Kulathī*	*Dolichos biflorus* Linn. Syn. *D. uniflorus* Lamk.
99.	Indian aconite	*Vatsanābha* (*Mīṭhāviṣa*)	*Aconitum ferox* Wall. ex Ser. Syn. *A. atrox* Walp.
100.	Indian berberry	*Dāruhaldī* (*Dāruharidrā*)	*Berberis aristata* DC. Syn. *B. macrophylla* K.Koch

S.No.	Common Names	*Hindi / Sanskrit* Names	Botanical Names
101.	Indian fig	*Gūlara* (*Udumbara*)	*Ficus glomerata* Roxb. Syn. *F. racemosa* Linn.
102.	Indian fleabane	*Rāsnā*	*Pluchea lanceolata* (DC.) Clarke Syn. *Berthelotia lanceolata* DC.
103.	Indian gooseberry	*Āṁvalā* (*Āmalakī*)	*Emblica officinalis* Gaertn. Syn. *Phyllanthus emblica* Linn.
104.	Indian hemp, Marijuana	*Bhāṅga* (*Bhaṅgā*)	*Cannabis sativa* Linn. Syn. *C. indica* Lam.
105.	Indian hog plum	*Amaṟā* (*Āmrātaka*)	*Spondias mangifera* Willd. Syn. *S. pinnata* (Linn. f.) Kurz
106.	Indian jalap	*Trivṛta* (*Niśotha*)	*Operculina turpethum* Linn. Syn. *Merremia turpethum* (Linn.) Silva Manso
107.	Indian jujuba	*Bera*	*Ziziphus jujuba* Mill. Syn. *Z. mauritiana* Lam.
108.	Indian kino tree	*Vijayasāra, asana*	*Pterocarpus marsupium* Roxb. Syn. *P. marsupium* f. *acuminata* (Prain) Prain
109.	Indian kudzu	*Vidārīkanda*	*Pueraria tuberosa* (Roxb. ex Willd.) DC. Syn. *Hedysarum tuberosum* Willd.
110.	Indian laburnum	*Amalatāsa* (*Āragvadha*)	*Cassia fistula* Linn. Syn. *C. excelsa* Kunth
111.	Indian mallow	*Atibalā*	*Abutilon indicum* (Linn.) Sw. Syn. *A. indicum* G. Don
112.	Indian millet	*Jūrṇa*	*Sorghum vulgare* (Linn.) Pers. Syn. *S. bicolor* (Linn.) Moench
113.	Indian nightshade	*Kaṭerī Baṟī*	*Solanum anguivi* Lam. Syn. *S. indicum* Linn.
114.	Indian valerian	*Tagara, sugandhabalā*	*Valeriana wallichii* DC. Syn. *V. jatamansi* Jones.
115.	Indian pennywort	*Maṇḍūkaparṇī*	*Centella asiatica* (Linn.) Urban Syn. *Hydrocotyle asiatica* Linn.
116.	Indian rosewood tree	*Śīśama* (*Śiṁśapa*)	*Dalbergia sissoo* Roxb. ex DC. Syn. *Amerimnon sissoo* (Roxb.) Kuntze
117.	Indian spikenard	*Jaṭāmāṁsī*	*Nardostachys jatamansi* DC. Syn. *N. grandiflora* DC.
118.	Indian spurge tree, Common milk hedge	*Thūhara, Snuhi, Sehuṇḍa*	*Euphorbia neriifolia* Linn. Syn. *E. ligularia* Roxb.
119.	Indian trumpet plant	*Sonāpāthā* (*Śyonāka*)	*Oroxylum indicum* (Linn.) Vent. Syn. *Bignonia indica* Linn.
120.	Jack tree	*Kaṭahala* (*Panasa*)	*Artocarpus integrifolia* Linn. f. Syn. *A. heterophyllus* Lam.
121.	Jasmine	*Camelī*	*Jasminum officinale* Linn.
122.	Java long pepper	*Cavya*	*Piper chaba* Hunter Syn. *P. retrofractum* Vahl
123.	Juniper	*Hapuṣā*	*Juniperus communis* Linn.
124.	Khorsan thorn	*Dhamāsā*	*Fagonia arabica* Linn. Syn. *F. cretica* Linn.
125.	Kidney bean	*Rājamāṣa* (*Lobiyā*)	*Vigna catjang* Walp. Syn. *V. unguiculata* (L.) Walp. ssp. *cylindrica*
126.	King's solomon seal	*Mahāmedā*	*Polygonatum cirrhifolium* (Wall.) Royle Syn. *Convallaria cirrhifolia* Wall.

S.No.	Common Names	*Hindi* / *Sanskrit* Names	Botanical Names
127.	Lady finger	*Bhiṇḍī*	*Hibiscus esculentus* Linn. Syn. *Abelmoschus esculentus* (Linn.) Moench.
128.	Lebbeck tree	*Śirīṣa* (*Sirasā*)	*Albizia lebbeck* (Linn.) Willd. Syn. *Acacia lebbek* (Linn.) Willd.
129.	Lemon	*Nimbū Jambīra*	*Citrus limon* (Linn.) Burm. f. Syn. *C. medica* Linn. var. *limonum*
130.	Lentil	*Masūra*	*Lens culinaris* Medik. Syn. *Ervum lens* Wall.
131.	Leptadave	*Jīvantī*	*Leptadenia reticulata* (Retz.) W. & A. Syn. *Gymnema aurantiacum* Wall. ex Hook. f.
132.	Lettuce	*Kāhū*	*Lactuca sativa* Linn.
133.	Linseed, Common flax	*Atasī*	*Linum usitatissimum* Linn. Syn. *L. humi* Mill.
134.	Licorice root	*Yaṣṭīmadhu, mulеṭhī*	*Glycyrrhiza glabra* Linn. Syn. *G. brachycarpa* Boiss.
135.	Lollipop plant	*Śivaliṅgī*	*Bryonopsis laciniosa* Linn. Syn. *Bryonia laciniosa* Linn.
136.	Long pepper	*Pippalī* (*Pīpara*)	*Piper longum* Linn.
137.	Lotus	*Kamala* (*Puṇḍarīka*)	*Nelumbo nucifera* Gaertn. Syn. *Nelumbium speciosum* Willd.
138.	Malabar nut	*Vāsā* (*Aḍūsā*)	*Adhatoda vasica* Nees Syn. *A. zeylanica* Medik.
139.	Malabar spinach	*Poi*	*Basella alba* var. *rubra* Linn.
140.	Malaxis	*Jīvaka*	*Crepidium acuminatum* (D. Don) Szlach. Syn. *Malaxis acuminata* D. Don
141.	Mango tree	*Āma* (*Āmra*)	*Mangifera indica* Linn. Syn. *M. austroyunnanensis* Hu
142.	Marjoram	*Maruvaka, Maruā*	*Origanum majorana* Linn. Syn. *Majorana hortensis* Moench
143.	Margosa tree	*Nīma* (*Nimba*)	*Azadirachta indica* (Linn.) A. Juss. Syn. *Melia azadirachta* Linn.
144.	Marking nut	*Bhilāvā* (*Bhallātaka*)	*Semecarpus anacardium* Linn. f.
145.	Mexican poppy	*Svaṇa Svarṇakṣīrī*	*Argemone mexicana* Linn. Syn. *A. vulgaris* Spach
146.	Mint	*Pudīnā*	*Mentha spicata* Linn. Syn. *M. viridis* Linn.
147.	Monkey jack	*Lakuca* (*Baṟahara*)	*Artocarpus lakoocha* Roxb. Syn. *A. ficifolius* W.T.Wang
148.	Muscle	*Mūsalī Śveta*	*Chlorophytum borivilianum* Santapau & Fernandes
149.	Mushroom	*Chatraka*	*Psalliota campestris* (Linn.) Fries. Syn. *Agaricus campestris* Linn.
150.	Musk melon	*Kharabūja* (*Daśāṅgula*)	*Cucumis melo* Linn. Syn. *C.acidus* Jacq.
151.	Mustard	*Sarasoṁ* (*Sarṣapa*)	*Brassica campestris* Linn. var. *sarson* Prain
152.	Myrobalan	*Haraṟa* (*Harītakī*)	*Terminalia chebula* (Gaertn.) Retz.
153.	Nut grass	*Nāgaramothā*	*Cyperus rotundus* Linn. Syn. *Pycreus rotundus* (Linn.) Hayek

S.No.	Common Names	*Hindi / Sanskrit* Names	Botanical Names
154.	Nutmeg	*Jāyaphala*	*Myristica fragrans* Houtt. Syn. *M. aromatica* Lam.
155.	Oat	*Yavaka*	*Avena sativa* Linn. Syn. *A. algeriensis* Trab.
156.	Olive	*Jaitūna*	*Olea europaea* Linn.
157.	Onion	*Pyāja (Palāṇḍu)*	*Allium cepa* Linn. Syn. *A. angolense* Baker
158.	Opium	*Aphīma (Ahiphena)*	*Papaver somniferum* Linn. Syn. *P. setigerum* DC.
159.	Orange	*Nāraṅgī*	*Citrus reticulata* Blanco Syn. *C. crenatifolia* Lush.
160.	Oregano, Wild marjoram	*Janglī maruā*	*Origanum vulgare* Hirtum
161.	Papaya	*Papītā (Eraṇḍa karrkaṭī)*	*Carica papaya* Linn. Syn. *C. citriformis* Jacq.
162.	Parsley	*Ajamodā*	*Petroselinum crispum* (Mill.) Fuss Syn. *Apium crispum* Mill.
163.	Pea	*Maṭara*	*Pisum sativum* Linn. Syn. *P.vulgare* Judz.
164.	Peach	*Āḍū (Āruka)*	*Prunus persica* (Linn.) Batsch Syn. *Persica vulgaris* Mill.
165.	Peacock's tail	*Mālatī*	*Aganosma dichotoma* (Roth) K. Schum. Syn. *A. caryophyllata* (Roxb. ex Sim.) G. Don
166.	Peanut, Ground nut	*Mūgaphalī (Bhū-Śimbī)*	*Arachis hypogaea* Linn. Syn. *A. nambyquara* Hoehne
167.	Pear	*Nāśapātī (Ṭaṅka)*	*Pyrus communis* Linn.
168.	Pearl millet	*Bājarā (Bjrānna)*	*Pennisetum glaucum* (L.) R.Br. Syn. *Pennisetum typhoides* (Burm.f.)Stapf. & Hubbard.
169.	Pellitory root	*Akarakarā*	*Anacyclus pyrethrum* DC. Syn. *A. officinarum* Heyne
170.	Phalsa	*Phālasā*	*Grewia asiatica* Linn. Syn. *G. subinaequalis* DC.
171.	Pigeon pea	*Arahara (Āḍhakī)*	*Cajanus cajan* (Linn.) Mullsp. Syn. *C.indicus* Spreng.
172.	Pineapple	*Anānāsa*	*Ananas comosus* (Linn.) Merr. Syn. *A. sativus* Schult. f.
173.	Pista, Pistachiu	*Pistā*	*Pistacia vera* Linn.
174.	Plum	*Ālūcā*	*Prunus domestica* Subsp. *insititia* (Linn.) Bonnier & Layens
175.	Pointed gourd	*Paravala (Paṭola)*	*Trichosanthes dioica* Roxb.
176.	Pomegranate	*Anāra (Dāṟima)*	*Punica granatum* Linn. Syn. *P. spinosa* Lam.
177.	Potato	*Ālū*	*Solanum tuberosum* Linn. Syn. *S. subandigena* Hawkes
178.	Prickly chaff flower	*Apāmārga Śveta*	*Achyranthes aspera* Linn. Syn. *A. sicula* Roth
179.	Pumpkin	*Kūṣmāṇḍa pita (Kumhaṟā)*	*Cucurbita maxima* Duch. ex Lam. Syn. *C. zapallito* Carriere
180.	Purging cotton, Purging nut	*Dantī*	*Baliospermum montanum* (Willd.) Muell. Arg. Syn. *B. axillare* Blume
181.	Putrajivaka	*Putrajīvaka*	*Drypetes roxburghii* (Wall.) Hurus Syn. *Putranjiva roxburghii* Wall.

S.No.	Common Names	*Hindi / Sanskrit* Names	Botanical Names
182.	Radish	*Mūlī* (*Mūlaka*)	*Raphanus sativus* Linn.
183.	Red leaved spinach	*Caulāī bheda* (*Māriṣa rakta*)	*Amaranthus gangeticus* Linn. Syn. *A. tricolor* Linn.
184.	Rhubarb	*Revandacīnī*	*Rheum emodi* Wall. ex Meissn. Syn. *R. australe* D.Don
185.	Rice	*Cāvala* (*Taṇḍula, Śāli*)	*Oryza sativa* Linn. Syn. *O. montana* Lour.
186.	Roscoe's Lily	*Kākolī*	*Roscoea purpurea* Smith
187.	Rose	*Gulāba*	*Rosa centifolia* Linn. Syn. *R. gallica* var. *centifolia* Regel
188.	Safflower	*Kusumbha* (*Barre*)	*Carthamus tinctorius* Linn. Syn. *C. glaber* Burm.f.
189.	Saffron	*Keśara*	*Crocus sativus* Linn.
190.	Sandal wood	*Candana Śvet*	*Santalum album* Linn.
191.	Scindapsus	*Gajapippalī*	*Scindapsus officinalis* (Roxb.) Schott
192.	Sesame	*Tila*	*Sesamum indicum* Linn. Syn. *S. orientale* Linn.
193.	Sesban	*Jayanti*	*Sesbania sesban* (Linn.) Merr. Syn. *S. aegyptiaca* Poir.
194.	Siberian tea	*Pāṣāṇa bheda* (*Patharcaṭṭā*)	*Bergenia ligulata* (Walll.) Engl. Syn. *B. ciliata* (Haw.) Sternb.
195.	Smooth leaved ponga	*Karañja*	*Derris indica* (Lam.) Bennet. Syn. *Pongamia pinnata* (Linn.) Merr.
196.	Snake cucumber	*Kakaṟī* (*Ervāru*)	*Cucumis utilissimus* Roxb. Syn. *C. melo* Linn. var. *utilissimus* Duth. & Full.
197.	Snakewood	*Kucalā latā*	*Strychnos colubrina* Linn.
198.	Soyabean	*Rājaśimbī Muleṭhī*	*Glycine max* Merrill. Syn. *G. hispida* Maxim.
199.	Spinach	*Pālaka* (*Palakyā*)	*Spinacia oleracea* Linn. Syn. *S. spinosa* Moench
200.	Sponge gourd	*Mahākośātakī* (*Dhāmārgava*)	*Luffa aegyptiaca* Mill. ex Hook. f.
201.	Stone breaker, Seed under leaf	*Bhūmyāmalakī* (*Tāmalakī*)	*Phyllanthus urinaria* Linn. Syn. *Diasperus urinaria* (Linn.) Kuntze
202.	Sunflower	*Suryamukhī*	*Helianthus annuus* Linn.
203.	Sugarcane	*Īkha*	*Saccharum officinarum* Linn. Syn. *S. occidentale* Sw.
204.	Swallow wort, Dead sea apple	*Arka rakta*	*Calotropis procera* (Ait.) R. Br. Syn. *Asclepias procera* Ait.
205.	Sweet flag	*Vacā* (*Ghoṟa vaca*)	*Acorus calamus* Linn.
206.	Sweet marjoram	*Maruvaka*	*Origanum jajorana* Linn.
207.	Sweet orange	Masaṁmī	*Citrus sinensis* (Linn.) Osbeck.
208.	Sweet potato	*Sitāluka*	*Ipomoea batatas* (Linn.) Lam.
209.	Tamarind	*Imalī* (*Amlikā*)	*Tamarindus indica* Linn. Syn. *T. officinalis* Hook.
210.	Tea	*Cāya*	*Camellia sinensis* (Linn.) Kuntze Syn. *C. thea* Link; *C. chinensis* (Sims) Kuntze

S.No.	Common Names	*Hindi / Sanskrit* Names	Botanical Names
211.	Thymol, Ajowan, Carom seed	*Ajavāyana* (*Yavānī*)	*Trachyspermun ammi* (Linn.) Sprague Syn. *Carum copticum* Benth. & Hook. f.
212.	Ticktree	*Śālaparṇī*	*Desmodium gangeticum* DC. Syn. *Hedysarum gangeticum* Linn.
213.	Tinospora	*Giloya, Guḍūcī, Amṛtā*	*Tinospora cordifolia* Miers Syn. *Menisprmum cordifolium* Willd.
214.	Tobacco	*Tambākū*	*Nicotiana tabacum* Linn. Syn. *N. chinensis* Fisch. ex Lehm.
215.	Toddy palm	*Tāla-Tāṟa*	*Borassus flabellifer* Linn. Syn. *B. flabelliformis* Murr.
216.	Tomato	*Ṭamāṭara*	*Lycopersicum esculentum* Mill.
217.	Turkish gram, Moth bean	*Moṭha* (*Makuṣṭha*)	*Phaseolus aconitifolius* Jacq. Syn. *Vigna aconitifolia* (Jacq.) Marec.
218.	Turmeric	*Haldī* (*Haridrā*)	*Curcuma longa* Linn. Syn. *C. domestica* Valeton.
219.	Turnip	*Śalajama*	*Brassica rapa* Linn.
220.	Velvet bean, Cowhage	*Keṁvṁāca, Kavñca, Ātmaguptā*	*Mucuna pruriens* (Linn.) DC. Syn. *M. prurita* Hook.
221.	Veronicalolia	*Nāgabalā*	*Grewia hirsuta* Vahl. Syn. *G. polygama* Mast.
222.	Vetiver	*Khasa* (*Uśīra*)	*Vetiveria zizanioides* (Linn.) Nash Syn. *Andropogon muricatus* Retz.
223.	Vomitting nut, Emetic nut	*Madanaphala* (*Mainaphala*)	*Randia spinosa* Bl. Syn. *R. dumetorum* Lam.
224.	Walnut	*Akharoṭa* (*Akṣaṭa*)	*Juglans regia* Linn. Syn. *J. orientis* Dode
225.	Water chestnut	*Siṁghāṟā*	*Trapa natans* Linn. var. *bispinosa* (Roxb) Makino Syn. *T .bispinosa* Roxb.
226.	Water hyssop	*Brāhmī Jalanīma*	*Bacopa monnieri* (Linn.) Pennel Syn. *Herpestis monniera* (L.) Rothm.
227.	Water melon	*Tarabūja Kālinda*	*Citrullus vulgaris* Schrad. Syn. *C. lanatus* (Thunb.) Mats. & Nakai
228.	Water-lily	*Kamala-Kumuda*	*Nymphaea alba* Linn. Syn. *N. occidentalis* Moss
229.	Wheat	*Gehūṁ* (*Godhūma*)	*Triticum sativum* Lam. Syn. *T. aestivum* Linn.
230.	White cinchona	*Kadama* (*Kadamba*)	*Anthocephalus cadamba* (Roxb.) Miq. Syn. *Nauclea cadamba* Roxb., *Neolamarckia cadamba* (Roxb.) Bosser
231.	White leadwort	*Citraka Śveta*	*Plumbago zeylanica* Linn. Syn. *P. scandens* Linn.
232.	Whorled solomon's seal	*Medā*	*Polygonatum verticillatum* (Linn.) Allioni Syn. *Convallaria verticillata* Linn.
233.	Wild orchid	*Sālamamiśrī*	*Eulophia dabia (*D. Don) Hochr. Syn. *E. campestris* Wall. ex Lindl.

S.No.	Common Names	*Hindi / Sanskrit* Names	Botanical Names
234.	Wild rice	*Nīvāra*	*Hygroryza aristata* Nees ex Wt. & Arn. Syn. *Leersia aristata* (Retz.) Roxb.
235.	Wintercherry	*Aśvagandhā*	*Withania somnifera* (Linn.) Dunal Syn. *Physalis flexuosa* Linn.
236.	Wood apple	*Kaitha* (*Kapittha*)	*Feronia elephantum* Correa Syn. *F. limonia* (Linn.) Swingle
237.	Woolly grass	*Darbha*	*Imperata cylindrica* Linn. Syn. *I. arundinacea* Cirillo.
238.	Yam	*Sūraṇa Kanda*	*Amorphophallus campanulatus* (Roxb.) Bl.ex Decne. Syn. *A . paeoniifolius* (Denst.) Nicols.
239.	Yellow berried nightshade	*Kaṭerī Choṭī* (*Kaṇṭakārī*)	*Solanum surattense* Burm. f. Syn. *S. xanthocarpum* Schrad. & Wendl.
240.	Yellow oleander	*Kanera*	*Thevetia peruviana* (Pers.) Schum. Syn. *T. neriifolia* Juss
241.	Yellow snake tree	*Pāṭalā*	*Stereospermum suaveolens* DC. Syn. *S. chelonoides* (Linn. f.) DC.